United Health Foundation

9900 Bren Road East
Minnetonka, MN 55343

August, 2004

Dear Colleague,

On behalf of United Health Foundation, I am pleased to provide you with this edition of *Clinical Evidence Mental Health*. This distribution stems from the ongoing partnership between our Foundation and the BMJ Publishing Group to provide our nation's physicians with the best available evidence for effective health care. Considerable feedback continues to indicate that physicians and other health professionals appreciate this evidence-based information and regularly use it to inform their clinical practice.

Over the years, *Clinical Evidence* has benefited from the scientific and clinical expertise of an extraordinary team of international experts, many of whom are from the United States. In recent years, as the evidence-based clinical literature has become more robust, so too have the challenges faced by the BMJ Publishing Group in organizing it into an efficient and convenient document. We hope that this updated and consolidated edition provides you with convenient access to useful information for your clinical practice.

In addition to this publication of *Clinical Evidence Mental Health,* the United Health Foundation has arranged for you to have free access to the online version of the complete edition of *Clinical Evidence*, which provides the evidence for the management of over 190 conditions. The complete on line edition can be viewed at www.clinicalevidence.com. Once there, click "Free Access – UHF".

I hope this edition of *Clinical Evidence Mental Health* will provide you with a resource that meaningfully supports your efforts to provide the best quality of care to your patients.

Sincerely,

William W. McGuire, M.D.
Chairman
United Health Foundation

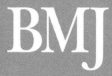

clinical
evidence
mental health

The international source of the best available evidence for effective mental health care

Reprinted from *Clinical Evidence*, Issue 11, 2004, published by the BMJ Publishing Group

Editorial Office
BMJ Publishing Group, BMA House, Tavistock Square, London, WC1H 9JR, United Kingdom.
Tel: +44 (0)20 7387 4499 • Fax: +44 (0)20 7383 6242 • www.bmjpg.com

Subscription prices for *Clinical Evidence*
Clinical Evidence and *Clinical Evidence Concise* (with companion CD-ROM) are both published six monthly (June/December) by the BMJ Publishing Group. The annual subscription rates (for June, Issue 11 and December, Issue 12) are:

Concise edition
Personal: £90 • €145 • US$145 • Can$200
Institutional: £190 • €305 • US$305 • Can$420
Student/nurse: £40 • €65 • US$65 • Can$90

Full edition
Personal: £100 • €160 • US$160 • Can$220
Institutional: £210 • €335 • US$335 • Can$460
Student/nurse: £45 • €70 • US$70 • Can$100

All individual subscriptions (personal, student, nurse) include online access at no additional cost. Institutional subscriptions are for print editions only. Institutions may purchase online site licences separately. For information on site licences and individual electronic subscriptions please visit the subscription pages of our website www.clinicalevidence.com or email us at CEsubscriptions@bmjgroup.com (UK and ROW) or clinevid@pmds.com (Americas). You may also telephone us or fax us on the following numbers:

UK and ROW Tel: +44 (0)20 7383 6270 • Fax: +44 (0)20 7383 6402
Americas Tel: +1 800 373 2897/240 646 7000 • Fax: +1 240 646 7005

Bulk subscriptions for societies and organisations
The Publishers offer discounts for any society or organisation buying bulk quantities for their members/specific groups. Please contact Miranda Lonsdale, Sales Manager (UK) at mlonsdale@bmjgroup.com or Maureen Rooney, Sales Manager (USA) at mrooney@bmjgroup.com.

Rights and permission to reproduce
For information on translation rights, please contact Daniel Raymond-Barker at draymond-barker@bmjgroup.com. To request permission to reprint all or part of any contribution in *Clinical Evidence Mental Health* please contact Polly Brown at pbrown@bmjgroup.com.

British Library Cataloguing in Publication Data. A catalogue record for this book is available from the British Library. ISBN 0-7279-1876-1.

Legal Disclaimer
The information contained in this publication, is intended for medical professionals. Categories presented in Clinical Evidence indicate a judgement about the strength of the evidence available to our authors prior to publication and the relative importance of benefits and harms.

We rely on our authors to confirm the accuracy of the information presented, and to describe generally accepted practices, and therefore we as the publisher, and our editors, cannot warrant its accuracy. Readers should be aware that professionals in the field may have different opinions. Because of this fact and also because of regular advances in medical research, we strongly recommend that readers independently verify specified treatments and drugs, including manufacturers' guidance. Also, the categories do not indicate whether a particular treatment is generally appropriate or whether it is suitable for a particular individual. Ultimately it is the readers' responsibility to make their own professional judgements, so to appropriately advise and treat their patients.

Description or reference to a product or publication does not imply endorsement of that product or publication, unless it is owned by the BMJ Publishing Group Limited.

To the fullest extent permitted by law, BMJ Publishing Group Limited and its editors, are not responsible for any losses, injury or damage caused to any person or property, (including under contract, by negligence, products liability or otherwise), whether they be direct or indirect, special, incidental or consequential, resulting from the application of the information in this publication.

Printed by Quebecor, Kingsport, Tennessee, USA

Designed by Pete Wilder, The Designers Collective, London, UK

Team and Advisors

Contents

Acknowledgements

The BMJ Publishing Group would like to thank United Health Foundation for their advice and support.

The BMJ Publishing Group thanks the following people and organisations for their advice and support: The Cochrane Collaboration, and especially Iain Chalmers, Mike Clarke, Phil Alderson, Peter Langhorne, and Carol Lefebvre; the National Health Service (NHS) Centre for Reviews and Dissemination, and especially Jos Kleijnen and Julie Glanville; the NHS, and especially Tom Mann, Sir John Patteson, Ron Stamp, Ben Toth, Veronica Fraser, Muir Gray, and Nick Rosen; the British National Formulary, and especially Dinesh Mehta, Eric Connor, and John Martin; Martindale: The Complete Drug Reference, and especially Sean Sweetman; the Health Information Research Unit at McMaster University, and especially Brian Haynes and Ann McKibbon; the United Health Foundation (UHF), and especially Reed Tuckson and Yvette Krantz; Bazian Ltd, and especially Anna Donald and Vivek Muthu; Paul Dieppe, Tonya Fancher, and Richard Kravitz who are working with Clinical Evidence to explore ways of presenting evidence on the usefulness of diagnostic test; previous staff who have contributed to this issue; the clinicians, epidemiologists, and members of patient groups who have acted as contributors, advisors, and peer reviewers; and members of our user panels: Lis Hawthorne and colleagues at Didcot Health Centre, Murray Lough and colleagues at Airdrie Health Centre, Alex Potter and colleagues at Clydebank Health Centre, Aimee Brame, Chris Clark, Gloria Daly, Hilary Durrant, Sarah Gwynne, James Harper, Diane Hickford, Sarosh Irani, Alison Kedward, Denise Knight, Sarah Lourenco, Vina Mayor, Michael Murphy, Ross Overshott, Deborah Rigby, and Catherine Tighe.

The BMJ Publishing Group values the ongoing support it has received from the global medical community for *Clinical Evidence*. We are grateful to the clinicians and patients who have taken part in focus groups, which are crucial to the development of *Clinical Evidence*. Finally, we would like to acknowledge the readers who have taken the time to send us their comments and suggestions.

The BMJ Publishing Group wishes to thank United Health Foundation for its efforts in providing educational funding which has allowed the wide dissemination of this valuable resource to millions of physicians and health professionals in the USA.

Clinical Evidence Mental Health

Welcome to this collection of mental health reprints from *Clinical Evidence*, a compendium of the best available evidence to guide clinical practice in specific mental health problems. This book is aimed primarily at psychiatrists, psychologists, nurses, social workers, and therapists working in a mental health setting.

There is sometimes a perception that an evidence-based approach is less applicable in mental health than in other areas of medicine — perhaps because of the importance of the patient's individual experience and narrative. However, in the same way that other areas of medicine are now recognising the value of individual experience and narrative, so it has become clear that many clinical questions and uncertainties in mental health are best answered using clinical epidemiology and informatics, the approaches on which evidence-based practice is founded. The goal of evidence-based practice is to integrate the best currently available evidence into clinical decision making. Evidence from randomised controlled trials and systematic reviews can best inform treatment decisions, but this evidence must be used judiciously and integrated with the values and preferences of the person with a mental health problem and their relatives.[1]

When the editors of *Clinical Evidence* first asked me to be their section adviser on mental health, I talked to several colleagues about the idea. Some of them felt that the task was doomed to failure because there was far too little reliable evidence about mental health. Not only did this turn out to be untrue, it also overlooked the benefit of evaluating evidence as a rational way of identifying areas in need of further and better research.[2] Trials in mental health tend to be short and of poor quality.[3,4] Most drug trials are conducted by the pharmaceutical industry and are aimed more at licensing bodies than at providing reliable information on which to base clinical practice.[5]

Despite these limitations, there is a huge amount of evidence that can helpfully inform clinical and policy decisions. Reluctance to use available research evidence probably has many origins, including practical difficulties in accessing high quality evidence and a fear that the evidence might go against many routine practices. The primary goal of clinical practice is to improve patients' outcomes. Evidence-based practice is simply a tool to identify approaches that are most likely to help. Most of the time, the evidence supports routine clinical practices.[6] However, on occasions, a careful examination of the evidence will suggest that certain interventions are less securely supported than had been thought, or even that they are harmful. At other times, the evidence may suggest that certain practices should be adopted more widely.

Crucial to successful evidence-based practice is the availability of high quality evidence — particularly summaries of the evidence. *Clinical Evidence Mental Health* provides access to reliable summaries of the current best evidence to answer specific clinical questions. A consequence of starting with the clinical question is that the evidence may often be limited. Where gaps are found, they are highlighted as areas of uncertainty; however, in many of the chapters included here, substantial evidence is available to guide clinical decisions. Numerical estimates of benefits and harms of specific interventions are provided whenever possible, as these can be useful when working out which interventions are most likely to help and least likely to harm.

John Geddes
Section Advisor for Mental Health
Senior Clinical Research Fellow/Honorary Consultant Psychiatrist

About Clinical Evidence

The inspiration for *Clinical Evidence* came in a phone call in 1995. Tom Mann and his colleagues at the NHS Executive asked the BMJ Publishing Group to explore the possibility of developing an evidence "formulary" along the lines of the *British National Formulary*. They recognised that clinicians were under increasing pressure to keep up to date and to base their practice more firmly on evidence, but that few had the necessary time or skills to do this. Their idea was to provide a pocketbook containing concise and regularly updated summaries of the best available evidence on clinical interventions. However, they didn't think that the NHS could develop such a formulary itself. "It would be marvellous", said Tom Mann, "if somebody would just do it." A small team at the BMJ set to work to produce a pilot version of what was then called the *Clinical Effectiveness Directory*.

Since that pilot, a great deal has changed. In collaboration with the American College of Physicians–American Society of Internal Medicine, we convened an international advisory board, held focus groups of clinicians, talked to patient support groups, and adopted countless good ideas from early drafts by our contributors. Throughout we kept in mind an equation set out by Slawson et al.[7] This states that the usefulness of any source of information is equal to its relevance, multiplied by its validity, divided by the work required to extract the information. In order to be as useful as possible, we aimed for high relevance, high validity, and low work in terms of the reader's time and effort. We also kept in mind principles of transparency and explicitness. Readers needed to understand where our information came from and how it was assembled.

A UNIQUE RESOURCE

Clinical Evidence is one of growing number of sources of evidence-based information for clinicians. But it has several features that make it unique.

- Its contents are driven by questions rather than by the availability of research evidence. Rather than start with the evidence and summarise what is there, we identify important clinical questions, and then search for and summarise the best available evidence to answer them.

- It identifies but does not try to fill important gaps in the evidence. In a phrase used by Jerry Osheroff, who has led much of the research on clinicians' information needs,[8] *Clinical Evidence* presents the dark as well as the light side of the moon. We feel that it is helpful for clinicians to know when their uncertainty stems from gaps in the evidence rather than gaps in their own knowledge.

- It is continuously updated, with full literature searches in each topic every twelve months. Print copies containing the latest version of each topic are published every six months and the website is refreshed, with new and updated content, every month.

- It specifically aims not to make recommendations. The experience of the clinical practice guideline movement has shown that it is nearly impossible to make recommendations that are appropriate in every situation. Differences in individual patients' baseline risks and preferences, and in the local availability of interventions, will always mean that the evidence must be individually interpreted rather than applied across the board. *Clinical Evidence* provides the raw material for developing locally applicable clinical practice guidelines, and for clinicians and patients to make up their own minds on the best course of action. We supply the evidence, you make the decisions.

COMPLEMENTARY BUT DIFFERENT

We are often asked how *Clinical Evidence* differs from two other high quality sources of evidence-based information: The *Cochrane Library*; and the evidence-based journals *ACP Journal Club, Evidence-Based Medicine, Evidence-Based Mental Health,* and *Evidence-Based Nursing*.

Clinical Evidence is complementary to but different from the work of the Cochrane Collaboration (www.cochrane.org), which produces and publishes high quality systematic reviews of controlled trials. *Clinical Evidence* has been called the friendly front end of the *Cochrane Library*, because it takes this and other high quality information and pulls it together in one place in a concise format. Many of our advisors and contributors are active members of the Cochrane Collaboration, and we are exploring closer ties between *Clinical Evidence* and the Collaboration in the way the evidence is searched for, summarised, and accessed by users.

Clinical Evidence is also complementary to but different from the evidence-based journals, which select and abstract the best and most clinically relevant articles as they appear in the world's medical literature. Together these journals form a growing archive of high quality abstracts of individual articles. *Clinical Evidence* takes a different approach. It begins not with the journals but with clinical questions. It is able to answer some. For others it simply reports that no good evidence was found.

A WORK IN PROGRESS

Clinical Evidence continues to evolve. We knew when we started that we were undertaking an enormous task, and the more we work on it, the more we realise its enormity. Although we have made every effort to ensure that the searches are thorough and that the appraisals of studies are objective (see Searching and appraising the literature), we will inevitably have missed some important studies. In order not to make unjustified claims about the accuracy of the information, we use phrases such as "we found no systematic review" rather than "there is no systematic review". In order to be as explicit as possible about the methods used for each contribution, we have asked each set of contributors to provide a brief methods section, describing the searches that were performed and how individual studies were selected.

Clinical Evidence is now a family of products, appearing in different formats and languages for different audiences. Our expectation is that *Clinical Evidence* will evolve further over the next few years, in response to the needs of clinicians and patients.

A guide to the text

SUMMARY PAGE

The summary page for each topic presents the questions addressed, key messages, and a list of the interventions covered (in alphabetical order), categorised according to whether we have found evidence that they are effective or not. We have developed categories of effectiveness based on those used in the Cochrane Collaboration's *A guide to effective care in pregnancy and childbirth*.[9] The categories we now use are explained in the table below:

TABLE	**Categorisation of treatment effects in *Clinical Evidence***
Beneficial	Interventions for which effectiveness has been demonstrated by clear evidence from RCTs, and for which expectation of harms is small compared with the benefits.
Likely to be beneficial	Interventions for which effectiveness is less well established than for those listed under "beneficial".
Trade off between benefits and harms	Interventions for which clinicians and patients should weigh up the beneficial and harmful effects according to individual circumstances and priorities.
Unknown effectiveness	Interventions for which there are currently insufficient data or data of inadequate quality.
Unlikely to be beneficial	Interventions for which lack of effectiveness is less well established than for those listed under "likely to be ineffective or harmful".
Likely to be ineffective or harmful	Interventions for which ineffectiveness or harmfulness has been demonstrated by clear evidence.

Fitting interventions into these categories is not always straightforward. For one thing, the categories represent a mix of several hierarchies: the size of benefit (or harm), the strength of evidence (RCT or observational data), and the degree of certainty around the finding (represented by the confidence interval). Another problem is that much of the evidence that is most relevant to clinical decisions relates to comparisons between different interventions rather than to comparison with placebo or no intervention. Where necessary, we have indicated the comparisons. A third problem is that interventions may have been tested, or found to be effective, in only one group of people, such as those at high risk of an outcome. Again, we have indicated this where possible. But perhaps most difficult of all has been trying to maintain consistency across different topics. We continue to work on refining the criteria for putting interventions under each category. Interventions that cannot be tested in an RCT for ethical or practical reasons are sometimes included in the categorisation table and are identified with an asterisk.

NEGATIVE FINDINGS

A surprisingly hard aspect to get right is the reporting of negative findings. Saying that there is no good evidence that a treatment works is not, of course, the same as saying that the treatment doesn't work. In trying to get this right, we may have erred too much on the side of caution; when in doubt, instead of saying, for example, that "the review found no difference", we say that "the review found no evidence of a difference". We recognise that to get this right, we need a better handle on the power of individual systematic reviews and trials to demonstrate statistically significant differences between groups, and better information on what constitutes clinically important differences in the major outcomes for each intervention.

In the meantime, we hope that the text makes a clear distinction between lack of benefit and lack of evidence of benefit.

OUTCOMES

Clinical Evidence focuses on outcomes that matter to patients, meaning those that patients themselves are aware of, such as symptom severity, quality of life, survival, disability, walking distance, and live birth rate. We are less interested in proxy outcomes such as blood lipid concentrations, blood pressure, or ovulation rates. Each topic includes a list of the main patient oriented outcomes, and where possible describes how these are measured. We have for the moment decided not to address the vexed question of what constitutes a clinically important change in an outcome, but we would welcome suggestions on how to do this.

EFFECTS, NOT EFFECTIVENESS

A key aim of *Clinical Evidence* is to emphasise the important trade offs between advantages and disadvantages of different treatment options. We therefore talk about the effects of interventions, both positive and negative, rather than the effectiveness, and for each question or intervention option we present data on benefits and harms under separate headings.

HARMS

Information about harms is often more difficult to synthesize than information about benefits.[10] Most controlled trials are designed to investigate benefits. Many either fail to document harms or present the information in a form that is difficult to analyse or interpret. When drugs are licensed they may have been used clinically in only a few thousand people; the absence of documented harms is not strong evidence that harms will not be discovered in the years after licensing.

Clinical Evidence recognises that the evidence about harms is often weaker than that about benefits. In an attempt to correct for this bias, *Clinical Evidence* has lowered the threshold for evidence to be included in the harms section. Much of the evidence for harms comes from observational studies ranging from prospective controlled cohort studies to case reports, and these are included when the harm is serious or when there is good corroborating evidence that the harm can be attributed to the treatment.

DRUG NAMES

Clinical Evidence has an international audience. Difficulties can arise when different names for the same drug are used in different parts of the world. We state the recommended or proposed International Name where possible and give only the generic or non-proprietary names of drugs rather than the brand names. Where an international name for a drug is not available we use the most common name (e.g. aspirin). A regularly updated table of equivalent drug names, put together by *Martindale: The Complete Drug Reference,*[11] is available on the *Clinical Evidence* website (www.clinicalevidence.com).

INFORMATION ON COST

We have decided not to include information on the cost or cost effectiveness of interventions. This is not because we believe cost to be unimportant, but because the question of what constitutes good evidence on cost is much disputed and because costs vary greatly both within and between countries. However, we believe that it will become increasingly untenable for clinicians to act without paying attention to the cost of treatments. Future companion publications of *Clinical Evidence* may provide relevant information on costs.

NUMERICAL DATA

Whenever possible, data are presented in the same form as in the original studies. However, sometimes we have changed the units or type of information in an attempt to present the results in a systematic and easily interpretable form.

AN INTERNATIONAL APPROACH

Clinical Evidence takes an international approach to the evidence. This means including drugs that are not licensed in some countries. It also means keeping in mind the practicalities of treating people in poorer countries, by covering some interventions even if they have been superseded (for example, single drug treatment for HIV infection as opposed to three drug treatment).

COMPETING INTERESTS

In line with the *BMJ*'s policy,[12] our aim is not to try to eliminate conflicts of interest but to make them explicit so that readers can judge for themselves what influence, if any, these may have had on the contributors' interpretation of the evidence. We therefore ask all contributors (and peer reviewers) to let us know about any potential competing interests, and we append any that are declared to the end of the contribution. Where the contributor gives no competing interests, we record "none declared".

EMAIL ALERTING SERVICE

If you wish to be notified by email about new topics, updates, or corrections, you can register for our alerting service on our website.

HOW TO USE THE INFORMATION IN CLINICAL EVIDENCE

The type of information contained in *Clinical Evidence* is necessary but not sufficient for the provision of effective, high quality health care. It is intended as an aid to clinical decision making, to be used in conjunction with other important sources of information. These other sources include estimates of people's baseline risk of a condition or outcome based on history, physical examination and clinical investigations; individual preferences; economic arguments; availability of treatments; and local expertise.

Some guidance on how to apply research evidence in practice is available on our website (www.clinicalevidence.com) and in appendix 2.

How Clinical Evidence is put together

The summaries in *Clinical Evidence* result from a rigorous process aimed at ensuring that they are both reliable and relevant to clinical practice.

SELECTING TOPICS

Clinical Evidence aims to cover common or important clinical conditions seen in primary and hospital care. To decide which conditions to cover we review national data on consultation rates, morbidity and mortality, we take account of national priorities for health care such as those outlined in the UK National Service Frameworks and in the US Institute of Medicine reports, and we take advice from generalist clinicians and patient groups. Our website (www.clinicalevidence.com) provides a list of conditions that we are planning to cover in future issues. Further suggestions are welcome.

SELECTING THE QUESTIONS

The questions in *Clinical Evidence* concern the benefits and harms of preventative and therapeutic interventions, with emphasis on outcomes that matter to patients. Questions are selected for their relevance to clinical practice by section advisors and contributors, in collaboration with primary care clinicians and patient groups. Each new issue of *Clinical Evidence* includes new questions as well as updates of existing questions. Readers can suggest new clinical questions using the feedback slips to be found at the back of the book and on the *Clinical Evidence* website (www.clinicalevidence.com), or by writing directly to *Clinical Evidence*.

SEARCHING AND APPRAISING THE LITERATURE

For each question, the literature is searched using the Cochrane Library, Medline, Embase and, occasionally, other electronic databases, looking first for good systematic reviews of RCTs; then for good RCTs published since the search date of the review. Where we find no good recent systematic reviews, we search for individual RCTs back to 1966. The date of the search is recorded in the methods section for each topic. Of the studies that are identified in the search, we select and summarise only a small proportion. The selection is done by critically appraising the abstracts of the studies identified in the search, a task performed independently by information scientists using validated criteria similar to those of Sackett et al[13] and Jadad.[14, 15] Where the search identifies more than one or two good reviews or trials, we select those we judge to be the most robust or relevant. Where we identify few or no good reviews or trials, we include other studies but highlight their limitations. Contributors, chosen for their clinical expertise in the field and their skills in epidemiology, are asked to review our selection of studies and to justify any additions or exclusions they wish to make.

Our search strategy and critical appraisal criteria are available on our website (www.clinicalevidence.com).

SUMMARISING THE EVIDENCE, PEER REVIEW, AND EDITING

The contributors summarise the evidence relating to each question. Each topic is then peer reviewed by the section advisors, by at least two external expert clinicians, and by an editorial committee, including external expert clinicians and epidemiologists. The revised text is then extensively edited by editors with clinical and epidemiological training, and data are checked against the original study reports. Bazian Ltd has authored several topics, as acknowledged in each, and has provided additional content and support.

FEEDBACK AND ERROR CORRECTIONS

Despite the extensive peer review and quality checks, we expect that the text will contain some errors and inconsistencies. Please let us know if you find any, either by using the comment card at the back of the book or by emailing us at CEfeedback@bmjgroup.com.

REFERENCES

1. Sackett DL, Rosenberg WM, Gray JA, et al. Evidence based medicine: what it is and what it isn't. *BMJ* 1996;312:71–72.
2. Geddes J. Asking structured and focused clinical questions: essential first step of evidence-based practice. *Evid Based Ment Health* 1999;2:35–36.
3. Johnson AL. Clinical trials in psychiatry. *Psychol Med* 1983;13:1–8.
4. Thornley B, Adams C. Content and quality of 2000 controlled trials in schizophrenia over 50 years. *BMJ* 1998;317:1181–1184.
5. Geddes JR. Prevention of relapse in schizophrenia. *N Engl J Med* 2002;346:56–58.
6. Geddes JR, Game D, Jenkins NE, et al. What proportion of primary psychiatric interventions are based on randomised evidence? *Qual Health Care* 1996;5:215–217.
7. Slawson DC, Shaughnessy AF, Bennett JH. Becoming a medical information master: feeling good about not knowing everything. *J Fam Pract* 1994;38:505–513.
8. Ely JW, Osheroff JA, Ebell MJ, et al. Analysis of questions asked by family doctors regarding patient care. *BMJ* 1999;319:358–361.
9. Enkin M, Keirse M, Renfrew M, et al. *A guide to effective care in pregnancy and childbirth.* Oxford: Oxford University Press, 1998.
10. Derry S, Loke YK, Aronson JK. Incomplete evidence: the inadequacy of databases in tracing published adverse drugs reactions in clinical trials. *BMC Medical Research Methodology* 2001;1:7. http://www.biomedcentral.com/1471-2288/1/7 (last accessed 1 June 2004).
11. Sweetman SC (Ed). *Martindale: The complete drug reference.* 33rd ed. London: Pharmaceutical Press, 2002. http://www.pharmpress.com (last accessed 1 June 2004) or contact martindale@rpsgb.org.uk
12. Smith R. Beyond conflicts of interest. *BMJ* 1998;317:219–292.
13. Sackett DL, Haynes RB, Guyatt GH, et al. *Clinical epidemiology: a basic science for clinical medicine.* 2nd ed. Boston: Little Brown, 1991.
14. Jadad A. Assessing the quality of RCTs: why, what, how and by whom? In: Jadad A (Ed.) *Randomised controlled trials.* London: BMJ Books, 1998:45–60.
15. Jadad AR, Moore RA, Carroll D, et al. Assessing the quality of reports of randomized controlled trials: is blinding necessary? *Control Clin Trials* 1996;17:1–12.

Glossary

Absolute risk (AR) The probability that an individual will experience the specified outcome during a specified period. It lies in the range 0 to 1, or is expressed as a percentage. In contrast to common usage, the word "risk" may refer to adverse events (such as myocardial infarction) or desirable events (such as cure).

Absolute risk increase (ARI) The absolute difference in risk between the experimental and control groups in a trial. It is used when the risk in the experimental group exceeds the risk in the control group, and is calculated by subtracting the AR in the control group from the AR in the experimental group. This figure does not give any idea of the proportional increase between the two groups: for this, relative risk (RR) is needed (see below).

Absolute risk reduction (ARR) The absolute difference in risk between the experimental and control groups in a trial. It is used when the risk in the control group exceeds the risk in the experimental group, and is calculated by subtracting the AR in the experimental group from the AR in the control group. This figure does not give any idea of the proportional reduction between the two groups: for this, relative risk (RR) is needed (see below).

Allocation concealment A method used to prevent selection bias by concealing the allocation sequence from those assigning participants to intervention groups. Allocation concealment prevents researchers from (unconsciously or otherwise) influencing which intervention group each participant is assigned to.

Applicability The application of the results from clinical trials to individual people. A randomised trial only provides direct evidence of causality within that specific trial. It takes an additional logical step to apply this result to a specific individual. Individual characteristics will affect the outcome for this person.

Baseline risk The risk of the event occurring without the active treatment. Estimated by the baseline risk in the control group.

Best evidence Systematic reviews of RCTs are the best method for revealing the effects of a therapeutic intervention.

Bias Systematic deviation of study results from the true results, because of the way(s) in which the study is conducted.

Blinding/blinded A trial is fully blinded if all the people involved are unaware of the treatment group to which trial participants are allocated until after the interpretation of results. This includes trial participants and everyone involved in administering treatment or recording trial results.

Block randomisation Randomisation by a pattern to produce the required number of people in each group.

Case control study A study design that examines a group of people who have experienced an event (usually an adverse event) and a group of people who have not experienced the same event, and looks at how exposure to suspect (usually noxious) agents differed between the two groups. This type of study design is most useful for trying to ascertain the cause of rare events, such as rare cancers.

Case series Analysis of series of people with the disease (there is no comparison group in case series).

Cluster randomisation A cluster randomised study is one in which a group of participants are randomised to the same intervention together. Examples of cluster randomisation include allocating together people in the same village, hospital, or school. If the results are then analysed by individuals rather than the group as a whole bias can occur.

Cohort study A non-experimental study design that follows a group of people (a cohort), and then looks at how events differ among people within the group. A study that examines a cohort, which differs in respect to exposure to some suspected risk factor (e.g. smoking), is useful for trying to ascertain whether exposure is likely to cause specified events (e.g. lung cancer). Prospective cohort studies (which track participants forward in time) are more reliable than retrospective cohort studies.

Completer analysis Analysis of data from only those participants who remained at the end of the study. Compare with intention to treat analysis, which uses data from all participants who enrolled (see below).

Confidence interval (CI) The 95% confidence interval (or 95% confidence limits) would include 95% of results from studies of the same size and design in the same population. This is close but not identical to saying that the true size of the effect (never exactly known) has a 95% chance of falling within the confidence interval. If the 95% confidence interval for a relative risk (RR) or an odds ratio (OR) crosses 1, then this is taken as no evidence of an effect. The practical advantages of a confidence interval (rather than a P value) is that they present the range of likely effects.

Controlled clinical trial (CCT) A trial in which participants are assigned to two or more different treatment groups. In Clinical Evidence, we use the term to refer to controlled trials in which treatment is assigned by a method other than random allocation. When the method of allocation is by random selection, the study is referred to as a randomised controlled trial (RCT; see below). Non-randomised controlled trials are more likely to suffer from bias than RCTs.

Controls In a controlled trial, controls refer to the participants in the comparison group, who may be allocated to placebo, no treatment, or a standard treatment. **Correlation coefficient** A measure of association that indicates the degree to which two variables change together in a linear relationship. It is represented by r, and varies between -1 and $+1$. When r is $+1$, there is a perfect positive relationship (when one variable increases, so does the other, and the proportionate difference remains constant). When r is -1 there is a perfect negative relationship (when one variable increases the other decreases, or vice versa, and the proportionate difference remains constant). This, however, does not rule out a relationship—it just excludes a linear relationship.

Crossover randomised trial A trial in which participants receive one treatment and have outcomes measured, and then receive an alternative treatment and have outcomes measured again. The order of treatments is randomly assigned. Sometimes a period of no treatment is used before the trial starts and in between the treatments (washout periods) to minimise interference between the treatments (carry over effects). Interpretation of the results from crossover randomised controlled trials (RCTs) can be complex.

Cross sectional study A study design that involves surveying a population about an exposure, or condition, or both, at one point in time. It can be used for assessing prevalence of a condition in the population.

Disability Adjusted Life Year (DALY) A method for measuring disease burden, which aims to quantify in a single figure both the quantity and quality of life lost or gained by a disease, risk factor, or treatment. The DALYs lost or gained are a function of the expected number of years spent in a particular state of health, multiplied by a coefficient determined by the disability experienced in that state (ranging from 0 [optimal health] to 1 [deaths]). Later years are discounted at a rate of 3 per year, and childhood and old age are weighted to count for less.

Effect size (standardised mean differences) In the medical literature, effect size is used to refer to a variety of measures of treatment effect. In Clinical Evidence it refers to a standardised mean difference: a statistic for combining continuous variables (such as pain scores or height), from different scales, by dividing the difference between two means by an estimate of the within group standard deviation.

Event The occurrence of a dichotomous outcome that is being sought in the study (such as myocardial infarction, death, or a four-point improvement in pain score).

Experimental study A study in which the investigator studies the effect of intentionally altering one or more factors under controlled conditions.

Factorial design A factorial design attempts to evaluate more than one intervention compared with control in a single trial, by means of multiple randomisations.

False negative A person with the target condition (defined by the gold standard) who has a negative test result.

False positive A person without the target condition (defined by the gold standard) who has a positive test result.

Fixed effects The "fixed effects" model of meta-analysis assumes, often unreasonably, that the variability between the studies is exclusively because of a random sampling variation around a fixed effect (see random effects below).

Hazard ratio (HR) Broadly equivalent to relative risk (RR); useful when the risk is not constant with respect to time. It uses information collected at different times. The term is typically used in the context of survival over time. If the HR is 0.5 then the relative risk of dying in one group is half the risk of dying in the other group.

Heterogeneity In the context of meta-analysis, heterogeneity means dissimilarity between studies. It can be because of the use of different statistical methods (statistical heterogeneity), or evaluation of people with different characteristics, treatments or outcomes (clinical heterogeneity). Heterogeneity may render pooling of data in meta-analysis unreliable or inappropriate.

Homogeneity Similarity (see heterogeneity above).

Incidence The number of new cases of a condition occurring in a population over a specified period of time.

Intention to treat (ITT) analysis Analysis of data for all participants based on the group to which they were randomised and not based on the actual treatment they received.

Likelihood ratio The ratio of the probability that an individual with the target condition has a specified test result to the probability that an individual without the target condition has the same specified test result.

Meta-analysis A statistical technique that summarises the results of several studies in a single weighted estimate, in which more weight is given to results of studies with more events and sometimes to studies of higher quality.

Morbidity Rate of illness but not death.

Mortality Rate of death.

Negative likelihood ratio (NLR) The ratio of the probability that an individual with the target condition has a negative test result to the probability that an individual without the target condition has a negative test result. This is the same as the ratio (1-sensitivity/specificity).

Negative predictive value (NPV) The chance of not having a disease given a negative test result (not to be confused with specificity, which is the other way round; see below).

Non-systematic review A review or meta-analysis that either did not perform a comprehensive search of the literature and contains only a selection of studies on a clinical question, or did not state its methods for searching and appraising the studies it contains.

Not significant/non-significant (NS) In *Clinical Evidence*, not significant means that the observed difference, or a larger difference, could have arisen by chance with a probability of more than 1/20 (i.e. 5%), assuming that there is no underlying difference. This is not the same as saying there is no effect, just that this experiment does not provide convincing evidence of an effect. This could be because the trial was not powered to detect an effect that does exist, because there was no effect, or because of the play of chance. If there is a potentially clinically important difference that is not statistically significant then do not say there was a non-significant trend. Alternative phrases to describe this type of uncertainty include, "Fewer people died after taking treatment x but the difference was not significant" or "The difference was not significant but the confidence intervals covered the possibility of a large beneficial effect" or even, "The difference did not quite reach significance."

Number needed to harm (NNH) One measure of treatment harm. It is the average number of people from a defined population you would need to treat with a specific intervention for a given period of time to cause one additional adverse outcome. NNH can be calculated as 1/ARI. In *Clinical Evidence*, these are usually rounded downwards.

Number needed to treat (NNT) One measure of treatment effectiveness. It is the average number of people who need to be treated with a specific intervention for a given period of time to prevent one additional adverse outcome or achieve one additional beneficial outcome. NNT can be calculated as 1/ARR (see appendix 2). In *Clinical Evidence*, NNTs are usually rounded upwards.

NNT for a meta-analysis Absolute measures are useful at describing the effort required to obtain a benefit, but are limited because they are influenced by both the treatment and also by the baseline risk of the individual. If a meta-analysis includes individuals with a range of baseline risks, then no single NNT will be applicable to the people in that meta-analysis, but a single relative measure (odds ratio or relative risk) may be applicable if there is no heterogeneity. In *Clinical Evidence*, an NNT is provided for meta-analysis, based on a combination of the summary odds ratio (OR) and the mean baseline risk observed in average of the control groups.

Odds The odds of an event happening is defined as the probability that an event will occur, expressed as a proportion of the probability that the event will not occur.

Odds ratio (OR) One measure of treatment effectiveness. It is the odds of an event happening in the experimental group expressed as a proportion of the odds of an event happening in the control group. The closer the OR is to one, the smaller the difference in effect between the experimental intervention and the control intervention. If the OR is greater (or less) than one, then the effects of the treatment are more (or less) than those of the control treatment. Note that the effects being measured may be adverse (e.g. death or disability) or desirable (e.g. survival). When events are rare the OR is analagous to the relative risk (RR), but as event rates increase the OR and RR diverge.

Odds reduction The complement of odds ratio (1-OR), similar to the relative risk reduction (RRR) when events are rare.

Open label trial A trial in which both participant and assessor are aware of the intervention allocated.

Placebo A substance given in the control group of a clinical trial, which is ideally identical in appearance and taste or feel to the experimental treatment and believed to lack any disease specific effects. In the context of non-pharmacological interventions, placebo is usually referred to as sham treatment (see sham treatment below).

Positive likelihood ratio (LR+) The ratio of the probability that an individual with the target condition has a positive test result to the probability that an individual without the target condition has a positive test result. This is the same as the ratio (sensitivity/1-specificity).

Positive predictive value (PPV) The chance of having a disease given a positive test result (not to be confused with sensitivity, which is the other way round; see below).

Power A study has adequate power if it can reliably detect a clinically important difference (i.e. between two treatments) if one actually exists. The power of a study is increased when it includes more events or when its measurement of outcomes is more precise.

Pragmatic study An RCT designed to provide results that are directly applicable to normal practice (compared with explanatory trials that are intended to clarify efficacy under ideal conditions). Pragmatic RCTs recruit a population that is representative of those who are normally treated, allow normal compliance with instructions (by avoiding incentives and by using oral instructions with advice to follow manufacturers instructions), and analyse results by "intention to treat" rather than by "on treatment" methods.

Prevalence The proportion of people with a finding or disease in a given population at a given time.

Publication bias Occurs when the likelihood of a study being published varies with the results it finds. Usually, this occurs when studies that find a significant effect are more likely to be published than studies that do not find a significant effect, so making it appear from surveys of the published literature that treatments are more effective than is truly the case.

P value The probability that an observed or greater difference occurred by chance, if it is assumed that there is in fact no real difference between the effects of the interventions. If this probability is less than 1/20 (which is when the P value is less than 0.05), then the result is conventionally regarded as being "statistically significant".

Quality Adjusted Life Year (QALY) A method for comparing health outcomes, which assigns to each year of life a weight from 1 (perfect health) to 0 (state judged equivalent to death) dependent on the individual's health related quality of life during that year. A total score of years multiplied by weight can then be compared across different interventions. There is disagreement about the best methods for measuring health-related quality of life.

Quasi randomised A trial using a method of allocating participants to different forms of care that is not truly random; for example, allocation by date of birth, day of the week, medical record number, month of the year, or the order in which participants are included in the study (e.g. alternation).

Random effects The "random effects" model assumes a different underlying effect for each study and takes this into consideration as an additional source of variation, which leads to somewhat wider confidence intervals than the fixed effects model. Effects are assumed to be randomly distributed, and the central point of this distribution is the focus of the combined effect estimate (see fixed effects above).

Randomised controlled trial (RCT) A trial in which participants are randomly assigned to two or more groups: at least one (the experimental group) receiving an intervention that is being tested and an other (the comparison or control group) receiving an alternative treatment or placebo. This design allows assessment of the relative effects of interventions.

Regression analysis Given data on a dependent variable and one or more independent variables, regression analysis involves finding the "best" mathematical model to describe or predict the dependent variable as a function of the independent variable(s). There are several regression models that suit different needs. Common forms are linear, logistic, and proportional hazards.

Relative risk (RR) The number of times more likely (RR > 1) or less likely (RR < 1) an event is to happen in one group compared with another. It is the ratio of the absolute risk (AR) for each group. It is analogous to the odds ratio (OR) when events are rare.

Relative risk increase (RRI) The proportional increase in risk between experimental and control participants in a trial.

Relative risk reduction (RRR) The proportional reduction in risk between experimental and control participants in a trial. It is the complement of the relative risk (1-RR).

Sensitivity The chance of having a positive test result given that you have a disease (not to be confused with positive predictive value [PPV], which is the other way around; see above).

Sensitivity analysis Analysis to test if results from meta-analysis are sensitive to restrictions on the data included. Common examples are large trials only, higher quality trials only, and more recent trials only. If results are consistent this provides stronger evidence of an effect and of generalisability.

Sham treatment An intervention given in the control group of a clinical trial, which is ideally identical in appearance and feel to the experimental treatment and believed to lack any disease specific effects (e.g. detuned ultrasound or random biofeedback).

Significant By convention, taken to mean statistically significant at the 5% level (see statistically significant below). This is the same as a 95% confidence interval not including the value corresponding to no effect.

Specificity The chance of having a negative test result given that you do not have a disease (not to be confused with negative predictive value [NPV], which is the other way around; see above).

Standardised mean difference (SMD) A measure of effect size used when outcomes are continuous (such as height, weight, or symptom scores) rather than dichotomous (such as death or myocardial infarction). The mean differences in outcome between the groups being studied are standardised to account for differences in scoring methods (such as pain scores). The measure is a ratio; therefore, it has no units.

Statistically significant Means that the findings of a study are unlikely to have arisen because of chance. Significance at the commonly cited 5% level ($P < 0.05$) means that the observed difference or greater difference would occur by chance in only 1/20 similar cases. Where the word "significant" or "significance" is used without qualification in the text, it is being used in this statistical sense.

Subgroup analysis Analysis of a part of the trial/meta-analysis population in which it is thought the effect may differ from the mean effect.

Systematic review A review in which specified and appropriate methods have been used to identify, appraise, and summarise studies addressing a defined question. It can, but need not, involve meta-analysis (see meta-analysis). In *Clinical Evidence*, the term systematic review refers to a systematic review of RCTs unless specified otherwise.

True positive A person with the target condition (defined by a gold standard) who also has a positive test result.

Validity The soundness or rigour of a study. A study is internally valid if the way it is designed and carried out means that the results are unbiased and it gives you an accurate estimate of the effect that is being measured. A study is externally valid if its results are applicable to people encountered in regular clinical practice.

Weighted mean difference (WMD) A measure of effect size used when outcomes are continuous (such as symptom scores or height) rather than dichotomous (such as death or myocardial infarction). The mean differences in outcome between the groups being studied are weighted to account for different sample sizes and differing precision between studies. The WMD is an absolute figure and so takes the units of the original outcome measure.

Anorexia nervosa

Search date April 2003

Janet Treasure and Ulrike Schmidt

QUESTIONS

INTERVENTIONS

Key Messages

- **Inpatient versus outpatient treatment setting (in people not requiring emergency intervention)** One small RCT found no significant difference between outpatient treatment and inpatient treatment for increasing weight and improving Morgan Russell scale global scores at 1, 2, and 5 years in people who did not need emergency intervention.

- **Oestrogen treatment (for prevention of fractures)** We found no good evidence about the effects of oestrogen treatment on fracture rates in people with anorexia. Two small RCTs found no significant difference between oestrogen and placebo or no treatment in bone mineral density in people with anorexia.

- **Psychotherapies** We found insufficient evidence from small RCTs to compare psychotherapies versus dietary counselling or versus each other.

- **Selective serotonin reuptake inhibitors** We found insufficient evidence from three small RCTs about effects of selective serotonin reuptake inhibitors compared with placebo or no treatment in people with anorexia.

- **Zinc** One small RCT found limited evidence that zinc may improve daily body mass index gain compared with placebo in people managed in an inpatient setting. However, we were unable to draw reliable conclusions from this small study.

- **Cisapride** One small RCT found no significant difference between cisapride and placebo in weight gain at 8 weeks. Use of cisapride has been restricted in many countries because of concern about cardiac irregularities, including ventricular tachycardia, torsades de pointes, and sudden death.

- **Cyproheptadine** One small RCT in an outpatient setting and two RCTs in inpatient settings found no significant difference between cyproheptadine and placebo for weight gain.

- **Neuroleptic drugs** We found no RCTs. The QT interval may be prolonged in people with anorexia nervosa, and many neuroleptic drugs (haloperidol, pimozide, sertindole, thioridazine, chlorpromazine, and others) also increase the QT interval. Prolongation of the QT interval may be associated with increased risk of ventricular tachycardia, torsades de pointes, and sudden death.

- **Tricyclic antidepressants** Two small RCTs found no evidence of benefit with amitriptyline compared with placebo. They found that amitriptyline was associated with more adverse effects, such as palpitations, dry mouth, and blurred vision.

DEFINITION   Anorexia nervosa is characterised by a refusal to maintain weight at or above a minimally normal weight (< 85% of expected weight for age and height, or body mass index [see glossary, p 10] < 17.5 kg/m^2), or a failure to show the expected weight gain during growth. In association with this, there is often an intense fear of gaining weight, preoccupation with weight, denial of the current low weight and its adverse impact on health, and amenorrhoea. Two subtypes of anorexia nervosa, binge–purge and restricting, have been defined.[1]

INCIDENCE/   A mean incidence in the general population of 19/100 000 a year in
PREVALENCE females and 2/100 000 a year in males has been estimated from 12 cumulative studies.[2] The highest rate was in female teenagers (age 13–19 years), where there were 50.8 cases/100 000 a year. A large cohort study screened 4291 Swedish school children, aged 16 years, by weighing and subsequent interview, and found the prevalence of anorexia nervosa (defined using DSM-III and DSM-III-R criteria) to be 7/1000 for girls and 1/1000 for boys.[3] Little is known of the incidence or prevalence in Asia, South America, or Africa.

AETIOLOGY/   Anorexia nervosa has been related to family, biological, social, and
RISK FACTORS cultural factors. Studies have found that anorexia nervosa is associated with a family history of anorexia nervosa (adjusted HR 11.4, 95% CI 1.1 to 89.0), of bulimia nervosa (adjusted HR 3.5, 95% CI 1.1 to 14.0),[4] depression, generalised anxiety disorder, obsessive compulsive disorder, or obsessive compulsive personality disorder (adjusted RR 3.6, 95% CI 1.6 to 8.0).[5] A twin study suggested that anorexia nervosa may be related to genetic factors but it was unable to estimate reliably the contribution of non-shared environmental factors.[6] Specific aspects of childhood temperament thought to be related include perfectionism, negative self evaluation, and extreme compliance.[7] Perinatal factors include prematurity, particularly if the baby was small for gestational age (prematurity: OR 3.2, 95% CI 1.6 to 6.2; small for gestational age: OR 5.7, 95% CI 1.1 to 28.7).[8]

PROGNOSIS   One prospective study followed up 51 people with teenage-onset anorexia nervosa, about half of whom received no or minimal treatment (< 8 sessions). After 10 years, 14/51 people (27%) had a persistent eating disorder, three (6%) had ongoing anorexia nervosa, and six (12%) had experienced a period of bulimia nervosa. People with anorexia nervosa were significantly more likely to have an affective disorder than controls matched for sex, age, and school (lifetime risk of affective disorder 96% in people with anorexia v 23% in controls; ARI 73%, 95% CI 60% to 85%). Obsessive compulsive disorder was, similarly, significantly more likely in people with anorexia nervosa compared with controls (30% v 10%; ARI 20%, 95% CI 10% to 41%). However, in 35% of people with obsessive compulsive disorder and anorexia nervosa, obsessive compulsive disorder preceded the anorexia. About half of all participants continued to have poor psychosocial functioning at 10 years (assessed using the Morgan Russell scale [see glossary, p 10] and Global Assessment of Functioning Scale).[9] A summary of treatment studies (68 studies published between 1953 and 1989, 3104 people, length of follow up 1–33 years) found that 43% of people recover completely (range 7–86%), 36% improve (range 1–69%), 20% develop a chronic eating disorder (range 0–43%), and 5% die from anorexia nervosa (range 0–21%).[10] Favourable prognostic factors include an early age at onset and a short interval between onset of symptoms and the beginning of treatment. Unfavourable prognostic factors include vomiting, bulimia, profound weight loss, chronicity, and a history of premorbid developmental or clinical abnormalities. The all cause standardised mortality ratio of eating disorders (anorexia nervosa and bulimia nervosa) has been estimated at 538, about three times higher than other psychiatric illnesses.[11] The average annual mortality was 0.59% a year in females in 10 eating disorder populations (1322 people) with a minimum follow up of 6 years.[12] The mortality was higher for people with lower weight and with older age at presentation. Young women with anorexia nervosa are at an increased risk of fractures later in life.[13]

AIMS OF INTERVENTION   To restore physical health (weight within the normal range and no sequelae of starvation, e.g. regular menstruation, normal bone mass), normal patterns of eating and attitudes towards weight and shape, and no additional psychiatric comorbidity (e.g. depression, anxiety, obsessive compulsive disorder); to reduce the impact of the illness on social functioning and quality of life.

OUTCOMES   The most widely used measure of outcome is the Morgan Russell scale,[14] which includes nutritional status, menstrual function, mental state, and sexual and social adjustment. Biological outcome criteria alone such as weight (body mass index or in relation to matched population weight) and menstrual function are used infrequently as outcome measures. RCTs do not usually have sufficient power or long enough follow up periods to examine mortality. Other validated outcome measures include eating symptom measures.[15–18] Bone mineral density is included as a proxy outcome for fracture risk.

METHODS   *Clinical Evidence* search and appraisal April 2003 and hand searches of reference lists of identified reviews. To be included, an RCT had to have at least 30 people and follow up greater than 75%. Results from each of the identified trials were extracted independently by the two reviewers. Any disagreements were discussed until a consensus was reached.

Mental health

OPTION PSYCHOTHERAPY

We found insufficient evidence from small RCTs to compare psychotherapies versus dietary counselling or versus each other.

Benefits: **Versus treatment as usual or dietary counselling:** We found no systematic review. We found three small RCTs of limited quality that compared different psychotherapies versus dietary counselling (see glossary, p 10) or treatment as usual. All three RCTs were carried out in an outpatient setting in people with a late age of onset and long duration of illness.[19–21] The largest RCT found significant improvements in weight gain for some psychotherapies compared with treatment as usual and for the proportion of people classified as recovered.[19] The second RCT found a significant improvement from baseline for cognitive therapy.[21] All people treated with dietary counselling either did not take up or withdrew from treatment and refused release of their results, making it impossible to compare the two groups. The third RCT found no difference in outcomes between the groups.[20] **Versus each other:** We found six small RCTs of limited quality that compared different psychotherapies (see glossary, p 10). Three of these were undertaken in an outpatient setting in people with an early age of onset and short illness duration.[22–24] Two of the RCTs were carried out in an outpatient setting in people with a later age of onset and longer duration of illness.[19,25] One RCT included people with early and late onset anorexia nervosa and with long and short duration of illness.[26,27] None of the RCTs found an overall significant difference between different psychotherapies.

Harms: The acceptability of the treatment varied among RCTs. Failure to take up treatment ranged from 0–30% and withdrawal from treatment ranged from 0–70% among RCTs but this may have been caused by different methods of case ascertainment. The proportion of people admitted for inpatient treatment (see glossary, p 10) also varied among RCTs, ranging from 0–36%. One death was attributed to anorexia nervosa in the control group in one outpatient RCT with a 1 year follow up.[19] Three deaths attributed to anorexia nervosa occurred in the 5 year follow up period of one inpatient based RCT.[27]

Comment: All the RCTs were small and had limited power to detect clinically important differences. The amount of therapeutic input varied considerably among and within the RCTs. There was variation in methods of recruitment, reporting of key results (e.g. withdrawal rates), and the description of participants' characteristics and selection. The people in the inpatient RCT covered a broad range of severity.[26]

OPTION TRICYCLIC ANTIDEPRESSANTS

Two small RCTs found no evidence of benefit with amitriptyline compared with placebo. They found that amitriptyline was associated with more adverse events, such as palpitations, dry mouth, and blurred vision.

Benefits: We found no systematic review. We found two small RCTs.[28,29] The first RCT (43 people, 5 of them outpatients, with early onset and short duration anorexia nervosa, mean age 16.6 years, mean 27% below average weight, mean duration of anorexia nervosa 1.5 years) compared amitriptyline versus placebo.[29] Participants could also receive various kinds of psychotherapy (see glossary, p 10). Eighteen people refused to participate and were used as a third comparison group. The RCT found no significant difference between the groups on any of the outcome scales measured at 5 weeks (> 50% improvement in global response 1/11 [9%] with amitriptyline v 1/14 [7%] with placebo; RR 1.2, 95% CI 0.1 to 16.7). The second RCT (72 women, mean age 20.6 years, mean 2.9 years' duration) compared amitriptyline (up to a maximum of 160 mg), cyproheptadine, and placebo.[29] It found no significant difference between amitriptyline and placebo for rate of weight gain.[29]

Harms: Adverse events more common with amitriptyline included increased perspiration (2/11 [18%] with amitriptyline v 0/14 [0%] with placebo), drowsiness (6/11 [55%] line v 0/14 [0%]), dry mouth (4/11 [36%] v 2/14 [14%]), blurred vision (1/11 [9%] v 0/14 [0%]), urinary retention (1/11 [9%] v 0/14 [0%]), hypotension (2/11 [18%] v 0/14 [0%]), and leukopenia (1/11 [9%] v 0/14 [0%]). Adverse events more common with placebo included palpitations (0/11 [0%] with amitriptyline v 1/14 [7%] with placebo) and dizziness (0/11 [0%] v 2/14 [14%]). The QT interval may be prolonged in people with anorexia nervosa[30] and tricyclic antidepressants (amitriptyline, protriptyline, nortriptyline, doxepin, and maprotiline) also increase the QT interval.[31–33] In an observational study (495 people with mental illness and 101 healthy controls) an increased risk of prolonged QT interval was seen with tricyclic antidepressant use, adjusting for age and other drug use (adjusted OR 2.6, 95% CI 1.2 to 5.6).[34] The RCT comparing amitriptyline with placebo found more adverse effects with amitriptyline than placebo. General harms of tricyclic antidepressants are described in the section on depression (see depressive disorders, p 114).

Comment: The RCTs were both of short duration. Prolongation of the QT interval may be associated with increased risk of ventricular tachycardia, torsades de pointes, and sudden death.[32,33] It is not clear if people in the second amitriptyline RCT also received psychotherapy.[29]

OPTION   **SELECTIVE SEROTONIN REUPTAKE INHIBITORS**

We found insufficient evidence from three small RCTs about effects of selective serotonin reuptake inhibitors compared with placebo or no treatment in people with anorexia.

Benefits: We found no systematic review. We found three small RCTs.[35–37] The first RCT (33 women; mean age 26.2 years; mean body mass index [see glossary, p 10] 15.0 kg/m^2; mean duration of anorexia nervosa 8.0 years) compared fluoxetine 60 mg versus placebo for the duration (mean 36 days) of inpatient treatment, which included individual and group psychotherapy (see glossary, p 10).[35] There were two early withdrawals from the fluoxetine group. The RCT found no significant differences in weight gain, eating symptoms, or depressive symptoms between the groups. The second RCT (39 women, binge–purge type anorexia excluded, mean age about 22 years, mean duration of anorexia nervosa 4–7 years) compared fluoxetine (starting dosage 20 mg/day) with placebo for 1 year. All women had been discharged from hospital after weight gain (minimum weight restoration was 75% of average body weight). Women were allowed additional psychotherapy. Women who had substantial and incapacitating symptoms were encouraged to withdraw from the study. Withdrawal rates were too high to draw reliable conclusions about effects, although withdrawal rate was significantly lower with fluoxetine compared with placebo (6/16 [37%] with fluoxetine v 16/19 [84%] with placebo; RR 0.45, 95% CI 0.23 to 0.86).[36] The third RCT (52 adults with moderately severe restricting anorexia nervosa [body mass index 15.8 kg/m^2]) compared citalopram (10 mg/day increasing to 20 mg/day) versus waiting list control for 12 weeks before the start of standard integrated dietary and psychiatric treatment.[37] Reliability was limited because withdrawal rates were high (7/26 [29.5%] with citalopram v 6/26 [23.1%] with control). The RCT found no significant difference in weight gain between citalopram and control. It found that self reported depressive symptoms (and some additional measures of comorbidity) improved in the citalopram group only (change in weight from baseline to 12 weeks: from 43.5 kg to 46.5 kg with citalopram v from 42.5 kg to 43.9 kg with control; P value not reported; Beck Depression Inventory: 14.5 to 7.3 with citalopram v 12.7 to 12.3 with control; P value not reported).

Harms: General harms of selective serotonin reuptake inhibitors are described in the section on depression (see depressive disorders, p 114). The RCT comparing citalopram with control did not report adverse effects or reasons for withdrawal.[37]

Comment: In the second RCT, four further women were excluded from the analysis. Three became aware of the treatment and one stopped taking medication before the end of 30 days.[36]

OPTION   **NEUROLEPTIC DRUGS**

We found no good evidence of benefit. Some neuroleptic drugs may prolong the QT interval.

Benefits: We found no systematic review and no RCTs.

Harms: General harms of neuroleptic drugs are described in the section on schizophrenia (see schizophrenia, p 224). The QT interval may be prolonged in people with anorexia nervosa[30,31] and many neuroleptic drugs (haloperidol, pimozide, sertindole, thioridazine, chlorpromazine, and others) may also increase the QT interval.[32,33] An observational study (495 people with mental illness and 101 healthy controls) found an increased risk of prolonged QT interval with high and very high dose neuroleptic use after adjusting for age and other drug use (high dose: adjusted OR 3.4, 95% CI 1.2 to 10.1; very high dose: adjusted OR 5.6, 95% CI 1.6 to 19.3).[34]

Comment: Prolongation of the QT interval may be associated with increased risk of ventricular tachycardia, torsades de pointes, and sudden death.[32,33]

OPTION   **ZINC**

One small RCT found limited evidence that zinc may improve daily body mass index gain compared with placebo in people managed in an inpatient setting. However, we were unable to draw reliable conclusions from this small study.

Benefits: We found no systematic review. We found one RCT (54 people aged > 15 years, mean body mass index (see glossary, p 10) 15.8 kg/m^2, mean duration of anorexia nervosa 3.7 years, admitted to 2 eating disorder units), which compared 100 mg zinc gluconate versus placebo.[38] All but three of the people had normal zinc levels before treatment. Treatment was continued until the individual had gained 10% of weight over the admission weight on two consecutive weeks. Ten people in the zinc group and nine in the placebo group did not complete the study. The RCT found that zinc significantly increased the daily rate of gain in body mass index compared with placebo (0.079 with zinc v 0.039 with placebo; P = 0.03).[38]

Harms: None reported.

Comment: The rationale for zinc supplements in people with normal zinc levels is unclear.

OPTION   **CYPROHEPTADINE**

One small RCT in an outpatient setting and two RCTs in inpatient settings found no significant difference between cyproheptadine and placebo for weight gain.

Benefits: We found no systematic review. We found three small RCTs. The first RCT (24 women in an outpatient setting) compared cyproheptadine with placebo.[39] It found no significant difference in response to treatment after 2 months. The second RCT (81 women in 3 specialised inpatient units) compared cyproheptadine versus placebo, and behaviour therapy versus no behaviour therapy.[40] The effect of behaviour therapy was not reported. There were no significant differences in weight gain between the cyproheptadine and placebo groups. The third RCT (72 women, mean age 20.6 years, mean 77% of target weight, mean duration of anorexia 2.9 years, at 2 specialised inpatient units) compared amitriptyline versus cyproheptadine (up to a maximum of 32 mg) and versus placebo.[29] It found no significant difference between cyproheptadine and placebo for rate of weight gain.

Harms: No harms were reported in the first two RCTs.[39,40] In the third RCT, on both day 7 and day 21, placebo exceeded the amitriptyline group in number of physical adverse events rated moderate or severe. Adverse effects were less frequent with cyproheptadine. No one had to be withdrawn from the protocol because of adverse effects.[29]

Comment: All three RCTs were of short duration.

OPTION	INPATIENT VERSUS OUTPATIENT TREATMENT SETTING IN ANOREXIA NERVOSA

One small RCT found no significant difference between outpatient treatment and inpatient treatment for increasing weight and improving Morgan Russell scale global scores at 1, 2, and 5 years in people who did not need emergency intervention.

Benefits: We found one systematic review (search date 1999) comparing inpatient treatment (see glossary, p 10) versus outpatient care.[41] The review identified one RCT, which had a 5 year follow up.[42,43] Ninety people referred with anorexia nervosa (mean age 22 years, weight loss 26% of matched population mean weight, mean duration 3.2 years) were randomised to four treatment groups: inpatient treatment, outpatient treatment (individual and family therapy [see glossary, p 10]), outpatient group therapy, and assessment interview only. Assessors were not blind to treatment allocation. Adherence to allocated treatment (defined as accepting allocation and at least 1 attendance at a treatment group or individual treatment session) differed significantly among groups (adherence rates: inpatient treatment 18/30 [60%], outpatient treatment [individual and family therapy] 18/20 [90%], outpatient group psychotherapy 17/20 [85%], and assessment interview only 20/20 [100%]). Treatment adherence differed significantly between outpatient and inpatient treatment (RR 1.5, 95% CI 1.1 to 2.0). Average acceptance of treatment also varied among groups (20 weeks' inpatient treatment, 9 outpatient sessions, and 5 group sessions). In the assessment interview only group, six people had no treatment of any kind in the first year and the others had treatment elsewhere (6 had inpatient treatment, 5 had outpatient hospital treatment, and 3 had at least weekly contact with their general practitioners). Six people in this group spent almost the entire year in treatment. There were no significant differences in mean weight or in the Morgan Russell scale (see glossary, p 10) global scores among any of the four groups at 1, 2, and 5 years. The proportion of people with a good outcome with inpatient treatment was 5/29 (17%) at 2 years and 9/27 (33%) at 5 years; with outpatient treatment (individual and family therapy) 4/20 (20%) at 2 years and 8/17 (47%) at 5 years; with outpatient group psychotherapy 5/19 (26%) at 2 years and 10/19 (53%) at 5 years; and with assessment interview only 2/20 (10%) at 2 years and 6/19 (32%) at 5 years.

Harms: One person died from anorexia nervosa between the assessment and the start of outpatient group treatment, and one of the people allocated to inpatient treatment died from anorexia nervosa within 5 years.[42,43]

Comment: The systematic review[41] was unable to draw meaningful conclusions from numerous case series because participant characteristics, treatments, mortality, and outcomes varied widely. People admitted for inpatient treatment had a lower mean weight than those treated as outpatients. One subsequent observational study (355 people with anorexia nervosa; 169 of whom had bulimic type anorexia nervosa; mean age 25 years; mean duration of illness 5.7 years; 75% available for 2.5 years' follow up) found that people with longer duration of illness had a higher likelihood of good outcome with longer than with briefer duration of inpatient treatment.[44] People with a shorter duration of illness had a higher likelihood of good outcome with briefer inpatient treatment. Median duration of inpatient treatment was 11.6 weeks for anorexia nervosa and 10.6 weeks for bulimic type anorexia nervosa.

OPTION CISAPRIDE

One small RCT found no significant difference between cisapride and placebo in weight gain at 8 weeks. Use of cisapride has been restricted in many countries because of concern about cardiac irregularities, including ventricular tachycardia, torsades de pointes, and sudden death.

Benefits: We found no systematic review. We found one small RCT (34 inpatients aged 18–40 years at 2 hospitals; mean duration 2.7 years; body mass index (see glossary, p 10) 15.1 kg/m^2) comparing cisapride 30 mg with placebo for 8 weeks.[45] The trial found no difference in weight gain (5.1 kg with cisapride v 5.7 kg with placebo; P > 0.05).

Harms: No adverse events were noted in this RCT. The QT interval in anorexia nervosa is prolonged even in the absence of medication. Therefore, cisapride, which may prolong the QT interval, is not recommended in anorexia nervosa. Use of cisapride has been restricted in many countries because of concern about cardiac irregularities, including ventricular tachycardia, torsades de pointes, and sudden death.[32,33]

Comment: Five people withdrew from the RCT and were not included in the analysis.

QUESTION What are the effects of interventions to prevent or treat complications of anorexia nervosa?

OPTION OESTROGEN TREATMENT

We found no good evidence about the effects of oestrogen treatment on fracture rates in people with anorexia. Two small RCTs found no significant difference between oestrogen and placebo or no treatment in bone mineral density.

Benefits: We found no systematic review. We found two RCTs.[46,47] The first RCT (48 women, mean age 23.7 years, mean duration of anorexia nervosa 4.0 years) compared hormone replacement therapy (conjugated oestrogens 0.625 mg on days 1–25 of each month plus medroxyprogesterone 5 mg on days 16–25) versus an oral contraceptive containing 35 µg ethinyl oestradiol versus no medication over 6 months.[46] All women maintained a calcium intake of 1500 mg using oral calcium carbonate. Spinal bone mineral density was measured at 6 monthly intervals. There was no significant difference in the final bone density at follow up of 0.5–3.0 years. The second RCT (60 women aged 18–38 years, mean weight 44.7 kg; body mass index (see glossary, p 10) 16.6 kg/m^2, duration of anorexia nervosa 2.3 years and with osteopenia at entry) compared four treatments: oral contraceptive alone (35 µg ethinyl oestradiol plus 0.4 mg norethindrone); placebo; recombinant human insulin-like growth factor-1 alone; and oral contraceptive plus recombinant human insulin-like growth factor-1.[47] In addition, all women received calcium 1500 mg/day and vitamin D 400 IU/day. The RCT found no significant difference between oral contraceptives and placebo in bone density at 9 months (hip density: P = 0.071; spine density: P = 0.21).

Harms:　In the first RCT comparing hormone replacement therapy with the oral contraceptive pill and placebo, three women withdrew from the oestrogen treatment; two because of adverse effects, and one because she had left the country.[46] One woman who was in the control group was unwilling to return for further testing.

Comment:　Improvements in bone mineral density may not reduce fracture risk.

GLOSSARY

Body mass index Weight (kg) divided by height (m) squared.

Dietary counselling Dieticians with experience of eating disorders discuss diet, mood, and daily behaviours.

Family therapy Treatment that includes members of the family of origin or the constituted family, and that addresses the eating disorder as a problem of family life.

Inpatient treatment This has been regarded as the standard approach to the management of anorexia nervosa.[48] One of the key components of inpatient treatment is refeeding, which is achieved through structured, supervised meals. Psychotherapy (of a variety of different types) and pharmacotherapy are included in many programmes.

Morgan Russell scale A widely used measure of outcome for anorexia nervosa that consists of two scores: an average outcome score and a general outcome score. The average outcome score is based on the outcome in five areas: nutritional status, menstrual function, mental state, sexual adjustment, and socioeconomic status.

Psychotherapy Different types of psychological treatments given individually or in groups are included here. These use psychodynamic, cognitive behavioural, or supportive techniques, or combinations of these.

REFERENCES

1. American Psychiatric Association. *Diagnostic and statistical manual of mental disorders (DSM-IV)*. 4th ed. Washington DC: APA, 1994.

2. Pawluck DE, Gorey KM. Secular trends in the incidence of anorexia nervosa: integrative review of population-based studies. *Int J Eat Disord* 1998;23:347–352.

3. Rastam M, Gillberg C, Garton M. Anorexia nervosa in a Swedish urban region. A population-based study. *Br J Psychiatry* 1989;155:642–646.

4. Strober M, Freeman R, Lampert C, et al. Controlled family study of anorexia nervosa and bulimia nervosa: evidence of shared liability and transmission of partial syndromes. *Am J Psychiatry* 2000;157:393–401.

5. Lilenfeld LR, Kaye WH, Greeno CG, et al. A controlled family study of anorexia nervosa and bulimia nervosa: psychiatric disorders in first-degree relatives and effects of proband comorbidity. *Arch Gen Psychiatry* 1998;55:603–610.

6. Wade TD, Bulik CM, Neale M, et al. Anorexia nervosa and major depression: shared genetic and environmental risk factors. *Am J Psychiatry* 2000;157:469–471.

7. Fairburn CG, Cooper Z, Doll HA, et al. Risk factors for anorexia nervosa: three integrated case-control comparisons. *Arch Gen Psychiatry* 1999;56:468–476.

8. Cnattingius S, Hultman CM, Dahl M, et al. Very preterm birth, birth trauma, and the risk of anorexia nervosa among girls. *Arch Gen Psychiatry* 1999;56:634–638.

9. Wentz E, Gillberg C, Gillberg IC, et al. Ten-year follow-up of adolescent-onset anorexia nervosa: psychiatric disorders and overall functioning scales. *J Child Psychol Psychiatry* 2001;42:613–622.

10. Steinhausen, H-C. The course and outcome of anorexia nervosa. In: Brownell K, Fairburn CG, eds. *Eating disorders and obesity: a comprehensive handbook*. New York: Guilford Press, 1995:234–237.

11. Harri, EC, Barraclough B. Excess mortality of mental disorder. *Br J Psychiatry* 1998;173:11–53.

12. Nielsen S, Møller-Madsen S, Isager T, et al. Standardized mortality in eating disorders: a quantitative summary of previously published and new evidence. *J Psychosom Res* 1998;44:413–434.

13. Lucas A, Melton L, Crowson C, et al. Long term fracture risk among women with anorexia nervosa: a population-based cohort study. *Mayo Clin Proc* 1999;74:972–977.

14. Morgan HG, Russell GF. Value of family background and clinical features as predictors of long-term outcome in anorexia nervosa: four-year follow-up study of 41 patients. *Psychol Med* 1975;5:355–371.

15. Cooper Z, Fairburn CG. The Eating Disorders Examination. A semi-structured interview for the assessment of the specific psychopathology of eating disorders. *Int J Eat Disord* 1987;6:1–8.

16. Garner DM. *Eating Disorder Inventory-2 (EDI-2): professional manual*. Odessa FL: Psychological Assessment Resources Inc, 1991.

17. Garner DM, Garfinkel PE. The eating attitudes test: an index of the symptoms of anorexia nervosa. *Psychol Med* 1979;9:273–279.

18. Henderson M, Freeman CPL. A self-rating scale for bulimia: the 'BITE'. *Br J Psychiatry* 1987;150:18–24.

19. Dare C, Eisler I, Russell G, et al. Psychological therapies for adult patients with anorexia nervosa: a randomised controlled trial of outpatient treatments. *Br J Psychiatry* 2001;178:216–221.

20. Hall A, Crisp AH. Brief psychotherapy in the treatment of anorexia nervosa. Outcome at one year. *Br J Psychiatry* 1987;151:185–191.

21. Serfaty MA. Cognitive therapy versus dietary counselling in the outpatient treatment of anorexia nervosa: effects of the treatment phase. *Eur Eat Dis Rev* 1999;7:334–350.

22. Eisler I, Dare C, Hodes M, et al. Family therapy for adolescent anorexia nervosa: the results of a controlled comparison of two family interventions. *J Child Psychol Psychiatry* 2000;41:727–736.

23. Robin AL, Siegel PT, Moye AW, et al. A controlled comparison of family versus individual therapy for adolescents with anorexia nervosa. *J Am Acad Child Adolesc Psychiatry* 1999;38:1482–1489.

24. Wallin U, Kronvall P, Majewski ML. Body awareness therapy in teenage anorexia nervosa: outcome after 2 years. *Eur Eat Dis Rev* 2000;8:19–30.

25. Treasure JL, Todd G, Brolly M, et al. A pilot study of a randomized trial of cognitive analytical therapy vs educational behavioral therapy for adult anorexia nervosa. *Behav Res Ther* 1995;33:363–367.

26. Russell GFM, Szmukler G, Dare C, et al. An evaluation of family therapy in anorexia nervosa and bulimia nervosa. *Arch Gen Psychiatry* 1987;44:1047–1056.

27. Eisler I, Dare C, Russell GFM, et al. Family and individual therapy in anorexia nervosa. A 5-year follow-up. *Arch Gen Psychiatry* 1997;54:1025–1030.

28. Biederman J, Herzog DB, Rivinus TM, et al. Amitriptyline in the treatment of anorexia nervosa: a double-blind, placebo-controlled study. *J Clin Psychopharmacol* 1985;5:10–16.

29. Halmi KA, Eckert E, LaDu TJ, et al. Anorexia nervosa. Treatment efficacy of cyproheptadine and amitriptyline. *Arch Gen Psychiatry* 1986;43:177–181.

30. Ackerman MJ. The long QT syndrome: ion channel diseases of the heart. *Mayo Clin Proc* 1998;73:250–269.

31. Becker A, Grinspoon SK, Klibanski A, et al. Current concepts: eating disorders. *N Engl J Med* 1999;340:1092–1098.

32. Yap Y, Camm J. Risk of torsades de pointes with non-cardiac drugs: doctors need to be aware that many drugs can cause QT prolongation. *BMJ* 2000;320:1158–1159.

33. Sheridan DJ. Drug-induced proarrhythmic effects: assessment of changes in QT interval. *Br J Clin Pharmacol* 2000;50:297–302.

34. Reilly JG, Ayis SA, Ferrier IN, et al. QTc interval abnormalities and psychotropic drug therapy in psychiatric patients. *Lancet* 2000;355:1048–1052.

35. Attia E, Haiman C, Walsh BT, et al. Does fluoxetine augment the inpatient treatment of anorexia nervosa? *Am J Psychiatry* 1998;155:548–551.

36. Kaye WH, Nagata T, Weltzin TE, et al. Double-blind placebo-controlled administration of fluoxetine in restricting- and restricting-purging-type anorexia nervosa. *Soc Biol Psych* 2001;49:644–652.

37. Fassino S, Leombruni P, Daga G, et al. Efficacy of citalopram in anorexia nervosa: a pilot study. *Eur Neuropsychopharmacol* 2002;12:453–459.

38. Birmingham CL, Goldner EM, Bakan R. Controlled trial of zinc supplementation in anorexia nervosa. *Int J Eat Disord* 1994;15:251–255.

39. Vigersky RA, Loriaux L. The effect of cyproheptadine in anorexia nervosa: a double blind trial. In: Vigersky RA, ed. *Anorexia nervosa*. New York: Raven Press, 1977:349–356.

40. Goldberg SC, Halmi KA, Eckert RC, et al. Cyproheptadine in anorexia nervosa. *Br J Psychiatry* 1979;134:67–70.

41. West Midlands Development and Evaluation Service. *In-patient versus out-patient care for eating disorders*. DPHE 1999 Report No 17. Birmingham: University of Birmingham, 1999. Search date 1999; primary sources Medline, Psychlit, The Cochrane Library, variety of internet sites, and hand searches of relevant editions of relevant journals and references from identified articles.

42. Crisp AH, Norton K, Gowers S, et al. A controlled study of the effect of therapies aimed at adolescent and family psychopathology in anorexia nervosa. *Br J Psychiatry* 1991;159:325–333.

43. Gowers S, Norton K, Halek C, et al. Outcome of outpatient psychotherapy in a random allocation treatment study of anorexia nervosa. *Int J Eat Disord* 1994;15:65–177.

44. Kächele H for the study group MZ-ESS. Eine multizentrische studie zu aufwand und erfolg bei psychodynamischer therapie von eßstörungen. *Psychother Med Psychol (Stuttg)* 1999;49:100–108.

45. Szmukler GI, Young GP, Miller G, et al. A controlled trial of cisapride in anorexia nervosa. *Int J Eat Disord* 1995;17:347–357.
46. Klibanski A, Biller BMK, Schoenfeld DA, et al. The effects of estrogen administration on trabecular bone loss in young women with anorexia nervosa. *J Clin Endocrinol Metab* 1995;80:898–904.
47. Grinspoon S, Thomas L, Miller K, et al. Effects of recombinant human IGF-I and oral contraceptive administration on bone density in anorexia nervosa. *J Clin Endocrinol Metab* 2002;87:2883–2891.
48. American Psychiatric Association. Practice guideline for the treatment of patients with eating disorders (revision). *Am J Psychiatry* 2000;157(suppl 1):1–39.

Janet Treasure
Psychiatrist
Institute of Psychiatry
Kings College London
London
UK

Ulrike Schmidt
Psychiatrist
South London and Maudsley NHS Trust
London
UK

Competing interests: None declared.

INTERVENTIONS

Key Messages

Mania

- **Lithium** One RCT in people with bipolar type I disorder experiencing a manic episode found that lithium increased the proportion of people who responded after 3–4 weeks compared with placebo. One systematic review found that lithium increased the proportion of people who had remission of manic symptoms at 3 weeks compared with chlorpromazine, and found no significant difference in symptoms at 3–6 weeks between lithium and haloperidol, olanzapine, valproate, lamotrigine, or clonazepam. One RCT found that lithium was less effective than risperidone in reducing manic symptoms at 4 weeks.

Lithium can cause a range of adverse effects. The RCTs provided insufficient evidence about how the adverse effects of lithium compared with those of other antipsychotic drugs.

- **Olanzapine** One systematic review in people with bipolar type I disorder found that olanzapine increased the proportion of people who responded at 3–6 weeks compared with placebo, both as monotherapy and as add on therapy to lithium or valproate, and found no significant difference in symptoms at 28 days between olanzapine and lithium. RCTs found that olanzapine was more effective in reducing symptoms than valproate, but was also more likely to cause adverse effects such as sedation and weight gain. The acceptability of olanzapine may be limited by weight gain.

- **Valproate** One systematic review in people with bipolar type I disorder experiencing a manic episode found that valproate increased the proportion of people who responded over 3 weeks compared with placebo. It found no significant difference in response at 1–6 weeks between valproate and lithium, haloperidol, or carbamazepine. It found that valproate was less effective in reducing manic symptoms than olanzapine, but was also less likely to cause adverse effects such as sedation and weight gain.

- **Carbamazepine** RCTs in people with bipolar type I disorder experiencing a manic episode found no significant difference in manic symptoms at 4–6 weeks between carbamazepine and lithium or valproate.

- **Clonazepam** We found no RCTs comparing clonazepam versus placebo in people with bipolar mania. RCTs in people with bipolar type I disorder experiencing a manic episode suggest that clonazepam may be as effective as lithium in improving manic symptoms at 1–4 weeks.

- **Haloperidol** We found no RCTs comparing haloperidol versus placebo in people with bipolar mania. RCTs in people with bipolar type I disorder experiencing a manic episode found no significant difference in manic symptoms at 1–3 weeks between haloperidol and lithium or valproate, although haloperidol was associated with more extrapyramidal adverse effects and sedation than valproate.

- **Risperidone** We found no RCTs comparing risperidone versus placebo in people with bipolar mania. One RCT in people with bipolar type I disorder experiencing a manic episode found that risperidone reduced manic symptoms at 4 weeks compared with lithium. It gave no information on adverse effects.

- **Chlorpromazine** One very small RCT in people with mania found limited evidence that chlorpromazine may improve manic symptoms over 7 weeks more than placebo or imipramine. One systematic review found that fewer people had remission of symptoms at 3 weeks with chlorpromazine than with lithium.

- **Lamotrigine** We found no RCTs comparing lamotrigine versus placebo in people with bipolar mania. One RCT in people with bipolar type I disorder experiencing a manic episode found no significant difference in manic symptoms at 4 weeks between lamotrigine and lithium.

Bipolar depression

- **Lamotrigine** One RCT in people with bipolar type I disorder experiencing a major depressive episode found that lamotrigine increased the proportion of people who responded over 7 weeks compared with placebo.

- **Antidepressants** Systematic reviews found that antidepressants improved depressive symptoms at the end of the trial (unspecified) compared with placebo. They found limited evidence that selective serotonin reuptake inhibitors were more effective than tricyclic antidepressants, and found no significant difference in symptoms between monoamine oxidase inhibitors and tricyclic antidepressants or between selective serotonin reuptake inhibitors and serotonin noradrenaline reuptake inhibitors. The reviews provided insufficient evidence to assess whether antidepressants induce bipolar mania.
- **Carbamazepine; lithium** One systematic review identified no RCTs of sufficient quality to assess these treatments in people with bipolar depression.
- **Psychological treatments; valproate** We found no RCTs of these treatments in people with bipolar depression.

Preventing relapse of mania or bipolar depression

- **Lithium** RCTs have found that lithium reduces relapse over 2 years compared versus placebo, and have found no significant difference in relapse between lithium and valproate, carbamazepine, or lamotrigine.
- **Carbamazepine** We found no RCTs comparing carbamazepine versus placebo in preventing relapse. One systematic review found no significant difference between carbamazepine and lithium in the proportion of people who relapsed over 1–3 years.
- **Education to recognise symptoms of relapse** One RCT found limited evidence that an educational programme to recognise symptoms of relapse reduced manic relapse over 18 months, but that it may increase depressive episodes.
- **Lamotrigine (bipolar depressive episodes)** Three RCTs have found that lamotrigine reduces relapse compared with placebo. However, secondary analyses in two of the RCTs suggested that lamotrigine protected against depressive relapse, but not manic relapse. RCTs have found no significant difference between lamotrigine and lithium in the proportion of people who relapse.
- **Valproate** One RCT found that valproate reduced relapse over 12 months compared with placebo. One systematic review found no significant difference between lithium and valproate in relapse over 12 months.
- **Antidepressant drugs** One systematic review provided insufficient evidence to assess antidepressants in preventing relapse of bipolar disorder.
- **Family focused psychoeducation** One RCT found that 21 sessions of family focused psychoeducation reduced relapse over 12 months compared with two family sessions plus crisis management.

DEFINITION Bipolar disorder (bipolar affective disorder, manic depressive disorder) is characterised by marked mood swings between mania (mood elevation) and bipolar depression that cause significant personal distress or social dysfunction, and are not caused by drugs or known physical disorder. **Bipolar type I disorder** is diagnosed when episodes of depression are interspersed with mania or mixed episodes. **Bipolar type II disorder** is diagnosed when depression is interspersed with less severe episodes of elevated mood that do not lead to dysfunction or disability (hypomania). Bipolar disorder has been subdivided in several further ways (see table 1, p 32).[1]

INCIDENCE/ PREVALENCE One 1996 cross-national community based study (38 000 people) found lifetime prevalence rates of bipolar disorder ranging from 0.3% in Taiwan to 1.5% in New Zealand.[2] It found that men and women were at similar risk, and that the age at first onset ranged from 19–29 years (average of 6 years earlier than first onset of major depression).

AETIOLOGY/ RISK FACTORS The cause of bipolar disorder is uncertain, although family and twin studies suggest a genetic basis.[3] The lifetime risk of bipolar disorder is increased in first degree relatives of a person with bipolar disorder (40–70% for a monozygotic twin; 5–10% for other first degree relatives). If the first episode of mania occurs in an older adult, it may be secondary mania due to underlying medical or substance induced factors.[4]

PROGNOSIS Bipolar disorder is a recurring illness and one of the leading causes of worldwide disability, especially in the 15–44 year age group.[5] One 4 year inception cohort study (173 people treated for a first episode of mania or mixed affective disorder) found that 93% of people no longer met criteria for mania at 2 years (median time to recover from a syndrome 4.6 weeks), but that only 36% had recovered to premorbid function.[6] It found that 40% of people had a recurrent manic (20%) or depressive (20%) episode within 2 years of recovering from the first episode. A meta-analysis, comparing observed suicide expected rates of suicide in an age and sex matched sample of the general population, found that the lifetime prevalence of suicide was about 2%, or 15 times greater than expected, in people with bipolar disorder.[7]

AIMS OF INTERVENTION To alleviate mania and bipolar depressive symptoms; to prevent relapse (see glossary, p 30) and suicide; to optimise social and occupational functioning; and to improve quality of life, with minimal adverse effects of treatment.

OUTCOMES Level of symptoms on rating scales (completed by clinician, patient, or both); proportion of people with clinically important response to treatment; time to remission; quality of life scores; social and occupational functioning scores; relapse; hospital admission; rates of suicide; frequency of adverse events; and clinical trial withdrawal rates. Commonly used instruments for assessing symptoms include the Young Mania Rating Scale, which rates 11 manic symptoms with a total score of 0–60; the Schedule for Affective Disorders Change Mania Sub Scale, which rates 18 manic items with a total score of 10–65; and the Hamilton Depression Rating Scale, which has both a 17 and a 21 item version. On these scales, a clinically important response to treatment is usually defined as a > 50% reduction in score from baseline.[8] A person is usually considered to be in remission if, at the end of trial, they score ≤ 12 on the Young Mania Rating Scale and ≤ 8 on the Hamilton Depression Rating Scale.[8] Quality of life is assessed by scales such as the SF-36, and social and occupational functioning on scales such as the Clinical Global Impression Scale.

METHODS *Clinical Evidence* search and appraisal April 2002, including a search for observational studies on adverse effects of treatments. The author also performed a search for systematic reviews in the Cochrane Library, Issue 3, 2003.

QUESTION What are the effects of treatments in mania?

OPTION LITHIUM

One RCT in people with bipolar type I disorder experiencing a manic episode found that lithium increased the proportion of people who responded after 3–4 weeks compared with placebo. One systematic review found that lithium increased the proportion of people who had remission of manic symptoms at 3 weeks compared with chlorpromazine, and found no significant difference in symptoms at 3–6 weeks between lithium and haloperidol, olanzapine, valproate, lamotrigine, or clonazepam. One RCT found that lithium was less effective than risperidone in reducing manic symptoms at 4 weeks. Lithium can cause a range of adverse effects. The RCTs provided insufficient evidence about how the adverse effects of lithium compared with those of other antipsychotic drugs.

Benefits: **Versus placebo:** We found one systematic review (search date 1999, 1 RCT, 179 people with bipolar type I disorder).[9] The RCT compared three treatments: lithium (36 people); valproate (69 people); and placebo (74 people). It found that lithium significantly increased the proportion of people who responded after 3–4 weeks compared with placebo (response defined as ≥ 50% improvement in mania score on the Schedule for Affective Disorders and Schizophrenia-Change [SADS-C]; 18/36 [50%] with lithium v 19/74 [27%] with placebo; RR 1.95, 95% CI 1.17 to 3.23; NNT 5, 95% CI 3 to 20). **Versus chlorpromazine:** We found one systematic review (search date 1999, 4 RCTs, 114 people with bipolar type 1 disorder).[9] It found that lithium significantly increased the proportion of people who had remission of symptoms at 3 weeks compared with chlorpromazine (remission not defined, 3 RCTs that assessed outcomes at 3 weeks: 23/57 [40%] with lithium v 7/57 [12%] with chlorpromazine; RR 1.96, 95% CI 1.02 to 3.77; NNT 4, 95% CI 3 to 9). **Versus haloperidol:** We found one systematic review (search date 1999, 2 RCTs, 50 people with bipolar type I disorder).[9] It found no significant difference between haloperidol and lithium in symptom scores at 3 weeks (assessed by the Brief Psychiatric Rating Scale [BPRS]: effect size −2.14, 95% CI −6.57 to +2.30). **Versus risperidone:** We found one systematic review (search date 1999, 1 RCT, 54 people with bipolar type I disorder).[9] It found that risperidone was significantly more effective than lithium in improving symptom severity score at 4 weeks (assessed by BPRS: effect size −2.79, 95% CI −4.22 to −1.36). **Versus olanzapine:** We found no systematic review but found one RCT (30 people with bipolar type I disorder).[10] It found no significant difference between lithium and olanzapine in Young Mania Rating Scale [YMRS] score at 28 days (13.2 with lithium v 10.2 with olanzapine; P = 0.315). **Versus valproate:** We found one systematic review (search date 2002, 3 RCTs, 158 people with bipolar type 1 disorder).[8] It found no significant difference between valproate and lithium in the proportion of people who failed to respond over 3–6 weeks (response defined as 50% reduction in mania score on the YMRS or the SADS-C; 45/97 [46%] with valproate v 26/61 [43%] with lithium; RR 1.05, 95% CI 0.74 to 1.50). **Versus**

carbamazepine: We found one systematic review (search date 1999, 3 RCTs, 176 people with bipolar type I disorder).[9] The review could not perform a meta-analysis of all three RCTs because of differences in outcomes assessed. The first RCT (105 people) found no significant difference in the proportion of people who responded over 4 weeks between lithium and carbamazepine (15/54 [28%] with lithium v 14/51 [27%] with carbamazepine; RR 1.01, 95% CI 0.54 to 1.88). The other two RCTs (71 people) found no significant difference in global severity of symptoms over 4 weeks between lithium and carbamazepine (assessed by Clinical Global Impression [CGI] scores: effect size +0.44, 95% CI –0.78 to +1.67).[9] **Versus lamotrigine:** We found no systematic review but found one RCT (30 people with bipolar type I disorder).[11] It found no significant difference between lithium and lamotrigine in YMRS scores at 4 weeks (mean 13.2 with lithium v 14.3 with lamotrigine; reported as non-significant; no further data reported). **Versus clonazepam:** We found one systematic review (search date 1999, 2 RCTs, 52 people with bipolar type I disorder).[9] The review could not perform a meta-analysis because the RCTs assessed different outcomes. The first RCT (12 people) found limited evidence that clonazepam improved some measures of mania more than lithium after 10 days treatment (mean motor activity score 1.8 with clonazepam v 2.8 with lithium; mean logorrhoea score 2.2 with clonazepam v 2.9 with lithium; CI not reported). The second RCT (40 people, unblinded) found no significant difference between lithium and clonazepam in symptom severity at 4 weeks assessed by BPRS (mean score 6.27 with lithium v 7.79 with clonazepam) or global severity of symptoms assessed by CGI Scale (mean score 2.07 with lithium v 1.68 with clonazepam; reported as non-significant, CI not reported) after 4 weeks.

Harms: **Versus placebo:** The RCT identified by the review found that lithium significantly increased the proportion of people who had adverse effects compared with placebo (33/36 [92%] with lithium v 58/74 [78%] with placebo; RR 1.17, 95% CI 1.00 to 1.37; NNH 8, 95% CI 4 to 334).[9] Adverse effects were not specified. **Versus chlorpromazine:** The review gave no information on adverse effects.[9] **Versus haloperidol:** The review gave no information on adverse effects.[9] **Versus risperidone:** The review gave no information on adverse effects.[9] **Versus olanzapine:** The RCT found no extrapyramidal adverse effects associated with lithium or olanzapine.[10] **Versus valproate:** The review found that valproate significantly reduced the proportion of people who had fever compared with lithium (1 RCT 1/69 [1%] with valproate v 5/36 [14%] with lithium; RR 0.10, 95% CI 0.01 to 0.86), but found no significant difference in the rates of other adverse events.[8] **Versus carbamazepine:** The review found no significant difference in adverse effects between lithium and carbamazepine (2 RCTs: 27/73 [37%] with lithium v 35/66 [53%] with carbamazepine; RR 0.71, 95% CI 0.49 to 1.02).[9] **Versus lamotrigine:** The RCT found no significant difference in adverse effects between lithium and lamotrigine, but it is likely to have been too small to detect a clinically important difference.[11] One person taking lithium withdrew because of a seizure and one person taking lamotrigine withdrew because of aggravation of diabetes. **Versus clonazepam:** The review gave no information on adverse effects.[9]

Comment: None.

OPTION	VALPROATE

One systematic review in people with bipolar type I disorder experiencing a manic episode found that valproate increased the proportion of people who responded over 3 weeks compared with placebo. It found no significant difference in response at 1–6 weeks between valproate and lithium, haloperidol, or carbamazepine. It found that valproate was less effective in reducing manic symptoms than olanzapine, but was also less likely to cause adverse effects such as sedation and weight gain.

Benefits: **Versus placebo:** We found one systematic review (search date 2002, 3 RCTs, 316 people with bipolar type I disorder).[8] It found that valproate significantly increased the proportion of people who responded over 3 weeks compared with placebo (response defined as 50% reduction in mania score on the Young Mania Rating Scale [YMRS] or the Schedule for Affective Disorders and Schizophrenia-Change [SADS-C]; proportion of people who failed to respond: 66/155 [42%] with valproate v 111/161 [69%] with placebo; RR of failing to respond 0.62, 95% CI 0.51 to 0.77).[8] **Versus lithium:** See benefits of lithium, p 17. **Versus haloperidol:** We found one systematic review (search date 2002, 1 RCT, 36 people with bipolar type I disorder).[8] The RCT found no significant difference in the proportion of patients who failed to respond over 6 days between valproate and haloperidol (11/21 [52%] with valproate v 10/15 [67%] with lithium; RR 0.79, 95% CI 0.46 to 1.35). **Versus olanzapine:** We found one systematic review (search date 2002, 2 RCTs, 363 people with bipolar type I disorder).[8] It found that people taking olanzapine had greater symptom reductions at the end of the trial (unspecified) than those taking valproate (symptoms assessed by the YMRS: WMD 2.81, 95% CI 0.83 to 4.79). One of the RCTs (251 people) found that olanzapine significantly increased the proportion of people who responded at the end of the trial (unspecified) compared with valproate (response defined as 50% reduction in YMRS; proportion of people who failed to respond: 77/123 [63%] with valproate v 57/125 [46%] with olanzapine; RR of failing to respond 1.27, 95% CI 0.99 to 1.62). **Versus carbamazepine:** We found one systematic review (2 RCTs, 59 people with bipolar type I disorder), which found no significant difference between valproate and carbamazepine in the proportion of people who failed to respond at 4–6 weeks (response defined with 50% reduction in mania score on the YMRS or the SADS-C; 11/30 [37%] with valproate v 16/29 [55%] carbamazepine; RR 0.66, 95% CI 0.38 to 1.16).[8]

Harms: **Versus placebo:** The review found no significant difference between valproate and placebo in the proportion of people who withdrew from the trial because of adverse effects (9/158 [6%] with valproate v 5/163 [3%] with placebo; RR 1.95, 95% CI 0.66 to 5.71), but found that people taking valproate were significantly more likely to suffer from dizziness (13/138 [9%] with valproate v 4/141 [3%] with placebo; RR 3.17, 95% CI 1.13 to 8.88).[8] No other adverse effects were more commonly reported with valproate than with placebo. **Versus lithium:** See harms of lithium, p 18. **Versus haloperidol:** The RCT found that valproate caused significantly fewer extrapyramidal adverse effects compared with haloperidol (0/21 [0%] with valproate v 8/15 [53%] with haloperidol; RR 0.04, 95% CI 0.00 to 0.69), dry mouth (1/21 [5%] with valproate v 3/15 [20%] with haloperidol; RR 0.24, 95% CI 0.03 to 2.07), and was less likely to cause sedation than haloperidol (1/21 [5%] with valproate v 4/15 [27%] with haloperidol; RR 0.18, 95% CI 0.02 to 1.44).[8] **Versus olanzapine:** The review found no significant difference between valproate and olanzapine in the proportion of patients who withdrew because of adverse events (1 RCT: 9/126 [7%] with valproate v 12/125 [10%] with olanzapine; RR 0.74, 95% CI 0.33 to 1.70) or had movement disorders (akathisia: WMD −0.02, 95% CI −0.27 to +0.23; abnormal involuntary movement: WMD −0.17, 95% CI −0.62 to +0.28).[8] It found that valproate caused significantly more nausea than olanzapine (1 RCT: 36/126 [28%] with valproate v 13/125 [10%] with olanzapine; RR 2.75, 95% CI 1.53 to 4.93), but caused less increased appetite (1 RCT: 3/126 [2%] with valproate v 15/125 [12%] with olanzapine; RR 0.20, 95% CI 0.06 to 0.67), weight gain (WMD −2.14 kg, 95% CI −2.65 kg to −1.62 kg), dry mouth (8/126 [6%] with valproate v 42/125 [34%] with olanzapine; RR 0.19, 95% CI 0.09 to 0.39), and sedation (2 RCTs: 44/189 [23%] with valproate v 76/182 [42%] with olanzapine; RR 0.55, 95% CI 0.41 to 0.76). **Versus carbamazepine:** One RCT (28 people) assessed adverse effects.[8] It found no significant difference in adverse effects between valproate and carbamazepine, but it is likely to have been underpowered to detect a clinically important difference.

Comment: None.

OPTION   CHLORPROMAZINE

One very small RCT in people with mania found limited evidence that chlorpromazine may improve manic symptoms over 7 weeks compared with placebo or imipramine. One systematic review found that fewer people had remission of symptoms at 3 weeks with chlorpromazine than with lithium.

Benefits: **Versus placebo:** We found one non-systematic review, which identified one very small RCT (13 people with mania) comparing three treatments: chlorpromazine, imipramine, and placebo.[12] It found that chlorpromazine significantly improved global outcome at 7 weeks compared with imipramine or placebo (assessed on a scale from −9 to +9 where +9 = improvement: +6.1 with chlorpromazine v +2.0 with imipramine v −2.8 with placebo; reported as significant; no further data reported). **Versus lithium:** See benefits of lithium, p 17.

Harms: **Versus placebo:** The non-systematic review gave no information on adverse effects.[12] **Versus lithium:** See harms of lithium, p 18.

Comment: The evidence for older antipsychotic drugs is sparse and there are currently no systematic reviews available. The drugs are, however, widely used in mania.

OPTION · HALOPERIDOL

We found no RCTs comparing haloperidol versus placebo in people with bipolar mania. RCTs in people with bipolar type I disorder experiencing a manic episode found no significant difference in manic symptoms at 1–3 weeks between haloperidol and lithium or valproate, although haloperidol was associated with more extrapyramidal adverse effects and sedation than valproate.

Benefits: **Versus placebo:** We found no systematic review and no RCTs comparing haloperidol versus placebo. **Versus lithium:** See benefits of lithium, p 17. **Versus valproate:** See benefits of valproate, p 19.

Harms: **Versus placebo:** We found no RCTs. **Versus lithium:** See harms of lithium, p 18. **Versus valproate:** See harms of valproate, p 19.

Comment: The evidence for older antipsychotics is sparse and there are currently no systematic reviews available. The drugs are, however, widely used in bipolar mania.

OPTION · RISPERIDONE

We found no RCTs comparing risperidone versus placebo in people with bipolar mania. One RCT in people with bipolar type I disorder experiencing a manic episode found that risperidone reduced manic symptoms at 4 weeks compared with lithium. It gave no information on adverse effects.

Benefits: **Versus placebo:** We found no systematic review and no RCTs. **Versus lithium:** See benefits of lithium, p 17.

Harms: **Versus placebo:** We found no RCTs. **Versus lithium:** See harms of lithium, p 18.

Comment: None.

OPTION · OLANZAPINE

One systematic review in people with bipolar type I disorder found that olanzapine increased the proportion of people who responded at 3–6 weeks compared with placebo, both as monotherapy and as add on therapy to lithium or valproate, and found no significant difference in symptoms at 28 days between olanzapine and lithium. RCTs found that olanzapine was more effective in reducing symptoms than valproate, but was also more likely to cause adverse effects such as sedation and weight gain. The acceptability of olanzapine may be limited by weight gain.

Benefits: **Versus placebo:** We found one systematic review (search date 2002, 6 RCTs, 1422 people with bipolar type I disorder).[13] It found that olanzapine significantly increased the proportion of people who responded over 3–4 weeks compared with placebo (response defined as 50% reduction in mania score on the Young Mania Rating Scale; 2 RCTs: proportion who failed to respond 56/125

[45%] with olanzapine v 89/129 [69%] with placebo; RR of failing to respond 0.64, 95% CI 0.52 to 0.81). It also found that adding olanzapine to lithium or valproate significantly increased the proportion of people who responded at 6 weeks compared with placebo (1 RCT; proportion who failed to respond: 80/229 [35%] with olanzapine v 64/115 [56%] with placebo; RR of failing to respond 0.63, 95% CI 0.49 to 0.80). **Versus lithium:** See benefits of lithium, p 17. **Versus valproate:** See benefits of valproate, p 19.

Harms: The review found that olanzapine, both as monotherapy and as add-on therapy to lithium or valproate, caused significantly more weight gain than placebo (3 RCTs, 581 people: WMD 2.27 kg, 95% CI 1.56 kg to 2.99 kg).[13] It found no significant difference in movement disorders between olanzapine and placebo (measured on the Barnes Akathisia Scale; 2 RCTs, 246 people: WMD −0.13, 95% CI −0.32 to +0.06), but found that olanzapine significantly increased somnolence (162/354 [46%] with olanzapine v 48/244 [20%] with placebo; RR 2.13, 95% CI 1.62 to 2.79), dry mouth (100/354 [28%] v 18/244 [7%]; RR 3.64, 95% CI 2.24 to 5.91), dizziness (54/354 [15%] v 16/244 [6%]; RR 2.37, 95% CI 1.39 to 4.04), muscle weakness (61/354 [17%] v 23/244 [9%]; RR 1.69, 95% CI 1.09 to 2.64), increased appetite (54/229 [23%] v 9/115 [8%]; RR 3.01, 95% CI 1.54 to 5.88), and speech disorder (15/229 [6%] with olanzapine v 1/115 [0.9%] with placebo; RR 7.53, 95% CI 1.01 to 56.32).**Versus lithium:** See harms of lithium, p 18. **Versus valproate:** See harms of valproate, p 19.

Comment: None.

OPTION   CARBAMAZEPINE

RCTs in people with bipolar type I disorder experiencing a manic episode found no significant difference in manic symptoms at 4–6 weeks between carbamazepine and lithium or valproate.

Benefits: **Versus placebo:** We found no RCTs. **Versus lithium:** See benefits of lithium, p 17. **Versus valproate:** See benefits of valproate, p 19.

Harms: **Versus placebo:** We found no RCTs. **Versus lithium:** See harms of lithium, p 18. **Versus valproate:** See harms of valproate, p 19.

Comment: None.

OPTION   LAMOTRIGINE

We found no RCTs comparing lamotrigine versus placebo in people with bipolar mania. One RCT in people with bipolar type I disorder experiencing a manic episode found no significant difference in manic symptoms at 4 weeks between lamotrigine and lithium.

Benefits: **Versus placebo:** We found no systematic review or RCTs comparing lamotrigine versus placebo in people with bipolar mania. **Versus lithium:** See benefits of lithium, p 17.

Harms: **Versus placebo:** We found no RCTs. **Versus lithium:** See harms of lithium, p 18.

Comment: None.

OPTION CLONAZEPAM

We found no RCTs comparing clonazepam versus placebo in people with bipolar mania. RCTs in people with bipolar type I disorder experiencing a manic episode suggest that clonazepam may be as effective as lithium in improving manic symptoms at 1–4 weeks.

Benefits: **Versus placebo:** We found no systematic review or RCTs comparing clonazepam versus placebo in people with bipolar mania. **Versus lithium:** See harms of lithium, p 18.

Harms: **Versus placebo:** We found no RCTs. **Versus lithium:** See harms of lithium, p 18.

Comment: None.

QUESTION **What are the effects of treatments in bipolar depression?**

OPTION PSYCHOLOGICAL TREATMENTS

We found no RCTs of psychological treatments in people with bipolar depression.

Benefits: We found no systematic review or RCTs in people with bipolar depression (see comment below).

Harms: We found no RCTs.

Comment: We found no RCTs of psychological interventions in bipolar depression. It is unclear if it is reasonable to extrapolate from the evidence for treatments for unipolar depression. It is likely that specific interventions will have some effect, but RCTs are needed to estimate the size of any benefits and harms of these treatments. See depressive disorders in adults, p 114.

OPTION ANTIDEPRESSANTS

Systematic reviews found that antidepressants improved depressive symptoms at the end of the trial (unspecified) compared with placebo. They found limited evidence that selective serotonin reupdate inhibitors were more effective that tricyclic antidepressants, and found no significant difference in symptoms between monoamine oxidase inhibitors and tricyclic antidepressants or between selective serotonin reuptake inhibitors and serotonin noradrenaline reuptake inhibitors. The reviews provided insufficient evidence to assess whether antidepressants induce bipolar mania.

Benefits: We found two systematic reviews of antipressents in people with bipolar depression or mixed unipolar/bipolar depression.[14,15] **Versus placebo:** The first review (search date not reported, 12 RCTs; 732 people with depressive disorder or mixed episode disorder with at least one previous episode of mania), published only as an abstract, found that people taking antidepressants (tricyclic antidepressants [TCAs], selective serotonin reuptake inhibitors [SSRIs], selective noradrenaline reuptake inhibitors [SNRIs], or monoamine oxidase inhibitors [MAOIs]) were significantly less likely to fail to respond to treatment at the end of the trial (unspecified) than people taking placebo (302 people: 87/180 [48%] v 92/122 [75%]; OR 0.30, 95% CI 0.18 to 0.48; NNT 4, 95% CI 3 to 7).[14] **Versus each other:** The first review found no significant difference between SSRIs and TCAs in the proportion of people who responded to treatment at the end of the trial (unspecified), although people taking SSRIs were less likely to fail to respond (31/65 [48%] v 44/69 [64%]; OR 0.53, 95% CI 0.27 to 1.04).[14] It also found no significant difference in the proportion of people who responded at the end of the trial (unspecified) between MAOIs and TCAs (54/109 [49%] v 54/103 [52%]; OR 0.89, 95% CI 0.52 to 1.52) or between SSRIs and SNRIs (19/34 [56%] v 21/35 [60%]; OR 0.85, 95% CI 0.33 to 2.17). The second review (search date 2000; 6 RCTs; 422 people with bipolar depression, 190 people with unipolar depression, about 25% taking lithium, carbamazepine, or valproate) also found similar responses to treatment among antidepressants, but did not quantify its conclusions.[15] **Versus adding lithium or valproate:** We found one small RCT (27 people with mania or bipolar depression receiving lithium or valproate), which compared the addition of paroxetine versus the addition of a second dose of lithium or valproate. It found no significant difference between groups in depressive or manic symptoms over 6 weeks (results presented graphically).[16]

Harms: **Versus each other:** The first review found that SSRIs were significantly less likely to induce mania than TCAs (OR 0.14, 95% CI 0.02 to 0.81).[14] The second review also concluded that tricyclic drugs were more likely to induce mania than other antidepressants, but did not quantify its conclusions.[15]

Comment: A systematic review of antidepressants in bipolar depression is in progress.[17] The evidence for treatment of unipolar depression (see depressive disorders in adults, p 114) is believed to be applicable, although the efficacy of the treatments may be different, and specific adverse effects such as antidepressant induced mania should be considered.

OPTION   LITHIUM

One systematic review identified no RCTs of sufficient quality to assess lithium in people with bipolar depression.

Benefits: We found one systematic review (search date 2000), which identified no RCTs of sufficient quality in people with bipolar depression (see comment below).[15]

Harms: We found no good RCTs.

Comment: The review identified one crossover trial in people with depression (52 people, 40 with bipolar depression).[15] Participants were randomised to 2 weeks of lithium and then crossed over to 6 days of placebo. The trial found that lithium improved symptoms in 32/40 (80%) people over 2 weeks, and that 12/32 (38%) of these relapsed when taking placebo. It found limited evidence that lithium did not induce more manic switching (see glossary, p 30) than placebo in bipolar depression.[15]

OPTION CARBAMAZEPINE

One systematic review identified no RCTs of sufficient quality to assess carbamazepine in people with bipolar depression.

Benefits: We found one systematic review (search date 2000), which identified no RCTs of sufficient quality in people with bipolar depression (see comment below).[15]

Harms: We found no good RCTs.

Comment: The review identified one crossover trial in people with depression (35 people, 24 with bipolar depression).[15] Participants were randomised to placebo before and after being crossed over to carbamazepine over 45 days. The trial found that carbamazepine improved symptoms in 62% of people over a mean 45 days. It found limited evidence that lithium did not induce more manic switching (see glossary, p 30) than placebo in bipolar depression.

OPTION VALPROATE

We found no RCTs of valproate in people with bipolar depression.

Benefits: We found no systematic review or RCTs of valproate in people with bipolar depression.

Harms: We found no RCTs.

Comment: None.

OPTION LAMOTRIGINE

One RCT in people with bipolar type I disorder experiencing a depressive episode found that lamotrigine increased the proportion of people who responded over 7 weeks compared with placebo.

Benefits: We found one systematic review (search date 2000),[15] which identified one RCT (195 people aged 19–75 years with bipolar type 1 disorder experiencing a major depressive episode).[18] The RCT compared three treatments: lamotrigine 200 mg daily, lamotrigine 50 mg daily, and placebo.[18] It found no significant difference between lamotrigine and placebo in Hamilton Depression Rating Scale score over 7 weeks, but found that lamotrigine 200 mg daily significantly improved Mongometry–Asberg Depression Rating Scale score (mean reduction −13.3 with lamotrigine v −7.8 with placebo; $P < 0.05$) and increased the proportion of people who responded to treatment (measured by Clinical Global Impression Scale scores: mean change 2.6 with lamotrigine v 3.3 with placebo; $P < 0.05$).

Harms: The RCT found that significantly more people had headache with lamotrigine compared with placebo (20/63 [32%] with lamotrigine 200 mg v 11/65 [17%]; $P < 0.05$).[18]

Comment: None.

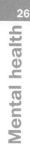

Mental health

OPTION PSYCHOLOGICAL TREATMENTS

One RCT found limited evidence that an educational programme to recognise symptoms of relapse reduced manic relapse over 18 months, but that it may increase depressive episodes. Another RCT found that 21 sessions of family focused psychoeducation reduced relapse over 12 months compared with two family sessions plus crisis management.

Benefits:
Education to recognise symptoms of relapse: We found one RCT (69 outpatients with bipolar disorder who had relapsed in the previous year) comparing an educational programme to recognise symptoms of relapse (see glossary, p 30) versus treatment as usual over 18 months.[19] It found that people in the educational programme were significantly less likely to suffer a manic relapse over 18 months compared with people receiving usual care (9/33 [27%] with educational programme v 20/35 [57%] with usual care; RR 0.48, 95% CI 0.25 to 0.86; NNT 4; 95% CI 2 to 16), but may have been more likely to suffer from a depressive episode (18/33 [55%] with educational programme v 13/35 [37%] with usual care; RR 1.47, 95% CI 0.87 to 2.54), although the difference was not significant. It found that, compared with usual care, the educational programme significantly improved social function from baseline at 18 months (measured on a 4 point scale assessing 8 areas of social activity where 0 is fair/good performance and 4 inability to carry out function; mean difference in score 1.97, 95% CI 0.71 to 3.23).[19] **Family focused psychoeducation:** We found one RCT (101 people with bipolar disorder who had recently recovered from an acute episode recruited from inpatient and outpatient facilities, all taking antipsychotic drugs) comparing 21 sessions of family focused pyschoeducation versus two family sessions plus crisis management over 12 months.[20] Family focused psychoeducation involved education about the symptoms, causes and treatment of bipolar disorder, education to recognise symptoms of relapse, preparation of a relapse prevention plan, and training in problem solving and communication skills. Crisis management involved emergency counselling sessions as needed, with a minimum of a monthly telephone call. The RCT found that family focused psychoeducation significantly reduced the proportion of people who relapsed over 12 months compared with family session plus crisis management (HR 1.47, CI not reported; P = 0.42).

Harms:
Education to recognise symptoms of relapse: The RCT found that, compared with usual care, education may increase depressive relapse; (see benefits above). **Family focused psychoeducation:** The RCT gave no information on harms.[20]

Comment: None.

OPTION LITHIUM

RCTs have found that lithium reduces relapse over 2 years compared with placebo, and have found no significant difference in relapse between lithium and valproate, carbamazepine, or lamotrigine.

Benefits: **Versus placebo:** We found three systematic reviews in people with bipolar disorder, unipolar disorder, or mixed unipolar/bipolar disorder,[21–23] and two subsequent RCTs.[24,25] The first review (search date not reported, 9 RCTs, 825 people with bipolar or unipolar disorder) found that lithium reduced the risk of relapse (see glossary, p 30) by 41% at up to 2 years compared with placebo (3 RCTs, 412 people with bipolar disorder: relapse as defined in the trial [including hospital admission or requiring additional medication]; 73/202 [36%] with lithium v 128/210 [61%] with placebo; RR 0.59, 95% CI 0.48 to 0.73).[21] The review found no significant difference between lithium and placebo in the proportion of people with bipolar or unipolar disorder who committed suicide, but it is likely to have been underpowered to detect a clinically important difference (4 RCTs, 0/186 [0%] v 2/189 [1%]; RR 0.32, 95% CI 0.03 to 2.98). The second review (search date not reported, 15 RCTs, including 8 identified by the first review, 558 people with bipolar disorder) found that, in people with bipolar disorder, there was an average 48% decrease in the absolute risk of relapse by the end of the trial (unspecified) with lithium compared with placebo.[22] The third review (search date 2000, 3 RCTs identified by the first review, 19 observational studies) assessed the effect of long term lithium treatment on suicide rates.[23] It found that people with bipolar or unipolar disorder treated with lithium had lower suicide rates compared with untreated people (159 v 876 deaths per 100 000 patient years of treatment; RR 8.85, 95% CI 4.12 to 19.1). Two subsequent RCTs (647 people aged 18 years or over with bipolar type I or type II disorder who had recently recovered from a manic or depressive/hypomanic episode and remained stable after an 8–16 week run in, during which they began taking lamotrigine and withdrew other psychotropic drugs), compared three treatments: lithium, lamotrigine, and placebo over 76 weeks.[24,25] Both RCTs found that, compared with placebo, lithium significantly increased the time to requirement of additional intervention for a manic or a depressive episode (median time to additional medication 24–42 weeks with lithium v 12–13 weeks with placebo: P = 0.05 in both RCTs). Secondary analyses in the RCTs suggested that lithium protected against manic but not depressive relapse. **Versus valproate:** We found one systematic review (search date not reported), which identified one RCT (372 people) comparing three treatments: lithium, valproate, and placebo.[26] It found no significant difference between lithium and valproate in relapse at 12 months (relapse defined as withdrawal due to episode of bipolar disorder; 12/187 [6%] v 9/91 [10%]; RR 0.8, 95% CI 0.5 to 1.2), but it is likely to have been too small to detect a clinically important difference. **Versus carbamazepine:** We found one systematic review (search date not reported, 10 RCTs, 572 people with unipolar or bipolar disorder) comparing lithium versus carbamazepine.[22] It found no significant difference between lithium and carbamazepine in the proportion of people who relapsed over 1–3 years (60% with lithium v 55% with carbamazepine; reported as non-significant; no further data reported; see comment below). **Versus lamotrigine:** We found no systematic review but found two RCTs comparing three treatments: lithium, lamotrigine, and placebo.[24,25] Both RCTs (647 people with bipolar type I or type II disorder who had recently recovered from a manic or depressive/hypomanic episode and remained stable after an 8–16 week run in, during which they began taking lamotrigine and withdrew other psychotropic drugs) found no significant difference between lithium and lamotrigine in the time to requirement of additional intervention for a mood episode (median time to additional medication 24–42 weeks with lithium v 20–29 weeks with lamotrigine: P > 0.05 in both RCTs). Secondary analysis in one of the RCTs suggested that lithium may significantly reduce manic relapse compared with lamotrigine (P = 0.092).[25]

Harms: **Versus placebo:** The first review found that significantly more people had overall adverse effects (not specified) with lithium than with placebo (160/233 [69%] with lithium v 112/225 [50%] with placebo; RR 1.4, 95% CI 1.2 to 1.6), and that lithium may increase hypothyroidism (7/158 [4%] with lithium v 0/152 [0%] with lithium; RR 5.1, 95% CI 0.9 to 27.7).[21] **Versus valproate:** The review found that valproate was significantly more likely than lithium to cause sedation (1 RCT: 78/187 [42%] with valproate v 24/91 [26%] with lithium; RR 1.6, 95% CI 1.1 to 2.3) and infection (1 RCT: 51/187 [27%] with valproate v 12/91 [13%] with lithium; RR 2.1, 95% CI 1.2 to 3.7), but significantly less likely to cause polyuria (15/187 [8%] with valproate v 17/91 [19%] with lithium; RR 0.4, 95% CI 0.2 to 0.8), thirst (11/187 [6%] with valproate v 14/91 [15%]; RR 0.4, 95% CI 0.2 to 0.8), and possibly diarrhoea (65/187 [35%] with valproate v 42/91 [46%] with lithium; RR 0.75, 95% 0.6 to 1.0).[26] **Versus carbamazepine:** The review gave no information on adverse effects.[22] One RCT (144 people with bipolar disorder) identified by the review found that, although more people taking carbamazepine than taking lithium withdrew from the trials (9/70 [13%] with carbamazepine v 4/74 [5%] with lithium; reported as non-significant; no further data reported), a significantly higher proportion of people taking lithium compared with carbamazepine had "slight or moderate" adverse effects over 2.5 years (61% v 21%; P < 0.001).[27] **Versus lamotrigine:** The first RCT found that lithium caused significantly fewer headaches than lamotrigine (4% v 20%; P = 0.02) but more diarrhoea (28% v 5%, P = 0.002).[24] The second RCT gave no information on adverse effects.[25]

Comment: **Versus carbamazepine:** The results of the review should be interpreted with caution as it combined trials of unipolar and bipolar disorder.[22]

| OPTION | VALPROATE |

One RCT found that valproate reduced relapse over 12 months compared with placebo. One systematic review found no significant difference between lithium and valproate in relapse over 12 months.

Benefits: **Versus placebo:** We found one systematic review (search date not reported, 1 RCT, 372 people with bipolar disorder) comparing three treatments: valproate, lithium, and placebo.[26] It found that lithium significantly reduced relapse (see glossary, p 30) over 12 months compared with placebo (relapse defined as withdrawal because of an episode of bipolar disorder; 45/187 [24%] with valproate v 36/94 [38%] with placebo; RR 0.6, 95% CI 0.4 to 0.9), but found no significant difference in time to relapse (P = 0.33; no further data reported). **Versus lithium:** See benefits of lithium, p 27.

Harms: **Versus placebo:** The review found that valproate was significantly more likely than placebo to cause tremor (RR 3.2, 95% CI 1.9 to 5.6); weight gain (RR 2.9, 95% 1.3 to 6.2); alopecia (RR 2.4, 95% CI 1.1 to 5.7), and nausea (RR 1.37, 95% CI 1.0 to 1.9).[26] **Versus lithium:** See harms of lithium, p 28.

Comment: None.

OPTION CARBAMAZEPINE

We found no RCTs comparing carbamazepine versus placebo in preventing relapse, but one systematic review found no significant difference between carbamazepine and lithium in the proportion of people who relapsed over 1–3 years.

Benefits: **Versus placebo:** We found no systematic review or RCTs comparing carbamazepine versus placebo in preventing relapse (see glossary, p 30). **Versus lithium:** See benefits of lithium, p 27.

Harms: **Versus placebo:** We found no RCTs. **Versus lithium:** See benefits of lithium, p 27.

Comment: A systematic review of the effects of carbamazepine in preventing relapse is in progress.[28]

OPTION LAMOTRIGINE

Three RCTs have found that lamotrigine reduces relapse compared with placebo. However, secondary analyses in two of the RCTs suggested that lamotrigine protected against depressive relapse, but not manic relapse. RCTs have found no significant difference between lamotrigine and lithium in the proportion of people who relapse.

Benefits: **Versus placebo:** We found no systematic review but found three RCTs.[24,25,29] Two RCTs (647 people aged 18 years or over with bipolar type I or type II disorder who had recently recovered from a manic episode or depressive/hypomanic episode and remained stable after 8–16 weeks during which they began taking lamotrigine and withdrew other psychotropic drugs) compared three treatments over 76 weeks: lamotrigine, lithium, and placebo (see comment below).[24,25] Both RCTs found that, compared with placebo, lamotrigine significantly increased the time to requiring additional medication for a manic or bipolar depressive episode (median time to additional medication 20–29 weeks with lamotrigine v 12–13 weeks with placebo; P = 0.05 in both RCTs). Secondary analyses suggested that lamotrigine reduced depressive but not manic relapse (see glossary, p 30).[24,25] The third RCT (182 people with rapid cycling bipolar disorder (see table 1, p 32) found no significant difference between lamotrigine and placebo in the time to requiring additional medication (P = 0.177, results presented graphically).[29] **Versus lithium:** See benefits of lithium, p 27.

Harms: **Versus placebo:** The RCTs gave no information on adverse effects.[24,25] The third RCT found no significant difference between lamotrigine and placebo in the proportion of people who had adverse effects, including nausea and headache (67% with lamotrigine v 68% with placebo, reported as non-significant, CI not reported).[29] **Versus lithium:** See benefits of lithium, p 27.

Comment: The first RCT is published only as an abstract.[24]

OPTION   ANTIDEPRESSANTS

One systematic review provided insufficient evidence to assess antidepressants in preventing relapse of bipolar disorder.

Benefits: We found one systematic review (search date 2000; 4 RCTs, 258 people with bipolar type I or type II disorder) comparing tricyclic antidepressants with placebo or lithium.[30] The review did not perform a meta-analysis. It provided a narrative overview of the studies and found no clear evidence that tricyclic antidepressants reduce relapse (see glossary, p 30) over 1–2 years compared with placebo. It suggested that tricyclic antidepressants may be less effective in preventing relapse over 1–2 years than lithium.

Harms: The review suggested that antidepressants may induce mood instability or manic episodes.[30]

Comment: None.

GLOSSARY

Manic switching involves onset of a manic episode shortly after treatment for a depressive episode. It may be more likely after treatment with antidepressants.
Relapse A return of symptoms to the extent that the disorder again meets criteria for the full syndromes. In practice, patients with bipolar disorder learn to recognise early warning signs and begin treatment before criteria are met. For this reason, relapse is often pragmatically defined as the need for drug treatment due to re-emergence of depressive or manic symptoms.

REFERENCES

1. American Psychiatric Association. *Diagnostic and statistical manual of mental disorders,* 4th ed. Washington, D.C.: American Psychiatric Association, 1994.
2. Weissman MM, Bland RC, Canino GJ, et al. Cross-national epidemiology of major depression and bipolar disorder. *JAMA* 1996;276:293–299.
3. Müller-Oerlinghausen B, Berghöfer A, Bauer M. Bipolar disorder. *Lancet* 2002;359:241–247.
4. Tohen M, Shulman KI, Satlin A. First-episode mania in late life. *Am J Psychiatry* 1994;151:130–132.
5. Murray CJ, Lopez AD. Global mortality, disability, and the contribution of risk factors: Global Burden of Disease Study. *Lancet* 1997;349:1436–1442.
6. Tohen M, Hennen J, Zarate C, et al. Harvard first episodes project: predictors of recovery and relapse. *Bipolar Disord* 2002;4(suppl 1):135–136.
7. Harris EC, Barraclough B. Suicide as an outcome for mental disorders. A meta-analysis. *Br J Psychiatry* 1997;170:205–208.
8. Macritchie K, Geddes JR, Scott J, et al. Valproate for acute affective episodes in bipolar disorder. In: The Cochrane Library, Issue 3, 2003. Oxford: Update Software. Search date 2002; primary sources Cochrane Collaboration Depression, Anxiety and Neurosis Review Group Controlled Trials Register, Cochrane Controlled Trials Register and hand searches of reference lists of relevant papers and textbooks and personal contact with authors of trials, experts and pharmaceutical companies.
9. Poolsup N, Li Wan Po A, de Oliveira IR. Systematic overview of lithium treatment in acute mania. *J Clin Pharm Ther* 2000;25:139–156. Search date 1999; primary sources Medline, Embase, Science Citation Index, the Cochrane Library and hand searches of reference lists of identified RCTs and reviews.
10. Berk M, Ichim M, Brook S. Olanzapine compared to lithium in mania: a double-blind randomized controlled trial. *Int Clin Psychopharmacol* 1999;14:339–343.
11. Ichim L, Berk M, Brook S. Lamotrigine compared with lithium in mania: a double-blind randomized controlled trial. *Ann Clin Psychiatry* 2000;12:5–10.
12. McElroy SL, Keck PE. Pharmacologic agents for the treatment of acute bipolar mania. *Biol Psychiatry* 2000;48:539–557.
13. Rendell JM, Gijsman HJ, Keck P, et al. Olanzapine alone or in combination for acute mania. In: The Cochrane Library, Issue 3, 2003. Oxford: Update Software. Search date 2002; primary sources The Cochrane Collaboration Depression, Anxiety and Neurosis Controlled Trials Register, The Cochrane Central Register of Controlled Trials, EMBASE, MEDLINE, CINAHL, and PsycINFO.

14. Gijsman HJ, Geddes JR, Rendell JM, et al. Systematic review of antidepressants for bipolar depression [abstract]. *J Psychopharmacol* 2001;15(suppl):A19. Search date not reported; primary sources Cochrane Collaboration Depression Anxiety and Neurosis Controlled Trials Register.

15. Nolen WA, Bloemkolk D. Treatment of bipolar depression: a review of the literature and a suggestion for an algorithm. *Neuropsychobiology* 2000;42(suppl 1):11–17. Search date 2000; primary sources Medline and hand searches of reference lists and recent congress abstracts books.

16. Young LT, Joffe RT, Robb JC, et al. Double-blind comparison of addition of a second mood stabilizer versus an antidepressant to an initial mood stabilizer for treatment of people with bipolar depression. *Am J Psychiatry* 2000;157:124–126.

17. Gijsman HJ, Rendell J, Geddes J, et al. Antidepressants for bipolar depression (protocol for a Cochrane Review). In: The Cochrane Library, Issue 3, 2003. Oxford: Update Software.

18. Calabrese JR, Bowden CL, Sachs GS, et al. A double-blind placebo controlled study of lamotrigine monotherapy in outpatients with bipolar 1 depression. *J Clin Psychiatry* 1999;60:79–88.

19. Perry A, Tarrier N, Morriss R, McCarthy E, Limb K. Randomised controlled trial of efficacy of teaching patients with bipolar disorder to identify early symptoms of relapse and obtain treatment. *BMJ* 1999;318:149–153.

20. Miklowitz DJ, Simoneau TL, George EL, et al. Family-focused treatment of bipolar disorder: 1-year effects of a psychoeducational program in conjunction with pharmacotherapy. *Biol Psychiatry* 2000;48:582–592.

21. Burgess S, Geddes J, Hawton K, et al. Lithium for maintenance treatment of mood disorders. In: The Cochrane Library, Issue 3, 2003. Oxford: Update Software. Search date not reported; primary sources Cochrane Collaboration Depression, Anxiety and Neurosis Review Group Specialised Register, Cochrane Controlled Trials Register and hand searches of reference lists of relevant papers, major textbooks of mood disorder and the journals Lithium and Lithium Therapy Monographs and personal communication with authors, other experts in the field and pharmaceutical companies.

22. Davis JM, Janicak PG, Hogan DM. Mood stabilizers in the prevention of recurrent affective disorders: a meta-analysis. *Acta Psychiatr Scand* 1999;100:406–417. Search date not reported; primary sources Medline, PsychLit, Pubmed and hand searches of reference lists of identified studies and personal communication with colleagues.

23. Tondo L, Hennen J, Baldessarini RJ. Lower suicide risk with long-term lithium treatment in major affective illness: a meta-analysis. *Acta Psychiatrica Scand* 2001;104:163–172. Search date 2000; primary sources Medline, Current Contents, PsychLit, Pubmed and hand searches of reference lists of relevant publications and contents lists and/or indices of leading international psychiatric research journals and personal communication with colleagues who have done research in the field.

24. Bowden CL, Calabrese JR, Sachs G, et al. A placebo-controlled 18-month trial of lamotrigine and lithium maintenance treatment in recently manic or hypomanic patients with bipolar 1 disorder. *Arch Gen Pshychiatry* 2003;60:392–400.

25. Bowden CL, Ghaemi N, Gyulai, et al. Lamotrigine delays mood episodes in recently depressed bipolar 1 patients. Am Psychiatr Assoc 2002.

26. Macritchie KAN, Geddes JR, Scott J, et al. Valproic acid, valproate and valproate semisodium in the maintenance treatment of bipolar disorder. In: The Cochrane Library, Issue 3, 2003. Oxford: Update Software. Search date not reported; primary sources Cochrane Collaboration Depression, Anxiety and Neurosis Review Group Specialised Register, Cochrane Controlled Trials Register, Embase, Medline, Lilacs, PsychLit, Psyndex and hand searches of reference lists of relevant papers, major textbooks on mood disorder, Comprehensive Psychiatry and relevant conference proceedings and personal communication with authors, other experts and pharmaceutical companies.

27. Greil W, Ludwig–Mayerhofer W, Erazo N, et al. Lithium versus carbamazepine in the maintenance treatment of bipolar disorders: a randomised study. *J Affect Disord* 43:151–161.

28. Bandeira CA, Lima MS, Geddes J, et al. Carbamazepine for bipolar affective disorders (protocol for a Cochrane Review). In: The Cochrane Library, Issue 3, 2003. Oxford: Update Software.

29. Calabrese, JR Suppes, T, Bowden, CL, et al. A double-blind, placebo-controlled, prophylaxis study of lamotrigine in rapid-cycling bipolar disorder. Lamictal 614 Study Group. *J Clin Psychiatry* 2000;61:841–850.

30. Ghaemi SN, Lenox MS, Baldessarini RJ. Effectiveness and safety of long-term antidepressant treatment in bipolar disorder. *J Clin Psychiatry* 2001;62:565–569. Search date 2000; primary sources Medline, HealthStar, Current Contents, PsychInfo and hand searches of bibliographies of identified reports and recent reviews.

John Geddes
Department of Psychiatry
University of Oxford
Oxford
UK

Competing interests: Sanofi-Synthelabo have donated supplies of Depakote and to the BALANCE trial of which JG in the principal investigator.

| TABLE 1 | DSM-IV classification of bipolar disorders (see text, p 15). Reprinted with permission from Elsevier (Müller-Oerlinghausen B, Berghöfer A, Bauer M Bipolar Disorder Lancet 2002; 359: 241–47).[1] |

DSM IV Category	Criteria	Course specifiers and examples
Bipolar I disorder	One or more manic or mixed episodes, usually accompanied by one or more major depressive episodes	To describe current (or most recent episode): mild, moderate, severe without psychotic features; severe with psychotic features; in partial or full remission; with catatonic features; with postpartum onset
		To describe current (or most recent) major depressive episode: chronic; with melancholic features; with atypical features
		To describe pattern of episodes: with or without full interepisode recovery; with seasonal pattern; with rapid cycling (> 4 episodes in previous 12 months)
Bipolar II disorder	Recurrent major depressive episodes with one or more hypomanic (milder than manic) episodes	To describe current (or most recent episode): hypomanic; depressed
		To describe current (or most recent) major depressive episode and pattern of episodes: see bipolar I disorder
Cyclothymic disorder	Chronic (> 2 years), fluctuating mood disturbance involving numerous periods of mild hypomanic and depressive symptoms that do not meet criteria for a major depressive episode	Over 2 years any symptom free intervals last no longer than 2 months
Bipolar disorder (not otherwise specified)	Disorders with bipolar features that do not meet criteria for any specific bipolar disorder	Examples: very rapid cycling (over days); recurrent hypomanias without depressive symptoms; indeterminate whether primary or secondary (due to a general medical condition or substance abuse)

Search date December 2002

Phillipa Hay and Josue Bacaltchuk

INTERVENTIONS

Key Messages

Antidepressants

- **Antidepressant medication (tricyclic antidepressants, monoamine oxidase inhibitors, and fluoxetine)** Systematic reviews and one subsequent RCT have found short term reduction in bulimic symptoms with tricyclic antidepressants, monoamine oxidase inhibitors, and fluoxetine. A further subsequent RCT found no significant difference in symptoms between moclobemide and placebo. One systematic review and one subsequent RCT found no significant difference in symptoms with antidepressants versus cognitive behavioural therapy.

- **Other antidepressants (venlafaxine, mirtazapine, and reboxetine)** We found no RCTs on the effects of venlafaxine, mirtazapine, and reboxetine.

- **Selective serotonin reuptake inhibitors (other than fluoxetine)** We found no good evidence on selective serotonin reuptake inhibitors other than fluoxetine.

- **Antidepressants as maintenance** We found insufficient evidence to assess the effects of antidepresssants for maintenance.

Psychotherapy

- **Cognitive behavioural therapy** One systematic review has found that cognitive behavioural therapy compared with remaining on a waiting list reduces specific symptoms of bulimia nervosa and improves non-specific symptoms such as depression. One systematic review found cognitive behavioural therapy compared with other psychotherapies improved abstinence from binge eating and depression scores at the end of treatment. One RCT in the review found that cognitive behavioural therapy compared with interpersonal psychotherapy reduced binge eating in the short term, but there was no significant difference in the longer term. One systematic review and one subsequent RCT found no significant difference in symptoms with cognitive behavioural therapy compared with antidepressants.

- **Other psychotherapies** One systematic review has found that non-cognitive behavioural psychotherapy increases abstinence from binge eating compared with waiting list controls. The systematic review found that the combined result for four specific psychotherapies, other than cognitive behavioural therapy, reduced bulimic symptoms compared with specified control psychotherapies, but the review included RCTs with weak methods, and the result was significant in only one of the four individual results. One systematic review found cognitive behavioural therapy compared with other psychotherapies improved abstinence from binge eating and depression scores at the end of treatment. One RCT in the review found that cognitive behavioural therapy compared with interpersonal psychotherapy reduced binge eating in the short term, but there was no significant difference in the longer term.

Combination treatment

- **Combination treatment (antidepressants plus psychotherapy)** One systematic review and one subsequent RCT found no significant difference between combination treatment (antidepressants plus psychotherapy) and antidepressants alone in binge frequency, depressive symptoms, and remission rates. The systematic review found that, compared with psychotherapy alone, combination treatment improved short term remission, but there was no significant difference in binge frequency and depressive symptoms. The systematic review found that combination treatment was with psychotherapy were associated with higher withdrawal rates compared with psychotherapy alone. One subsequent RCT of cognitive behavioural therapy in a self help form plus fluoxetine found limited evidence that combined treatment reduced bulimic symptoms compared with cognitive behavioural therapy alone. A second subsequent RCT found no significant difference in symptoms between group based CBT, fluoxetine, and their combination.

DEFINITION   Bulimia nervosa (see glossary, p 43) is an intense preoccupation with body weight and shape, with regular episodes of uncontrolled overeating of large amounts of food (binge eating — see glossary, p 43) associated with use of extreme methods to counteract the feared effects of overeating. If a person also meets the diagnostic criteria for anorexia nervosa, then the diagnosis of anorexia nervosa takes precedence.[1] Bulimia nervosa can be difficult to identify because of extreme secrecy about binge eating and purgative behaviour. Weight may be normal but there is often a history of anorexia nervosa or restrictive dieting. Some people alternate between anorexia nervosa and bulimia nervosa. Some RCTs included participants with subthreshhold bulimia nervosa or a related eating disorder, binge eating disorder. Where possible, only results relevant to bulimia nervosa are reported in this review.

INCIDENCE/   In community based studies, the prevalence of bulimia nervosa is
PREVALENCE between 0.5% and 1.0% in young women, with an even social class distribution.[2-4] About 90% of people diagnosed with bulimia nervosa are women. The numbers presenting with bulimia nervosa in industrialised countries increased during the decade that followed its recognition in the late 1970s and "a cohort effect" is reported in community surveys,[2,5,6] implying an increase in incidence. The prevalence of eating disorders such as bulimia nervosa is lower in

non-industrialised populations,[7] and varies across ethnic groups. African-American women have a lower rate of restrictive dieting than white American women, but have a similar rate of recurrent binge eating.[8]

AETIOLOGY/ RISK FACTORS Young women from the developed world who restrict their dietary intake are at greatest risk of developing bulimia nervosa and other eating disorders. One community based case control study compared 102 people with bulimia nervosa with 204 healthy controls and found higher rates of the following in people with the eating disorder: obesity, mood disorder, sexual and physical abuse, parental obesity, substance misuse, low self esteem, perfectionism, disturbed family dynamics, parental weight/shape concern, and early menarche.[9] Compared with a control group of 102 women who had other psychiatric disorders, women with bulimia nervosa had higher rates of parental problems and obesity.

PROGNOSIS A 10 year follow up study (50 people with bulimia nervosa from a trial of mianserin treatment) found that 52% had fully recovered, and only 9% continued to experience full symptoms of bulimia nervosa.[10] A larger study (222 people from a trial of antidepressants and structured, intensive group psychotherapy) found that, after a mean follow up of 11.5 years, 11% still met criteria for bulimia nervosa, whereas 70% were in full or partial remission.[11] Short term studies found similar results: about 50% of people made a full recovery, 30% made a partial recovery, and 20% continued to be symptomatic.[12] There are few consistent predictors of longer term outcome. Good prognosis has been associated with shorter illness duration, a younger age of onset, higher social class, and a family history of alcohol abuse.[10] Poor prognosis has been associated with a history of substance misuse,[13] premorbid and paternal obesity,[14] and, in some studies, personality disorder.[15-18] One study (102 people) of the natural course of bulimia nervosa found that 31% still had the disorder at 15 months and 15% at 5 years.[19] Only 28% received treatment during the follow up period. In an evaluation of response to cognitive behavioural therapy, early progress (by session 6) best predicted outcome.[20] A subsequent systematic review of the outcome literature found no consistent evidence to support early intervention and a better prognosis.[21]

AIMS OF INTERVENTION To reduce symptoms of bulimia nervosa; to improve general psychiatric symptoms; to improve social functioning and quality of life.

OUTCOMES Frequency of binge eating, abstinence from binge eating, frequency of behaviours to reduce weight and counter the effects of binge eating, severity of extreme weight and shape preoccupation, severity of general psychiatric symptoms, severity of depression, improvement in social and adaptive functioning, remission rates, relapse rates, and withdrawal rates.

METHODS *Clinical Evidence* search and appraisal December 2002 and hand search of reference lists from identified reviews.

QUESTION What are the effects of treatments for bulimia nervosa in adults?

OPTION COGNITIVE BEHAVIOURAL THERAPY

One systematic review has found that cognitive behavioural therapy compared with remaining on a waiting list reduces specific symptoms of bulimia nervosa and improves non-specific symptoms such as depression. One systematic review found cognitive behavioural therapy compared with other psychotherapies improved abstinence from binge eating and depression scores at the end of treatment. One RCT in the review found that cognitive behavioural therapy compared with interpersonal psychotherapy reduced binge eating in the short term, but there was no significant difference in the longer term. One systematic review and one subsequent RCT found no significant difference in symptoms with cognitive behavioural therapy compared with antidepressants.

Benefits: We found one systematic review (search date 2002, 34 RCTs).[22] It included RCTs of other binge eating disorders, although most studies were of people with bulimia nervosa (see glossary, p 43) (18 RCTs in people with bulimia nervosa characterised by purging behaviour).[22] The review reported data separately for bulimia nervosa and other disorders of binge eating. Unless otherwise specified, results reported here refer only to analyses of people with bulimia nervosa. **Versus waiting list controls:** One systematic review (search date 2002; individual analyses included a maximum of 10 RCTs and 735 people) found that cognitive behavioural therapy (CBT — see glossary, p 43) compared with remaining on a waiting list significantly increased the proportion of people abstaining from binge eating at the end of the trial (3 RCTs; RR 0.62, 95% CI 0.47 to 0.83), significantly reduced mean bulimic symptom scores (6 RCTs; SMD −0.85, 95% CI −1.14 to −0.57), and mean depression scores (3 RCTs; SMD −1.13, 95% CI −1.60 to −0.67).[22] It found no significant difference, in a mixed population, between CBT and remaining on the waiting list in weight at the end of treatment (3 RCTs, 1 with bulimia nervosa participants; SMD +0.12, 95% CI −0.23 to +0.46, 135 people). The review found insufficient evidence about other outcomes, such as social functioning. **Versus placebo medication:** One subsequent RCT (91 people) found no significant difference in efficacy between unguided manual based self help CBT and placebo medication.[23] **Versus other psychotherapies:** See table 1, p 46. The systematic review (search date 2002) found that CBT compared with other psychotherapies significantly improved abstinence from binge eating (6 RCTs, 448 people; RR 0.78, 95% CI 0.70 to 0.87) and depression scores at the end of treatment (6 RCTs, 206 people; SMD −0.66, 95% CI −0.94 to −0.37).[22] For all RCTs (including both binge eating disorder and bulimia nervosa participants) CBT plus exposure therapy (see glossary, p 43) was not significantly more effective than CBT alone (3 RCTs, 168 people; RR for abstinence from binge eating 0.87, 95% CI 0.65 to 1.16). Depression scores were significantly lower at the end of treatment with CBT plus exposure therapy compared with CBT alone (4 RCTs, 145 people;

SMD 0.45, 95% CI 0.11 to 0.79). CBT in a full or less intensive form was not significantly superior to CBT in a pure self help form (see glossary, p 44) (5 RCTs, 264 people; RR 0.92, 95% CI 0.82 to 1.03). One RCT included in the review (220 people) compared classic CBT versus interpersonal psychotherapy (see glossary, p 43) for bulimia nervosa that involved purging.[24] It found that CBT significantly improved abstinence from binge eating at the end of treatment (19 individual sessions conducted ≥ 20 weeks; intention to treat analysis; 29% with CBT v 6% with interpersonal psycho-therapy; P < 0.01). However, the difference was not significant at 4, 8, and 12 months of follow up, with improvement in both groups from baseline. We found one subsequent RCT (125 people with bulimia nervosa), which compared four sessions of CBT versus motivational enhancement therapy (see glossary, p 43).[25] It found no significant differences between CBT and motivational enhance-ment therapy in engaging participants or the chance of achieving a clinically significant reduction in binge frequency (17/25 [68%] v 23/43 [53%]; RR 1.3, 95% CI 0.9 to 1.9). However, results were reported only on the first 4 weeks of treatment, which was prior to all people receiving a further 8 weeks of individual or group CBT. **Versus antidepressants:** See benefits of antidepressants, p 39. **Versus combination treatment:** See benefits of combination treatment, p 42.

Harms: The systematic review (search date 2002) found that the RCTs did not report details of adverse effects.[22] It found no significant difference in completion rates between interventions,[22] suggesting no major difference in acceptability. However, it could not exclude infrequent serious adverse effects.[22] An observational study found that group psychotherapy offered very soon after presentation was sometimes perceived as threatening.[10]

Comment: We found a second systematic review in German, which is awaiting translation, and may be included in a future *Clinical Evidence* update.[26] One systematic review (search date 2002)[22] defined CBT as psychotherapy that uses the techniques and models specified by Wilson and Fairburn,[27] but it did not specify the number of sessions or specialist expertise (classical CBT for bulimia nervosa specifies 19 individual sessions over 20 weeks conducted by trained thera-pists[27]). Effect sizes for CBT were large, but over 50% of people were still binge eating at the end of treatment.[22] Further research is needed to evaluate the specific and non-specific effects of CBT and other psychotherapies, to explore individual characteristics (such as readiness to change) that may predict response, and to explore the long term effects of treatment. Waiting list or delayed treatment control groups are subject to bias because it is not possible to "blind" someone to the knowledge they are not in the active treatment group. It is difficult to interpret the clinical importance of the statistically significant changes in depression scores. Further limitations are that the quality of trials was variable (e.g. 57% were not blinded).[22] Sample sizes were often small. None of the studies measured harms rigorously. Two further analyses[28,29] found limited observational evidence that motivation and compliance factors may influence outcomes. One study[28] performed additional analyses in an RCT of CBT versus interpersonal psychotherapy.[24] It found that "stage of change", or psychological motivation and greater readiness to change, was not related to non-completion, but was associated with a good outcome in those who completed interpersonal psychotherapy. The second RCT examined the effects of compliance on outcome in 62 people randomised to guided self help or to full CBT for 16 weeks.[29] At 6 months' follow up, but not the end of treatment, binge eating abstinence rates were greater in those who had completed two or more of the CBT exercises (P = 0.04; CI not reported). Stricter inclusion criteria in the review removed previously included RCTs in people with binge eating disorders other than bulimia nervosa.[22] **Versus antidepressants:** See antidepressants, p 39.

OPTION   **OTHER PSYCHOTHERAPIES**

One systematic review has found that non-cognitive behavioural psychotherapy increases abstinence from binge eating compared with waiting list controls. The systematic review found that the combined result for four specific psychotherapies, other than cognitive behavioural therapy, reduced bulimic symptoms compared with specified control psychotherapies. However, the review included RCTs with weak methods, and the result was significant in only one of the four individual results. One systematic review found cognitive behavioural therapy compared with other psychotherapies improved abstinence from binge eating and depression scores at the end of treatment. One RCT in the review found that CBT compared with interpersonal psychotherapy reduced binge eating in the short term, but there was no significant difference in the longer term.

Benefits:
Versus waiting list controls: We found one systematic review (search date 2002),[22] which also included studies of other binge eating (see glossary, p 43) syndromes. It found that, for bulimia nervosa (see glossary, p 43) participants only, non-cognitive behavioural psychotherapies (e.g. hypnobehavioural therapy and interpersonal psychotherapy — see glossary, p 43) compared with waiting list control significantly increased abstinence from binge eating (3 RCTs, 124 people; RR 0.67, 95% CI 0.55 to 0.81) and reduced the number of people who did not achieve remission (4 RCTs, 162 people; RR 0.63, 95% CI 0.53 to 0.75). **Versus a control therapy:** The systematic review included four RCTs in which psychotherapies other than cognitive behavioural therapy were compared with a control therapy.[22] One compared nutritional counselling with stress management; one compared guided imagery with self monitoring; one was a three-armed RCT comparing self psychology (the active treatment), cognitive orientation (see glossary, p 43), and a control nutritional counselling therapy, and the fourth compared interpersonal psychotherapy with behavioural therapy alone. The combined results for psychotherapy, for participants with bulimia nervosa, significantly reduced bulimic symptoms compared with a control treatment (4 RCTs, 163 people; SMD −0.64 95% CI −1.00 to −0.29).[22] However, in only one trial was the individual result significant. **Versus antidepressants:** See antidepressants, p 39. **Versus cognitive behavioural therapy:** See benefits of cognitive behavioural therapy, p 36. **Versus combination treatment:** See combination treatment, p 41. We found one subsequent RCT, which is awaiting translation.[30]

Harms: The systematic review (search date 2002) found that the RCTs did not report details of adverse effects.[22] It found no significant difference in completion rates between interventions,[22] suggesting no major difference in acceptability. However, it could not exclude infrequent serious adverse effects.[22] An observational study found that group psychotherapy offered very soon after presentation was sometimes perceived as threatening.[10] Non-cognitive behavioural psychotherapies include a large number of options, and it remains unclear which therapies are most effective.

Comment: The quality of trials was variable, few were blinded, sample sizes were small, and none of the studies measured harms rigorously (see comment under cognitive behavioural therapy, p 37). Waiting list or delayed treatment control groups are subject to bias because it is not possible to "blind" someone to the knowledge they are not in the active treatment group. Stricter inclusion criteria in the review removed previously included RCTs in people with binge eating disorders other than bulimia nervosa.[22]

OPTION   ANTIDEPRESSANTS

Systematic reviews and one subsequent RCT have found short term reduction in bulimic symptoms with tricyclic antidepressants, monoamine oxidase inhibitors, and fluoxetine. A further subsequent RCT found no significant difference in symptoms between moclobemide and placebo. One systematic review and one subsequent RCT found no significant difference in symptoms or relapse rates with antidepressants versus cognitive behavioural therapy. One systematic review and one subsequent RCT found no significant difference between combination treatment (antidepressants plus psychotherapy) and antidepressants alone in binge frequency, depressive symptoms, and remission rates. We found no RCTs on the effects of venlafaxine, mirtazapine, and reboxetine. We found no good evidence on selective serotonin reuptake inhibitors other than fluoxetine. We found insufficient evidence to assess the effects of antidepresssants for maintenance.

Benefits: We found two systematic reviews (search date 2001[31] and 2000[32]), three additional RCTs of longer term maintenance (not primary treatment studies),[33–35] and one subsequent RCT.[36] **Versus placebo:** We found one systematic review comparing antidepressants with placebo.[31] It found that antidepressants reduced bulimic symptoms.[31] The review (search date 2001; antidepressants were imipramine [5 RCTs], amitriptyline [1 RCT], desipramine [5 RCTs], phenelzine [2 RCTs], isocarboxazid [1 RCT], brofaromine [1 RCT], fluoxetine [5 RCTs], mianserin [1 RCT], bupropion [1 RCT], and trazodone [1 RCT]) found significantly more frequent short term remission of bulimic episodes with antidepressants (9 RCTs, 777 people, 20% v 8% with placebo; pooled RR 0.87, 95% CI 0.81 to 0.93).[31] The review found no significant difference in effect between different classes of antidepressants, but there were too few RCTs to exclude a clinically important difference (see table 2, p 46). Most RCTs were of tricyclic antidepressants or monoamine oxidase inhibitors; fluoxetine was the only selective serotonin reuptake inhibitor included in the reviews.[31] The first subsequent, four armed RCT (91 women) compared fluoxetine

60 mg daily, placebo, self help cognitive behavioural therapy manual, and fluoxetine plus a self help manual.[23] It found a significantly greater reduction with fluoxetine compared with placebo in vomiting and binge eating symptoms at week 4 (P < 0.05). Remission rates after a 16 week treatment period with fluoxetine were 16%, and were not reported for placebo. The second subsequent RCT (78 women with bulimia nervosa [see glossary, p 43]) compared moclobemide (a reversible monoamine oxidase inhibitor) 600 mg daily versus placebo.[36] It reported no significant differences in weekly binge and vomiting episodes, Hamilton depression scores, and scores on three self report measures of eating disorder symptoms between those randomised to active drug or placebo, among the 52 women who completed the RCT. It was not possible to provide quantified results, as insufficient data were provided. Remission rates were not reported. We found no RCTs on the effects of other selective serotonin reuptake inhibitors (sertraline, paroxetine, and citaopram), venlafaxine, mirtazapine, and reboxetine. **Versus psychotherapy:** We found one systematic review (search date 2000, 5 RCTs) of antidepressants versus psychotherapy (all CBT RCTs) and one subsequent RCT.[32,37] We found another trial comparing fluoxetine with psychotherapy, which is awaiting translation.[38] The systematic review found no significant difference in remission rates, bulimic symptom severity (4 RCTs), or depression symptom severity at the end of the trials (3 RCTs).[32] A subsequent RCT (53 people) compared three treatments: group based CBT, fluoxetine 60 mg daily, and CBT plus fluoxetine.[37] Completer only analysis found no significant differences in 1 month abstinence from binge eating at the end of treatment (5/19 with CBT v 2/16 with fluoxetine; RR 2.11, 95% CI 0.47 to 9.43) or in 1 month absence from self induced vomiting (7/19 with CBT, 1/16 with fluoxetine; RR 5.9, 95% CI 0.81 to 42.99).[37] **Versus combination treatment:** See combination treatment, p 41. **Antidepressants as maintenance:** We found two small RCTs of maintenance treatment.[33,34] The first very small RCT (9 people who had responded well to despiramine over the previous 24 weeks) compared continuation of desipramine versus placebo.[33] It found no significant difference between treatments (relapse: 1/5 [20%] with desipramine v 2/4 [50%] with placebo; RR 0.4, 95% CI 0.1 to 3.0). The second very small RCT (9 women who had responded well to imipramine over the previous 10 weeks) compared continuation of imipramine versus placebo.[34] It found no significant difference in relapse (relapse: 2/3 [67%] with imipramine v 5/6 [83%] with placebo; RR 0.8, 95% CI 0.3 to 1.9).[34]

Harms: One systematic review (search date 2000) found that withdrawal significantly increased with antidepressants compared with psychotherapy (4 RCTs, 189 people; AR 40% v 18%; RR 2.18, 95% CI 1.09 to 4.35).[32] One subsequent RCT (53 people) found no significant difference in withdrawals with fluoxetine compared with CBT and with combined treatment (42% with CBT, 25% with fluoxetine; RR 1.68, 95% CI 0.62 to 4.57; and 33% with combined treatment; RR 1.33, 95% CI 0.46 to 3.89).[37] The authors thought this might be due to cultural differences because psychotherapy is rarely offered as part of a treatment trial in Germany. A second systematic review (search date 2001) found significantly increased withdrawal in people taking antidepressants compared with placebo (12 RCTs, 1123 people, 10.5% with any antidepressant v 5.1% with placebo; RR 1.83, 95% CI 1.13 to 2.95; NNH 7, 95% CI 4 to 18).[31] It found no significant difference in withdrawal due to adverse effects between and within classes of antidepressants. It found that withdrawal due to any cause was more likely with tricyclic antidepressants than with placebo (6 RCTs, 277 people, 29% with tricyclic v 14% with placebo; RR 1.93, 95% CI 1.15 to 3.25), but was more likely with placebo than with selective serotonin reuptake inhibitors (3 RCTs, 706 people, 37% with a selective serotonin reuptake inhibitor v 40% with placebo; RR 0.83, 95% CI 0.68 to 0.99). We found one RCT examining specific adverse effects. One found significant increases in reclining and standing blood pulse rate, lying systolic and diastolic blood pressure, and greater orthostatic effects on blood pressure with desipramine versus placebo.[39] Cardiovascular changes were well tolerated and few people withdrew because of these effects. Meta-analyses of two double blind RCTs of fluoxetine versus placebo found no significant difference in the incidence of suicidal acts or ideation in people treated with fluoxetine versus placebo.[40] However, the overall incidence of events was low (suicide attempts 1.2%, none fatal; emergent suicidal ideation 3.1%). The third subsequent RCT did not report on withdrawal or adverse events.[23]

Comment: We found no consistent predictors of response to treatment. We found no good evidence for the efficacy of other selective serotonin reuptake inhibitors apart from fluoxetine of the "newer" antidepressants venlafaxine, reboxetine, and mirtazapine. One review commented on the lack of follow up.[31] The second subsequent RCT found no differences between active and placebo groups in withdrawal rates because of adverse events, and no changes in blood pressure in those on moclobemide despite reports in food diaries of a high consumption of tyramine-containing foods.[36] The RCTs of maintenance both made multiple randomisations and compared a number of different groups. This meant that there were very few people in the groups for maintenance treatment.

OPTION COMBINATION TREATMENT

One systematic review and one subsequent RCT found no significant difference between combination treatment (antidepressants plus psychotherapy) and antidepressants alone in binge frequency, depressive symptoms, and remission rates. The systematic review found that, compared with psychotherapy alone, combination treatment improved short term remission, but there was no significant difference in binge frequency and depressive symptoms. The systematic review found that combination treatment with psychotherapy was associated with higher withdrawal rates compared with psychotherapy alone. One subsequent RCT of cognitive behavioural therapy in a self help form plus fluoxetine found limited evidence that combined treatment reduced bulimic symptoms compared with cognitive behavioural therapy alone. A second subsequent RCT found no significant difference in symptoms between group based CBT, fluoxetine, and their combination.

Benefits: **Versus antidepressants alone:** We found one systematic review (search date 2000, 7 RCTs, 247 people)[32] and one subsequent RCT comparing combination treatment (antidepressants plus psychotherapy) versus antidepressants alone.[37] The systematic review found that combination treatment compared with antidepressants alone did not significantly improve binge frequency, depressive symptoms, and short term remission rates, although outcomes were better with combination treatment (binge frequency 4 RCTs; SMD +0.34, 95% CI −0.05 to +0.73; depressive symptoms 3 RCTs; SMD +0.24, 95% CI −0.14 to +0.62; short term remission rates 4 RCTs, 141 people, 42% with combined treatment v 23% with antidepressants alone; RR 1.40, 95% CI 0.98 to 1.99).[32] The subsequent RCT (53 people) compared three treatments: group based cognitive behavioural therapy (CBT); fluoxetine 60 mg daily; and CBT plus fluoxetine (see option, p 39).[37] Completer only analysis found no significant difference in 1 month abstinence from binge eating (2/16 with fluoxetine v 3/18 with combination; RR 1.05, 95% CI 0.80 to 1.30) or in 1 month abstinence from self induced vomiting (1/16 with fluoxetine v 1/18 with combination; RR 0.99, 95% CI 0.84 to 1.18). **Versus psychotherapy alone:** We found one systematic review (search date 2000, 7 RCTs, 343 people)[32] and two subsequent RCTs comparing combination treatment (antidepressants plus psychotherapy) versus antidepressants alone.[23,37] The systematic review found that combination treatment compared with psychotherapy alone significantly increased short term remission (6 RCTs, 257 people, 49% v 36%; RR 1.21, 95% CI 1.02 to 1.45) but found no significant difference in depressive symptoms or in frequency of binge eating (see glossary, p 43) (6 RCTs; SMD +0.12, 95% CI −0.21 to +0.46).[32] The first subsequent RCT found that people who received both the self help manual and fluoxetine 60 mg daily had the greatest reduction in bulimic symptoms compared with those in the placebo, fluoxetine, or self help only arms, but significance was not reported.[23] Remission rates did not differ significantly across the three active treatment arms. The second subsequent RCT (53 people) compared three treatments: group based CBT; fluoxetine 60 mg daily; and CBT plus fluoxetine.[37] Completer only analysis found no significant difference in 1 month abstinence from binge eating (5/19 with CBT v 3/18 with combination; RR 1.58, 95% CI 0.44 to 5.67), or in 1 month abstinence from self induced vomiting (7/19 with CBT v 1/18 with combination; RR 6.63, 95% CI 0.90 to 48.69).

Harms: The review found no significant difference in withdrawal rates between combination treatment and antidepressants alone (4 RCTs, 196 people, 34% with combination treatment v 41% with antidepressants alone; RR 1.19, 95% CI 0.69 to 2.05).[32] Withdrawal rates were significantly lower with psychotherapy alone compared with combination treatments (6 RCTs, 295 people, 16% v 30%; RR 0.57, 95% CI 0.38 to 0.88).[32] The subsequent RCT[37] did not find higher non-completion rates when CBT was combined with fluoxetine.

Comment: Modest effect sizes in these analyses may be clinically relevant, but the small number and size of trials limit conclusions.

GLOSSARY

Binge eating Modified from DSM-IV.[1] Eating, in a discrete period (e.g. hours), a large amount of food, accompanied by a lack of control over eating during the episode.

Bulimia nervosa The American Psychiatric Association DSM-IV[1] criteria include recurrent episodes of binge eating; recurrent inappropriate compensatory behaviour to prevent weight gain; frequency of binge eating and inappropriate compensatory behaviour both, on average, at least twice a week for 3 months; self evaluation unduly influenced by body shape and weight; and disturbance occurring not exclusively during episodes of anorexia nervosa. Types of bulimia nervosa, modified from DSM-IV[1], are purging: using self induced vomiting, laxatives, diuretics, or enemas; non-purging: fasting, exercise, but not vomiting or other abuse as for the purging type. Many studies however evaluate efficacy for samples that may include participants with subthreshold bulimia nervosa or binge eating disorder. Where possible, only data of bulimia nervosa participants are reported in this review.

Cognitive behavioural therapy In bulimia nervosa this uses three overlapping phases. Phase one aims to educate the person about bulimia nervosa. People are helped to increase regularity of eating, and resist urge to binge or purge. Phase two introduces procedures to reduce dietary restraint (e.g. broadening food choices). In addition, cognitive procedures supplemented by behavioural experiments are used to identify and correct dysfunctional attitudes and beliefs, and avoidance behaviours. Phase three is the maintenance phase. Relapse prevention strategies are used to prepare for possible future set backs.[41]

Cognitive orientation therapy The cognitive orientation theory aims to generate a systematic procedure for exploring the meaning of a behaviour around themes, such as avoidance of certain emotions. Therapy for modifying behaviour focuses on systematically changing beliefs related to themes, not beliefs referring directly to eating behaviour. No attempt is made to persuade the people that their beliefs are incorrect or maladapative.[42]

Dialectical behaviour therapy A type of behavioural therapy that views emotional dysregulation as the core problem in bulimia nervosa, with binge eating and purging understood as attempts to influence, change, or control painful emotional states. Patients are taught a repertoire of skills to replace dysfunctional behaviours.[43]

Exposure therapy In bulimia nervosa this is a modification of the exposure and response prevention therapy developed for obsessive compulsive disorder. It involves exposure to food, for example, and then psychological prevention strategies to control weight behaviour, such as vomiting after eating until the urge or compulsion to vomit has receded.[44]

Hypnobehavioural psychotherapy Uses a combination of behavioural techniques, such as self monitoring to change maladaptive eating disorders, and hypnotic techniques to reinforce and encourage behaviour change.

Interpersonal psychotherapy In bulimia nervosa, this is a three phase treatment. Phase one analyses in detail the interpersonal context of the eating disorder. This leads to the formulation of an interpersonal problem area, which forms the focus of the second stage, which is aimed at helping the person make interpersonal changes. Phase three is devoted to the person's progress and an exploration of ways to handle future interpersonal difficulties. At no stage is attention paid to eating habits or body attitudes.[24]

Motivational enhancement therapy (MET) This is based on a model of change with focus on stages of change. Stages of change represent constellations of intentions and behaviours through which individuals pass as they move from having a problem to doing something to resolve it. People in "precontemplation" show no intention to change. People in "contemplation" acknowledge they have a problem

Mental health

and are thinking about change, but have not yet made a commitment to change. People in the third "action" stage are actively engaged in overcoming their problem, and people in "maintenance" work to prevent relapse. Transition from one stage to the next is sequential, but not linear. The aim of MET is to help people move from earlier stages into "action, utilising cognitive and emotional strategies". There is an emphasis on the therapeutic alliance. With precontemplators, the therapist explores perceived positive and negative aspects of their behaviours. Open-ended questions are used to elicit client expression, and reflective paraphrase is used to reinforce key points of motivation. During a session following structured assessment, most of the time is devoted to explaining feedback to the client. Later in MET, attention is devoted to developing and consolidating a change plan.[45]

Pure self help cognitive behavioural therapy A modified form of cognitive behavioural therapy, in which a treatment manual is provided for people to proceed with treatment on their own, or with support from a non-professional. "Guided self help" usually implies that the support person may or may not have some professional training, but is usually not a specialist in eating disorders.

Self psychology therapy This approaches bulimia nervosa as a specific case of the pathology of the self. The treated person cannot rely on people to fulfil their needs such as self esteem. They rely instead on a substance, food, to fulfil personal needs. Therapy progresses when the people move to rely on humans, starting with the therapist.[42]

REFERENCES

1. American Psychiatric Association. *Diagnostic and statistical manual of mental disorders* 4th ed. Washington DC: American Psychiatric Press, 1994.

2. Bushnell JA, Wells JE, Hornblow AR, et al. Prevalence of three bulimic syndromes in the general population. *Psychol Med* 1990;20:671–680.

3. Garfinkel PE, Lin B, Goering P, et al. Bulimia nervosa in a Canadian community sample: prevalence, co-morbidity, early experiences and psychosocial functioning. *Am J Psychiatry* 1995;152:1052–1058.

4. Gard MCE, Freeman CP. The dismantling of a myth: a review of eating disorders and socioeconomic status. *Int J Eat Disord* 1996;20:1–12.

5. Hall A, Hay PJ. Eating disorder patient referrals from a population region 1977–1986. *Psychol Med* 1991;21:697–701.

6. Kendler KS, Maclean C, Neale M, et al. The genetic epidemiology of bulimia nervosa. *Am J Psychiatry* 1991;148:1627–1637.

7. Choudry IY, Mumford DB. A pilot study of eating disorders in Mirpur (Pakistan) using an Urdu version of the Eating Attitude Test. *Int J Eat Disord* 1992;11:243–251.

8. Striegel-Moore RH, Wifley DE, Caldwell MB, et al. Weight-related attitudes and behaviors of women who diet to lose weight: a comparison for black dieters and white dieters. *Obes Res* 1996;4:109–116.

9. Fairburn CG, Welch SL, Doll HA, et al. Risk factors for bulimia nervosa: a community-based case-control study. *Arch Gen Psychiatry* 1997;54:509–517.

10. Collings S, King M. Ten year follow-up of 50 patients with bulimia nervosa. *Br J Psychiatry* 1994;164:80–87.

11. Keel PK, Mitchell JE, Davis TL, et al. Long-term impact of treatment in women diagnosed with bulimia nervosa *Int J Eat Disord* 2002;31:151–158.

12. Keel PK, Mitchell JE. Outcome in bulimia nervosa. *Am J Psychiatry* 1997;154:313–321.

13. Keel PK, Mitchell JE, Miller KB, et al. Long-term outcome of bulimia nervosa. *Arch Gen Psychiatry* 1999;56:63–69.

14. Fairburn CG, Norman PA, Welch SL, et al. A prospective study of outcome in bulimia nervosa and the long-term effects of three psychological treatments. *Arch Gen Psychiatry* 1995;52:304–312.

15. Coker S, Vize C, Wade T, et al. Patients with bulimia nervosa who fail to engage in cognitive behaviour therapy. *Int J Eat Disord* 1993;13:35–40.

16. Fahy TA, Russell GFM. Outcome and prognostic variables in bulimia. *Int J Eat Disord* 1993;14:135–146.

17. Rossiter EM, Agras WS, Telch CF, et al. Cluster B personality disorder characteristics predict outcome in the treatment of bulimia nervosa. *Int J Eat Disord* 1993;13:349–358.

18. Johnson C, Tobin DL, Dennis A. Differences in treatment outcome between borderline and nonborderline bulimics at 1-year follow-up. *Int J Eat Disord* 1990;9:617–627.

19. Fairburn C, Cooper Z, Doll H, et al. The natural course of bulimia nervosa and binge eating disorder in young women. *Arch Gen Psychiatry* 2000:57:659–665.

20. Agras WS, Crow SJ, Halmi KA, et al. Outcome predictors for the cognitive behavior treatment of bulimia nervosa: data from a multisite study. *Am J Psychiatry* 2000;157:1302–1308.

21. Reas DL, Schoemaker C, Zipfel S, et al. Prognostic value of duration of illness and early intervention in bulimia nervosa: a systematic review of the outcome literature. *Int J Eat Disord* 2001;30:1–10. Search date 1999; primary sources; not stated.

22. Hay PJ, Bacaltchuk J. Psychotherapy for bulimia nervosa and binging. In: The Cochrane Library, Issue 1, 2003. Oxford: Update Software. Search date 2002; primary sources Medline, Extramed, Embase, Psychlit, Current Contents, Lilacs,

Scisearch, The Cochrane Controlled Trials Register 1997, The Cochrane Collaboration Depression and Anxiety Trials Register, hand search of *Int J Eat Disord* since its first issue, citation lists in identified studies and reviews, and personal contacts.

23. Mitchell JE, Fletcher L, Hanson K, et al. The relative efficacy of fluoxetine and manual-based self-help in the treatment of outpatients with bulimia nervosa. *J Clin Psychopharmacol* 2001;21:298–304.

24. Agras WS, Walsh BT, Fairburn CG, et al. A multicenter comparison of cognitive-behavioral therapy and interpersonal psychotherapy. *Arch Gen Psychiatry* 2000; 54:459–465.

25. Treasure JL, Katzman M, Schmidt U, et al. Engagement and outcome in the treatment of bulimia nervosa: first phase of a sequential design comparing motivation enhancement therapy and cognitive behavioural therapy. *Behav Res Ther* 1999;37:405–418.

26. Leichsenring von F Zur. Wirksamkeit tiefenpsychologisch fundierter und psychodynamischer Therapie. Eine ubersicht unter berucksichtigung von kriterien der evidence-based medicine. *Z Psychosom Med Psychother* 2002;48:139–162.

27. Wilson GT, Fairburn CG. Treatments for eating disorders. In: Nathan PE, Gorman JM, eds. *A Guide to Treatments that Work.* New York: Oxford University Press, 1998:501–530.

28. Wolk SL, Devlin MJ. Stage of change as a predictor of response to psychotherapy for bulimia nervosa. *Int J Eat Disord* 2001;30:96–100.

29. Thiels C, Schmidt U, Troop N, et al. Compliance with a self-care manual in guided self-change for bulimia nervosa. *Eur Eat Disord Rev* 2001;9:115–122.

30. Eizaguirre E, et al. Un ensayo controlado de intervenciones familiares en trastornos alimentarios *An Psiquiatria (Madrid)* [in Spanish] 2000;16:322–336.

31. Bacaltchuk J, Hay P. Antidepressants versus placebo for people with bulimia nervosa. In: The Cochrane Library Issue 1, 2003. Oxford: Update Software. Search date 2001; primary sources Medline, Extramed, Embase, Psychlit, Current Contents, Lilacs, Scisearch, The Cochrane Controlled Trials Register, The Cochrane Collaboration Depression and Anxiety Trials Register, hand search of citation lists in identified studies and reviews, and personal contact.

32. Bacaltchuk J, Hay P. Antidepressants versus psychological treatments and their combination for people bulimia nervosa (Cochrane Review). Cochrane Library Issue 1, 2003. Oxford: Update Software. Search date 2000; primary sources Medline, Extramed, Embase, Psychlit, Current Contents, Lilacs, Scisearch, Cochrane Controlled Trials Register, Cochrane Collaboration Depression

and Anxiety Trials Register, hand search of *Int J Eat Disord* since its first issue, citation lists of identified studies and reviews, and personal contacts.

33. Walsh BT, Hadigan CM, Devlin MJ, et al. Long-term outcome of antidepressant treatment for bulimia nervosa. *Am J Psychiatry* 1991;148:1206–1212.

34. Pyle RL, Mitchell JE, Eckert ED, et al. Maintenance treatment and 6-month outcome for bulimic patients who respond to initial treatment. *Am J Psychiatry* 1990;147:871–875.

35. Agras WS, Rossiter EM, Arnow B, et al. One-year follow-up of psychosocial and pharmacologic treatments for bulimia nervosa. *J Clin Psychiatry* 1994;55:179–183.

36. Carruba MO, Cuzzolaro M, Riva L, et al. Efficacy and tolerability of moclobemide in bulimia nervosa: a placebo-controlled trial. *Int Clin Psychopharmacol* 2001;16:27–32.

37. Jacobi C, Dahme B, Dittman R Cognitive-behavioural, fluoxetine and combined treatment for bulimia nervosa: short- and long-term results. *Eur Eat Disord* 2002;10:179–198.

38. Campanelli M. Cecinella confronto tra gli effetti della terapia farmacologica con fluoxetine e las psicoterapia nel trattamento della bulimia nervosa [in Italian]. *Minerva Psichiatr* 2002 43(suppl 1):1–24.

39. Walsh BT, Hadigan CM, Wong LM. Increased pulse and blood pressure associated with desipramine treatment of bulimia nervosa. *J Clin Psychopharmacol* 1992;12:163–168.

40. Wheadon DE, Rampey AH, Thompson VL, et al. Lack of association between fluoxetine and suicidality in bulimia nervosa. *J Clin Psychiatry* 1992;53:235–241.

41. Fairburn CG, Marcus MD, Wilson GT. Cognitive-behavioral therapy for binge eating and bulimia nervosa: a comprehensive treatment manual. In :Fairburn CG, Wilson GT, eds. *Binge eating: nature, Assessment, and Treatment.* New York: Guilford Press, 1993:361–404.

42. Bachar E, Latzer Y, Kreitler S, et al. Empirical comparison of two psychological therapies. Self psychology and cognitive orientation in the treatment of anorexia and bulimia. *J Psychother Pract Res* 1999;8:115–128.

43. Safer DL, Telch CF, Agras WS. Dialectical behavior therapy for bulimia nervosa. *Am J Psychiatry* 2001;158:632–634.

44. Leitenberg H, Rosen J, Gross J, et al. Exposure plus response-prevention treatment of bulimia nervosa. *J Consult Clin Psychol* 1988;56:535–541.

45. Schmidt U, Treasure J, eds. *Clinician's guide to getting better bit(e) by bit(e)*. Hove: Psychology Press, 1997.

Phillipa Hay

Psychiatrist

University of Adelaide, Adelaide, Australia

Josue Bacaltchuk

Psychiatrist

Federal University of Sao Paulo, Sao Paulo, Brazil

Competing interests: PH has received reimbursement for attending symposia from Solvay Pharmaceuticals, Bristol-Myers Squibb, and Pfizer Pharmaceuticals, and for educational training of family doctors from Bristol-Myers Squibb, Pfizer Pharmaceuticals, and Lundbeck, and has been funded by Jansenn-Cilag to attend symposia. JB none declared.

TABLE 1 Comparison of remission rates between cognitive behaviour therapy or other active psychotherapy and comparison group (see text, p 36).[22]

Comparison	Number of RCTs	Number of people	Absolute remission rates	RR of not remitting (95% CI)
CBT v waiting list	3	122	43% v 5%	0.62 (0.47 to 0.83)
CBT v other psychotherapy	6	448	37% v 20%	0.78 (0.70 to 0.87)
CBT-M v other psychotherapy	3	316	33% v 16%	0.81 (0.69 to 0.95)
Other psychotherapy v waiting list	3	124	37% v 3%	0.67 (0.55 to 0.81)

CBT, cognitive behavioural therapy (broadly definied); CBT-M, cognitive behavourial therapy — manualised.[44]

TABLE 2 Comparison of remission rates between active drug and placebo by class of antidepressant (see text, p 39).[31]

Class: drug(s)	Number of RCTs	Number of people	Absolute remission rates	RR (95% CI)
TCA: desipramine, imipramine	3	132	21% v 9%	0.90 (0.79 to 1.04)
SSRI: fluoxetine	2	420	19% v 11%	0.91 (0.83 to 0.99)
MAOI: phenylzine, isocarboxacid	2	98	24% v 6%	0.81 (0.68 to 0.96)
Other: bupropion, trazodone	2	127	17% v 8%	0.86 (0.76 to 0.94)

MAOI, monoamine oxidase inhibitor; SSRI, selective serotonin reuptake inhibitor; TCA, tricyclic antidepressant.

Search date March 2003

Steven Reid, Trudie Chalder, Anthony Cleare, Matthew Hotopf, and Simon Wessely

INTERVENTIONS

Key Messages

- **Cognitive behavioural therapy** One systematic review found that cognitive behavioural therapy administered by highly skilled therapists in specialist centres improved quality of life and physical functioning compared with standard medical care or relaxation therapy. One additional multicentre RCT found that cognitive behavioural therapy administered by less experienced therapists may also be effective compared with guided support groups or no interventions.

- **Graded aerobic exercise** RCTs have found that a graded aerobic exercise programme improves measures of fatigue and physical functioning compared with flexibility and relaxation training or general advice. One RCT has found that an educational package to encourage graded exercise improved measures of physical functioning, fatigue, mood, and sleep at 1 year compared with written information alone.

- **Dietary supplements** One small RCT found no significant difference between a nutritional supplement (containing multivitamins, minerals, and coenzymes) and placebo in fatigue severity or functional impairment at 10 weeks.

- **Evening primrose oil** One small RCT found no significant difference between evening primrose oil and placebo in depression scores at 3 months.

- **Magnesium (intramuscular)** One small RCT found that intramuscular magnesium injections improved symptoms at 6 weeks compared with placebo. However, we were unable to draw reliable conclusions from this small study.

- **Antidepressants; corticosteroids; oral nicotinamide adenine dinucleotide** RCTs found insufficient evidence about the effects of these interventions in people with chronic fatigue syndrome.

- **Immunotherapy** Small RCTs found limited evidence that immunoglobulin G modestly improved physical functioning and fatigue at 3–6 months compared with placebo, but it was associated with considerable adverse effects. Small

RCTs found insufficient evidence on the effects of interferon alfa or aciclovir compared with placebo. One RCT found that staphylococcus toxoid improved symptoms at six months compared with placebo, although it is associated with local reaction and could cause anaphylaxis.

- **Prolonged rest** We found no RCTs on the effects of prolonged rest. Indirect observational evidence in healthy volunteers and in people recovering from a viral illness suggests that prolonged rest may perpetuate or worsen fatigue and symptoms.

DEFINITION Chronic fatigue syndrome (CFS) is characterised by severe, disabling fatigue and other symptoms, including musculoskeletal pain, sleep disturbance, impaired concentration, and headaches. Two widely used definitions of CFS, from the US Centers for Disease Control and Prevention[1] and from Oxford, UK,[2] were developed as operational criteria for research (see table 1, p 61). There are important differences between these definitions. The UK criteria insist upon the presence of mental fatigue, whereas the US criteria include a requirement for several physical symptoms, reflecting the belief that CFS has an underlying immunological or infective pathology.

INCIDENCE/ PREVALENCE Community and primary care based studies have reported the prevalence of CFS to be 0–3%, depending on the criteria used.[3,4] Systematic population surveys have found similar prevalences of CFS in people of different socioeconomic status and in all ethnic groups.[4,5]

AETIOLOGY/ RISK FACTORS The cause of CFS is poorly understood. Women are at higher risk than men (RR 1.3–1.7 depending on diagnostic criteria used).[6]

PROGNOSIS Studies have focused on people attending specialist clinics. A systematic review of studies of prognosis (search date 1996) found that children with CFS had better outcomes than adults: 54–94% of children showed definite improvement (after up to 6 years' follow up), whereas 20–50% of adults showed some improvement in the medium term and only 6% returned to premorbid levels of functioning.[7] Despite the considerable burden of morbidity associated with CFS, we found no evidence of increased mortality. The systematic review found that outcome was influenced by the presence of psychiatric disorders (depression and anxiety) and beliefs about causation and treatment.[7]

AIMS OF INTERVENTION To reduce levels of fatigue and associated symptoms, to increase levels of activity, and to improve quality of life.

OUTCOMES Severity of symptoms and their effects on physical function and quality of life. These outcomes are measured in several different ways: the medical outcomes survey short form general health survey (SF-36),[8] a rating scale measuring limitation of physical functioning caused by ill health (score range 0–100, where 0 = limited in all activities and 100 = able to carry out vigorous activities); the Karnofsky scale,[9] a modified questionnaire originally developed for the rating of quality of life in people undergoing chemotherapy for malignancy; the Beck Depression Inventory,[10] a checklist for quantifying depressive symptoms; the sickness impact profile,[11] a measure of the influence of symptoms on social and physical functioning; the Chalder fatigue scale,[12] a rating scale measuring subjective fatigue (score range 0–11, where scores ≥ 4 = excessive fatigue); the clinical global impression scale,[13] a validated measure of overall change compared with baseline at study onset, with seven possible scores from "very much worse" (score 7) to "very much better" (score 1); the checklist individual strength fatigue subscale (score range 8 (no fatigue at all) to 56 (maximally fatigued)[14]; and self reported severity of symptoms and levels of activity, the Nottingham health profile[15] contains questions in six categories: energy, pain perception, sleep patterns, sense of social isolation, emotional reactions, and physical mobility (weighted scores give maximum 100 for answer yes to all questions, and minimum 0 for someone with no complaints).

METHODS *Clinical Evidence search and appraisal March 2003.*

QUESTION **What are the effects of treatments?**

OPTION **ANTIDEPRESSANTS**

RCTs found insufficient evidence about the effects of antidepressants in people with chronic fatigue syndrome.

Benefits:
We found one systematic review (search date 2000), which did not report quantified results.[16] **Fluoxetine:** The review identified two RCTs.[17,18] The first RCT (107 depressed and non-depressed people with chronic fatigue syndrome [CFS]) compared fluoxetine versus placebo for 8 weeks.[17] It found that fluoxetine significantly improved the Beck Depression Inventory compared with placebo (mean difference between fluoxetine and placebo in improvement in Beck Depression Inventory –0.19, 95% CI –0.35 to –0.02), but the difference may not be clinically important. It found no significant difference between fluoxetine and placebo in the sickness impact profile (mean difference between fluoxetine and placebo measured by fatigue subscale of Checklist Individual Strength –0.16, 95% CI –0.64 to +0.31).[19] The second RCT (136 people with CFS) compared four groups: fluoxetine plus graded exercise; drug placebo plus graded exercise; fluoxetine plus general advice to exercise; and drug placebo plus general advice to exercise. It found no significant difference in the level of fatigue, although modest improvements in measures of depression were seen at 12 weeks (Hospital Anxiety and Depression scale, mean change 1.1, 95% CI 0.03 to 2.2).[18,20] **Phenelzine:** The review identified one RCT.[16,21] The RCT (30 people with CFS) compared phenelzine versus placebo, using a modified Karnofsky scale and other outcome measures (including functional status questionnaire, profile of mood states, Centres for Epidemiological Study of Depression fatigue severity scale, and symptom severity checklist).[20] This study concluded that there was a pattern of improvement across several measures (significance tests for individual measures not carried out). **Moclobemide:** The review identified one RCT but did not report quantified results.[16,22] The RCT (90 people with CFS) compared moclobemide (450–600 mg daily) versus placebo.[22] It found that moclobemide was associated with a non-significant increase in subjectively reported global improvement (moclobemide 24/47 [51%] v placebo 14/43 [33%]; OR 2.16, 95% CI 0.9 to 5.1), and a

non-significant improvement in the clinician rated Karnofsky scale. **Sertraline versus clomipramine:** We found one RCT comparing sertraline versus clomipramine in people with CFS.[23] It found no significant difference between sertraline and clomipramine. There was no placebo group, which makes it difficult to draw useful conclusions.

Harms: **Fluoxetine:** One RCT assessed separately the symptoms (which could be attributed to either CFS or to known adverse effects of fluoxetine) before starting treatment, after 2 weeks, after 6 weeks, and at the end of treatment (week 8). It found that fluoxetine increased complaints of tremor and perspiration compared with placebo at 8 weeks (tremor: $P = 0.006$; perspiration: $P = 0.008$).[16] It found no significant difference between fluoxetine and placebo at 2 and 6 weeks. It found that fluoxetine increased withdrawal due to adverse effects (9/54 [17%] v 2/53 [4%]).[17] The second RCT also found increased withdrawal rates with fluoxetine (24/68 people [36%] with fluoxetine withdrew v 16/69 people [24%] with placebo).[18] **Phenelzine:** Three of 15 people (20%) who took phenelzine withdrew because of adverse effects compared with none who took placebo.[21] **Sertraline versus clomipramine:** The RCT provided no information on adverse effects.[23]

Comment: Clinical trials were performed in specialist clinics. **Fluoxetine:** The first RCT[17] used a shorter duration of treatment and studied people with a longer duration of illness compared with the second RCT.[18]

OPTION   CORTICOSTEROIDS

Four RCTs found insufficient evidence about the effects of corticosteroids compared with placebo in people with chronic fatigue syndrome.

Benefits: We found one systematic review (search date 2000), which did not report quantified results.[16] **Fludrocortisone:** The systematic review[16] identified two RCTs.[24,25] The first large RCT (100 people with chronic fatigue syndrome [CFS] and neurally mediated hypotension) compared fludrocortisone (titrated to 0.1 mg daily) versus placebo for 9 weeks. It found no significant difference on a self rated global scale of "wellness" (recorded improvement of ≥ 15 points: fludrocortisone 14% v placebo 10%; $P = 0.76$; raw data not provided).[24] The second randomised crossover trial (20 people), which measured change in symptom severity (visual analogue scale of symptoms from 0–10 corresponding to "no problem" to "could not be worse") and functional status (using the SF-36) for 6 weeks. It found no significant difference between fludrocortisone and placebo.[25] **Hydrocortisone:** The review identified two RCTs.[16,26,27] The first RCT (65 people) compared hydrocortisone (25–35 mg daily) versus placebo for 12 weeks. It found that hydrocortisone significantly improved a self rated scale of "wellness" (recorded improvement of ≥ 5 points: hydrocortisone 53% v placebo 29%; $P = 0.04$). Other self rating scales did not show significant benefit (Beck Depression Inventory: hydrocortisone −2.1 v placebo −0.4, $P = 0.17$; activity scale: hydrocortisone 0.3 v placebo 0.7, $P = 0.32$; sickness impact profile: hydrocortisone −2.5 v placebo −2.2; $P = 0.85$).[26] The second RCT (32 people, crossover design) compared a lower dose of hydrocortisone (5 or 10 mg daily) versus placebo for 1 month. It found that hydrocortisone improved fatigue in the short term compared with placebo (self report fatigue scale: hydrocortisone 28% v placebo 9%; results before crossover not provided).[27]

Harms: **Fludrocortisone:** In the first RCT, fludrocortisone increased withdrawal rates due to adverse events compared with placebo (12/50 [24%] v 4/50 [8%]; RR 3, 95% CI 1.04 to 8.67; NNT 6, 95% CI 3 to 8).[24] Four people withdrew from the trial because of worsening symptoms.[25] **Hydrocortisone:** One RCT (25–35 mg daily doses of hydrocortisone) found that 12 people (40%) experienced adrenal suppression (assessed by measuring cortisol levels).[26] Another RCT (5 or 10 mg daily doses of hydrocortisone) reported minor adverse effects in up to 10% of participants. Three people on hydrocortisone had exacerbation of acne and nervousness, and one person on placebo had an episode of fainting.[27]

Comment: The RCTs used different reasons for their choice of active treatment. The use of fludrocortisone, a mineralocorticoid, was based on the hypothesis that CFS is associated with neurally mediated hypotension.[28] The use of hydrocortisone, a glucocorticoid, in the other RCTs was based on evidence of underactivity of the hypothalamic–pituitary–adrenocortical axis in some people with CFS.[29] Any benefit from low dose glucocorticoids seems to be short lived, and higher doses are associated with adverse effects.

| OPTION | ORAL NICOTINAMIDE ADENINE DINUCLEOTIDE |

One small RCT found insufficient evidence about the effects of oral nicotinamide adenine dinucleotide compared with placebo in people with chronic fatigue syndrome.

Benefits: We found one systematic review (search date 2000), which did not report quantified results.[16] It identified one poor quality randomised crossover trial (35 people), which compared nicotinamide adenine dinucleotide (10 mg daily) with placebo for 4 weeks.[30] Of the 35 people, two were excluded for non-compliance and seven were excluded for using psychotropic drugs. It found that nicotinamide adenine dinucleotide significantly improved scores on a self devised 50 item symptom rating scale compared with placebo (8/26 people [30%] attained a 10% improvement with nicotinamide adenine dinucleotide v 2/26 people [8%] with placebo; P < 0.05, calculated by authors).

Harms: Minor adverse effects (loss of appetite, dyspepsia and flatulence) were reported on active treatment but did not lead to cessation of treatment.[30]

Comment: The RCT had a number of problems with its methods, including the use of inappropriate statistical analyses, the inappropriate exclusion of people from the analysis, and lack of numerical data preventing independent analysis of the published results.[31]

OPTION	EXERCISE

RCTs have found that a graded aerobic exercise programme improves measures of fatigue and physical functioning compared with flexibility training and relaxation training or general advice. One RCT found that an educational package to encourage graded exercise improved measures of physical functioning, fatigue, mood, and sleep at 1 year compared with written information alone.

Benefits: We found one systematic review (search date 2000), which did not report quantified results.[16] **Graded aerobic exercise:** The review identified two RCTs.[18,32] One RCT (66 people) compared graded aerobic exercise (active intervention) versus flexibility and relaxation training (control intervention) over 12 weeks.[32] All participants undertook individual weekly sessions supervised by an exercise physiologist. The aerobic exercise group built up their level of activity to 30 minutes of exercise a day (walking, cycling, swimming up to a maximum oxygen consumption of 60% of V_{O2}max). People in the flexibility and relaxation training group were taught stretching and relaxation techniques (maximum 30 minutes daily, 5 days/week) and were specifically told to avoid any extra physical activities. It found that Aerobic exercise increased reports of feeling "better" or "very much better" and improved physical fatigue and physical functioning compared with control (clinical global impression scale: 52% v 27%, P = 0.04; Chalder fatigue scale: –8.4 v –3.1, P = 0.004; SF-36 scale: 20.5 v 8.0, P = 0.01). The second RCT (136 people) compared four groups (graded aerobic exercise plus fluoxetine; graded aerobic exercise plus drug placebo; general advice plus fluoxetine; general advice plus drug placebo) over 24 weeks.[18] The graded exercise groups were given specific advice to undertake preferred aerobic exercise (such as walking, jogging, swimming, or cycling) for 20 minutes three times a week up to an energy expenditure of 75% of V_{O2}max. The general advice (exercise placebo) groups were not given any specific advice on frequency, intensity, or duration of aerobic activity they should be undertaking. It found that Graded exercise reduced fatigue at 26 weeks compared with general advice (Chalder fatigue scale < 4: 12/67 [18%] v 4/69 [6%]; RR 3.1, 95% CI 1.05 to 9.10; NNT 9, 95% CI 5 to 91). **Educational intervention:** The review[16] identified one RCT (148 people).[33] The RCT compared three types of educational interventions to encourage graded exercise with written information only (control group).[33] The participants in the three educational intervention groups received two treatment sessions, two telephone follow ups, and an educational package that provided an explanation of symptoms and encouraged home based exercise. One group received seven additional follow up telephone calls and another received seven additional face to face sessions over 4 months. People in the written information group received advice and an information booklet that encouraged graded activity but gave no explanation for the symptoms. The RCT found that the educational interventions improved physical functioning, fatigue, mood, sleep, and disability (self reported) compared with written information only. The RCT found no significant difference between the educational interventions (mean for 3 educational intervention groups *v* written information, SF-36 subscale: ≥ 25 or an increase of ≥ 10, 1 year after randomisation, 69% *v* 6%, P < 0.001; Chalder fatigue scale: 3 *v* 10, P < 0.001; Hospital Anxiety and Depression scale: depression 4 *v* 10, P < 0.001; anxiety 7 *v* 10, P < 0.01).

Harms: None of the RCTs reported data on adverse effects, and we found no evidence that exercise is harmful in people with chronic fatigue syndrome. The second aerobic exercise RCT found no significant difference in withdrawal rates between exercise and no exercise (25/68 [37%] with exercise *v* 15/69 [22%] without exercise; RR 1.7, 95% CI 0.98 to 2.9).[18] The reasons for the withdrawals from the graded exercise groups were not stated.

Comment: Experience suggests that symptoms of chronic fatigue syndrome may be exacerbated by overly ambitious or overly hasty attempts at exercise.

OPTION   PROLONGED REST

We found no RCTs on the effects of prolonged rest. Indirect observational evidence in healthy volunteers and in people recovering from a viral illness suggests that prolonged rest may perpetuate or worsen fatigue and symptoms.

Benefits: We found no systematic review or RCTs of prolonged rest in people with chronic fatigue syndrome.

Harms: We found no direct evidence of harmful effects of rest in people with chronic fatigue syndrome. We found observational evidence, which suggested that prolonged inactivity may perpetuate or worsen fatigue and is associated with symptoms in both healthy volunteers[34] and people recovering from viral illness.[35]

Comment: It is not clear that evidence from people recovering from viral illness can be extrapolated to people with chronic fatigue syndrome.

OPTION   DIETARY SUPPLEMENTS

One small RCT found no significant difference between a nutritional supplement (containing multivitamins, minerals, and coenzymes) and placebo in fatigue severity or functional impairment at 10 weeks.

Benefits: We found one RCT (53 people who fulfilled US Centers for Disease Control and Prevention criteria for chronic fatigue syndrome with high fatigue severity and high disability scores; duration of illness ranged from 2 to 12 years) that compared a polynutrient supplement (containing several vitamins, minerals and coenzymes, taken twice daily) versus placebo for 10 weeks.[36] It found no significant difference between treatment in fatigue severity or functional impairment (change in Checklist Individual Strength fatigue subscale from baseline to 10 weeks: 51.4 to 48.6 with supplements *v* 51.3 to 48.2 with placebo; difference 2.16, 95% CI −4.30 to +4.39; Sickness Impact Scale < 750 at 10 weeks: 4% with supplements *v* 12% with placebo).

Harms: Three people (11%) on active treatment withdrew because of nausea.[36]

Comment: The RCT may have been too small to detect a clinically important difference.[36]

OPTION   MAGNESIUM

One small RCT found that intramuscular magnesium injections improved symptoms at 6 weeks compared with placebo. However, we were unable to draw reliable conclusions from this small study.

Benefits: We found one systematic review (search date 2000), which did not report quantified results.[16] The review identified one RCT (32 people with chronic fatigue syndrome, but not magnesium deficiency; see comment), which compared weekly intramuscular injections of magnesium sulphate 50% versus placebo (water for injection) for 6 weeks.[37] It found that magnesium improved overall benefit, energy, pain, and emotional reactions compared with placebo (overall benefit: 12/15 [80%] v 3/17 [18%]; RR 4.5, 95% CI 1.6 to 13.1; NNT 2, 95% CI 2 to 4; energy P = 0.002; pain: P = 0.001; and emotional reactions: P = 0.013).

Harms: The RCT reported no adverse effects.

Comment: In the RCT, plasma and whole blood magnesium were normal and only the red blood cell concentrations of magnesium were slightly lower than the normal range.[37] Three subsequent case control studies have not found a deficiency of magnesium in people with chronic fatigue syndrome.[38–40] In these three studies, magnesium was in the normal range and no different from controls without chronic fatigue syndrome. However, none of the studies state how the normal range was established, so it is difficult to say if they are equivalent.

OPTION   EVENING PRIMROSE OIL

One small RCT found no significant difference between evening primrose oil and placebo in depression scores at 3 months.

Benefits: We found one systematic review (search date 2000), which did not report quantified results.[16] The review identified one RCT (50 people with chronic fatigue syndrome according to Oxford, UK, diagnostic criteria), which compared evening primrose oil (4 g daily) with placebo for 3 months.[41] It found no significant difference between treatments in depression scores (Beck Depression Inventory), physical symptoms, or participant assessment (at 3 months 46% were improved with placebo v 29% with evening primrose oil; P = 0.09; figures were not presented in a manner that allowed RR with CI to be calculated).

Harms: The RCT reported no adverse effects.

Comment: One RCT (63 people) compared evening primrose oil (4 g daily) versus placebo in people with a diagnosis of postviral fatigue syndrome.[42] This diagnosis was made on the basis of overwhelming fatigue, myalgia, and depression, which had been present for at least 1 year, and all had been preceded by a febrile illness. At 3 months, 33/39 (85%) of the people on active treatment had improved compared with 4/24 (17%) on placebo — a significant benefit (P < 0.0001). The difference in outcome may be partly explained by participant selection: the study in people with chronic fatigue syndrome used currently accepted diagnostic criteria.[41] Also, whereas the RCT in people with postviral fatigue syndrome used liquid paraffin as a placebo,[42] the chronic fatigue syndrome RCT used sunflower oil, which is better tolerated and less likely to affect the placebo response adversely.[41]

OPTION	IMMUNOTHERAPY

Small RCTs found limited evidence that immunoglobulin G modestly improved physical functioning and fatigue at 3–6 months compared with placebo, but it was associated with considerable adverse effects. Small RCTs found insufficient evidence on the effects of interferon alfa or aciclovir compared with placebo. One RCT found that staphylococcus toxoid improved symptoms at six months compared with placebo, although it is associated with local reaction and could cause anaphylaxis.

Benefits: We found one systematic review (search date 2000), which did not report quantified results.[16] **Immunoglobulin G:** The review identified four relevant RCTs comparing immunoglobulin G versus placebo for 6 months.[43–46] The first RCT (30 people) compared monthly intravenous injections of immunoglobulin G (1 g/kg) versus placebo (albumin).[43] After 6 months, no large differences were found in measures of fatigue (self reported symptom severity) or in physical and social functioning (SF-36). It found that placebo significantly improved social function compared with immunoglobulin G (dichotomous figures not reported). The second RCT (49 people) compared monthly intravenous immunoglobulin G (2 g/kg) with intravenous placebo (a maltose solution) for 3 months.[44] It found that immunoglobulin G significantly increased the proportion of people who improved in terms of a physician rated assessment of symptoms and disability compared with placebo (10/23 [44%] v 3/26 [11%]; P = 0.03). The third RCT (99 adults) compared three doses of immunoglobulin G (0.5, 1, or 2 g/kg) versus placebo (albumin).[45] It found no significant difference in quality of life, scores on visual analogue scales, or changes in hours spent in non-sedentary activities. The fourth RCT (71 adolescents aged 11–18 years) compared immunoglobulin G (1 g/kg) with placebo (a solution of maltose plus albumin).[46] Three infusions were given 1 month apart. The RCT found that immunoglobulin G significantly improved mean functional outcome (assessed using the mean of clinician ratings from four areas of the participants' activities) compared with placebo (proportion of people who achieved improvement of ≥ 25% at 6 months: 26/36 [52%] with immunoglobin v 15/34 [31%] with placebo, RR 1.6, 95% CI 1.1 to 2.5). However, both groups showed significant improvements from baseline, which continued to the 6 month assessment after treatment. **Other treatments:** We found one systematic review (search date 2000)[16] and one subsequent RCT.[47] The review identified two RCTs (30 people) comparing interferon alfa with placebo.[48,49] The first RCT identified by the review only found treatment benefit on subgroup analysis of people with isolated natural killer cell dysfunction.[48] The second randomised crossover trial identified by the review did not present results in a manner that allowed clear interpretation of treatment effect.[49] Other RCTs in the review found no significant difference between placebo and aciclovir,[50] dialysable leucocyte extract (in a factorial design with cognitive behavioural therapy),[51] or terfenadine.[52] The subsequent RCT (100 women who met both the ACS criteria for fibromyalgia and the US Centers for Disease Control and Prevention criteria for chronic fatigue syndrome and had functional impairment > 6 months) compared weekly subcutaneous injections of staphylococcus toxoid (dose increased weekly from 0.1 to 1.0 mL, followed by 1.0 mL doses every 4 weeks) versus placebo.[47] It found that staphylococcus toxoid significantly improved the clinical global impression of change scale at 26 weeks compared with placebo (minimally improved, much improved or very much improved: 32/49 [65%] with toxoid v 9/49 [18%] with placebo; P < 0.001).

Harms: **Immunoglobulin G:** In the first RCT, adverse effects judged to be worse than pretreatment symptoms in either group included gastrointestinal complaints (18 people), headaches (23 people), arthralgia (6 people), and worsening fatigue. Of these symptoms, only headaches differed significantly between the groups (immunoglobulin G 14/15 [93%] v placebo 9/15 [60%]). Six participants (3 immunoglobulin G, 3 placebo) were considered to have major adverse effects. Adverse events by treatment group were only reported for headache.[43] **Other treatments:** In the RCT comparing interferon alfa 2/13 (15%) people taking active treatment developed neutropenia.[48] The RCT comparing staphylococcus toxoid with placebo found no significant difference in reported adverse effects, excluding local reactions (13/49[26%] with toxoid v 7/49 [14% with placebo, P = 0.14).[47] All those receiving the toxoid had a local reaction at the injection site.

Comment: **Immunoglobulin G:** The first two RCTs differed in that the second used twice the dose of immunoglobulin G, did not require participants to fulfil the operational criteria (similar but not identical to US Centers for Disease Control and Prevention criteria) for chronic fatigue syndrome, and made no assessments of them during the study, instead waiting until 3 months after completion.[44] **Other treatments:** Terfenadine, particularly at high blood concentrations, is associated with rare hazardous cardiac arrhythmias.[53] The RCT that compared staphylococcus toxoid with placebo only included women who also had a diagnosis of fibromyalgia.[47]

OPTION **COGNITIVE BEHAVIOURAL THERAPY**

One systematic review found that cognitive behavioural therapy administered by highly skilled therapists in specialist centres improved quality of life and physical functioning compared with standard medical care or relaxation therapy. One additional multicentre RCT found that cognitive behavioural therapy administered by less experienced therapists may also be effective compared with guided support groups or no interventions.

Benefits: We found two systematic reviews (search dates 1998[54] and 2000[16]). The first review[54] identified three RCTs that met the reviewers' inclusion criteria (all participants fulfilled accepted diagnostic criteria for chronic fatigue syndrome [CFS] and the trials used adequate randomisation and controls).[51,55,56] The second review identified one additional RCT that met inclusion criteria, but the review did not report quantified results.[17,57] The first RCT (90 people with CFS according to Australian diagnostic criteria that are similar to US Centers for Disease Control and Prevention [CDC] criteria) identified by the reviews evaluated cognitive behavioural therapy (CBT) and immunological therapy (dialysable leucocyte extract) using a factorial design.[51] Cognitive behavioural therapy was given every 2 weeks for six sessions of 30–60 minutes each, and people were encouraged to exercise at home and feel less helpless. The comparison group received standard medical care. The trial found no significant difference in quality of life measures (Karnofsky scale and symptom report on a visual analogue scale) between CBT and standard medical care. The second RCT (60 people with CFS according to Oxford, UK, diagnostic criteria) identified by the reviews compared CBT with normal general practice care in people attending a secondary care centre.[56] It found that CBT significantly improved quality of life (Karnofsky scale) at 12 months compared with those receiving standard medical care (final score > 80: 22/30 [73%] with CBT v 8/30 [27%] with placebo; RR 2.75, 95% CI 1.54 to 5.32; NNT 3, 95% CI 2 to 5). The active treatment consisted of a cognitive behavioural assessment, followed by 16 weekly sessions of behavioural experiments, problem solving activity, and re-evaluation of thoughts and beliefs that inhibited a return to normal functioning. The third RCT (60 people with CFS according to CDC diagnostic criteria in people attending a secondary care centre) identified by the reviews compared CBT with relaxation therapy.[55] It found that CBT significantly improvement physical functioning compared with relaxation therapy (improvement based on predefined absolute or relative increases in the SF-36 score: 19/30 [63%] with CBT v 5/30 [17%] with relaxation; RR 3.7, 95% CI 2.37 to 6.31; NNT 3, 95% CI 1 to 7). Improvement continued over 6–12 months' follow up. Cognitive behavioural therapy was given in 13 weekly sessions. A 5 year follow up study of 53 (88%) of the original participants found that more people rated themselves as "much improved" or "very much improved" with CBT compared with relaxation therapy (17/25 [68%] with CBT v 10/28 [36%] with relaxation therapy; RR 1.9, 95% CI 1.1 to 3.4; NNT 4, 95% CI 2 to 19).[58] More people treated with CBT met the authors' criteria for complete recovery at 5 years, but the difference was not significant (17/31 [55%] with CBT v 7/22 [32%] with relaxation therapy; RR 1.7, 95% CI 0.9 to 3.4). The additional multicentre RCT identified by the second review (278 people with CFS according to CDC criteria) compared CBT, guided support groups, or no intervention.[57] The CBT consisted of 16 sessions over 8 months administered by 13 therapists with no previous experience of treating CFS. The guided support groups were similar to CBT in terms of treatment schedule, with the participants receiving non-directive support from a social worker. At 8 months' follow up, the RCT found that more people in the CBT group met the criteria for clinical improvement for fatigue severity (checklist individual strength) and self reported improvement in fatigue compared with the guided support and no treatment groups (fatigue severity: CBT v support group, 27/83 [33%] v 10/80 [13%], RR 2.6, 95% CI 1.3 to 5.0; CBT v no intervention 27/83 [33%] v 8/62 [13%], RR 2.5, 95% CI 1.2 to 5.2; self reported improvement: CBT v support group 42/74 [57%] v 12/71 [17%], RR 3.4, 95% CI 1.9 to 5.8; CBT v no intervention 42/74 [57%] v 23/78 [30%], RR 1.9, 95% CI 1.3 to 2.9). The results were not corrected for multiple comparisons.

Harms: No harmful effects were reported.

Comment: The effectiveness of CBT for CFS outside of specialist settings has been questioned. The results of the multicentre RCT suggest that cognitive behavioural therapy may be effective when administered by less experienced therapists with adequate supervision. The trial had a high withdrawal rate (25% after 8 months), especially in the CBT and guided support groups. Although the presented confidence intervals are not adjusted for multiple comparisons, the results would remain significant after any reasonable adjustment. The authors commented that the results were similar after intention to treat analysis, but these results were not presented.[57] A randomised trial that comparing CBT and non-directive counselling found that both interventions were of benefit in the management of people who consulted their family doctor because of fatigue symptoms.[59] In this study, 28% of the sample conformed to CDC criteria for CFS.

REFERENCES

1. Fukuda K, Straus S, Hickie I, et al. The chronic fatigue syndrome: a comprehensive approach to its definition and study. Ann Intern Med 1994;121:953–959.

2. Sharpe M, Archard LC, Banatvala JE. A report — chronic fatigue syndrome: guidelines for research. J R Soc Med 1991;84:118–121.

3. Wessely S, Chalder T, Hirsch S, et al. The prevalence and morbidity of chronic fatigue and chronic fatigue syndrome: a prospective primary care study. Am J Public Health 1997;87:1449–1455.

4. Steele L, Dobbins JG, Fukuda K, et al. The epidemiology of chronic fatigue in San Francisco. Am J Med 1998;105(suppl 3A):83–90.

5. Lawrie SM, Pelosi AJ. Chronic fatigue syndrome in the community: prevalence and associations. Br J Psychiatry 1995;166:793–797.

6. Wessely S. The epidemiology of chronic fatigue syndrome. Epidemiol Rev 1995;17:139–151.

7. Joyce J, Hotopf M, Wessely S. The prognosis of chronic fatigue and chronic fatigue syndrome: a systematic review. QJM 1997;90:223–233. Search date 1996; primary sources Medline, Embase, Current Contents, and Psychlit.

8. Stewart AD, Hays RD, Ware JE. The MOS short-form general health survey. Med Care 1988;26:724–732.

9. Karnofsky DA, Burchenal JH, MacLeod CM. The clinical evaluation of chemotherapeutic agents in cancer. New York: Columbia University Press; 1949:191–206.

10. Beck AT, Ward CH, Mendelson M, et al. An inventory for measuring depression. Arch Gen Psychiatry 1961;4:561–571.

11. Bergner M, Bobbit RA, Carter WB, et al. The sickness impact profile: development and final revision of a health status measure. Med Care 1981;19:787–805.

12. Chalder T, Berelowitz C, Pawlikowska T. Development of a fatigue scale. J Psychosom Res 1993;37:147–154.

13. Guy W. ECDEU assessment manual for psychopharmacology. Rockville: National Institute of Mental Health, 1976:218 222.

14. Vercoulen JH, Swanink CM, Fennis JF, et al. Dimensional assessment of chronic fatigue syndrome. J Psychosom Res 1994;38:383–392.

15. Hunt SM, McEwen J, McKenna SP. Measuring health status: a new tool for clinicians and epidemiologists. J Roy Coll Gen Prac 1985;35:185–188.

16. Whiting P, Bagnall A-M, Sowden A, et al. Interventions for the treatment and management of chronic fatigue syndrome: A systematic review. JAMA 2001;286:1360–1368. Search date 2000; primary sources Medline, Embase, Psychlit, ERIC, Current Contents, Internet searches, bibliographies from the retrieved references, individuals and organisations through a website dedicated to the review, and members of advisory panels.

17. Vercoulen J, Swanink C, Zitman F. Randomised, double-blind, placebo-controlled study of fluoxetine in chronic fatigue syndrome. Lancet 1996;347:858–861.

18. Wearden AJ, Morriss RK, Mullis R, et al. Randomised, double-blind, placebo controlled treatment trial of fluoxetine and a graded exercise programme for chronic fatigue syndrome. Br J Psychiatry 1998;172:485–490.

19. Vercoulen JHMM, Swanink CMA, Galama JMD, et al. Dimensional assessment of chronic fatigue syndrome. *J Psychosom Res* 1994;38:383–392.

20. Zigmond AS, Snaith RP. The Hospital Anxiety and Depression Scale (HAD). *Acta Psychiatr Scand* 1983;67:361–370.

21. Natelson BH, Cheu J, Pareja J, et al. Randomised, double blind, controlled placebo-phase in trial of low dose phenelzine in the chronic fatigue syndrome. *Psychopharmacology* 1996;124:226–230.

22. Hickie IB, Wilson AJ, Murray Wright J, et al. A randomized, double-blind, placebo-controlled trial of moclobemide in patients with chronic fatigue syndrome. *J Clin Psychiatry* 2000;61:643–648.

23. Behan PO, Hannifah H. 5-HT reuptake inhibitors in CFS. *J Immunol Immunopharmacol* 1995;15:66–69.

24. Rowe PC, Calkins H, DeBusk K, et al. Fludrocortisone acetate to treat neurally mediated hypotension in chronic fatigue syndrome. *JAMA* 2001;285:52–59.

25. Peterson PK, Pheley A, Schroeppel J, et al. A preliminary placebo-controlled crossover trial of fludrocortisone for chronic fatigue syndrome. *Arch Intern Med* 1998;158:908–914.

26. McKenzie R, O'Fallon A, Dale J, et al. Low-dose hydrocortisone for treatment of chronic fatigue syndrome. *JAMA* 1998;280:1061–1066.

27. Cleare AJ, Heap E, Malhi G, et al. Low-dose hydrocortisone in chronic fatigue syndrome: a randomised crossover trial. *Lancet* 1999;353:455–458.

28. Bou-Holaigah I, Rowe P, Kan J, et al. The relationship between neurally mediated hypotension and the chronic fatigue syndrome. *JAMA* 1995;274:961–967.

29. Demitrack M, Dale J, Straus S, et al. Evidence for impaired activation of the hypothalamic-pituitary-adrenal axis in patients with chronic fatigue syndrome. *J Clin Endocrinol Metab* 1991;73:1224–1234.

30. Forsyth LM, Preuss HG, MacDowell AL, et al. Therapeutic effects of oral NADH on the symptoms of patients with chronic fatigue syndrome. *Ann Allergy Asthma Immunol* 1999;82:185–191.

31. Colquhoun D, Senn S. Re: Therapeutic effects of oral NADH on the symptoms of patients with chronic fatigue syndrome. *Ann Allergy Asthma Immunol* 2000;84:639–640.

32. Fulcher KY, White PD. A randomised controlled trial of graded exercise therapy in patients with the chronic fatigue syndrome. *BMJ* 1997;314:1647–1652.

33. Powell P, Bentall RP, Nye FJ, et al. Randomised controlled trial of patient education to encourage graded exercise in chronic fatigue syndrome. *BMJ* 2001;322:387–390.

34. Sandler H, Vernikos J. *Inactivity: physiological effects.* London: Academic Press, 1986.

35. Dalrymple W. Infectious mononucleosis: 2. Relation of bed rest and activity to prognosis. *Postgrad Med* 1961;35:345–349.

36. Brouwers FM, van der Werf S, Bleijenberg G, et al. The effect of a polynutrient supplement on fatigue and physical activity of patients with chronic fatigue syndrome: a double-blind randomized controlled trial. *QJM* 2002;95:677–683.

37. Cox IM, Campbell MJ, Dowson D. Red blood cell magnesium and chronic fatigue syndrome. *Lancet* 1991;337:757–760.

38. Clague JE, Edwards RHT, Jackson MJ. Intravenous magnesium loading in chronic fatigue syndrome. *Lancet* 1992;340:124–125.

39. Hinds G, Bell NP, McMaster D, et al. Normal red cell magnesium concentrations and magnesium loading tests in patients with chronic fatigue syndrome. *Ann Clin Biochem* 1994;31:459–461.

40. Swanink CM, Vercoulen JH, Bleijenberg G, et al. Chronic fatigue syndrome: a clinical and laboratory study with a well matched control group. *J Intern Med* 1995;237:499–506.

41. Warren G, McKendrick M, Peet M. The role of essential fatty acids in chronic fatigue syndrome. *Acta Neurol Scand* 1999;99:112–116.

42. Behan PO, Behan WMH, Horrobin D. Effect of high doses of essential fatty acids on the postviral fatigue syndrome. *Acta Neurol Scand* 1990;82:209–216.

43. Peterson PK, Shepard J, Macres M, et al. A controlled trial of intravenous immunoglobulin G in chronic fatigue syndrome. *Am J Med* 1990;89:554–560.

44. Lloyd A, Hickie I, Wakefield D, et al. A double-blind, placebo-controlled trial of intravenous immunoglobulin therapy in patients with chronic fatigue syndrome. *Am J Med* 1990;89:561–568.

45. Vollmer-Conna U, Hickie I, Hadzi-Pavlovic D, et al. Intravenous immunoglobulin is ineffective in the treatment of patients with chronic fatigue syndrome. *Am J Med* 1997;103:38–43.

46. Rowe KS. Double-blind randomized controlled trial to assess the efficacy of intravenous gammaglobulin for the management of chronic fatigue syndrome in adolescents. *J Psychiatr Res* 1997;31:133–147.

47. Zachrisson O, Regland B, Jahreskog M, et al. Treatment with staphylococcus toxoid in fibromyalgia/chronic fatigue syndrome – a randomised controlled trial. *Eur J Pain* 2002;6:455–466.

48. See DM, Tilles JG. Alpha interferon treatment of patients with chronic fatigue syndrome. *Immunol Invest* 1996;25:153–164.

49. Brook M, Bannister B, Weir W. Interferon-alpha therapy for patients with chronic fatigue syndrome. *J Infect Dis* 1993;168:791–792.

50. Straus SE, Dale JK, Tobi M, et al. Acyclovir treatment of the chronic fatigue syndrome. Lack of efficacy in a placebo-controlled trial. *N Engl J Med* 1988;319:1692–1698.

51. Lloyd A, Hickie I, Boughton R, et al. Immunologic and psychological therapy for patients with chronic fatigue syndrome. *Am J Med* 1993;94:197–203.

52. Steinberg P, McNutt BE, Marshall P, et al. Double-blind placebo-controlled study of efficacy of oral terfenadine in the treatment of chronic fatigue syndrome. *J Allergy Clin Immunol* 1996;97:119–126.

53. Medicines Control Agency (UK). *Current Problems in Pharmacovigilance,* Volume 23, September 1997.

54. Price JR, Couper J. Cognitive behaviour therapy for CFS. In: The Cochrane Library, Issue 2. Oxford: Update Software, 2002. Search date 1998; primary sources Medline, Embase, Biological Abstracts, Sigle, Index to Theses of Great Britain and Ireland, Index to Scientific and Technical Proceedings, Science Citation Index, Trials Register of the Depression, Anxiety and Neurosis Group, citation lists, and personal contacts.

55. Deale A, Chalder T, Marks I, et al. Cognitive behaviour therapy for chronic fatigue syndrome: a randomized controlled trial. *Am J Psychiatry* 1997;154:408–414.

56. Sharpe M, Hawton K, Simkin S, et al. Cognitive behaviour therapy for chronic fatigue syndrome: a randomized controlled trial. *BMJ* 1996;312:22–26.

57. Prins JB, Bleijenberg G, Bazelmans E, et al. Cognitive behaviour therapy for chronic fatigue syndrome: a multicentre randomised controlled trial. *Lancet* 2001;357:841–847.

58. Deale A, Husain K, Chalder T, et al. Long-term outcome of cognitive behaviour therapy versus relaxation therapy for chronic fatigue syndrome: a 5-year follow-up study. *Am J Psychiatry* 2001;158:2038–2042.

59. Ridsdale L, Godfrey E, Chalder T, et al. Chronic fatigue in general practice: is counselling as good as cognitive behaviour therapy? A UK randomised trial. *Br J Gen Pract* 2001;51:19–24.

Steven Reid
Consultant Liaison Psychiatrist
St Mary's Hospital
London
UK

Trudie Chalder
Reader

Anthony Cleare
Senior Lecturer

Matthew Hotopf
Reader

Simon Wessely
Professor of Epidemiological and
Liaison Psychiatry

Guy's, King's and St Thomas' School of
Medicine and Institute of Psychiatry
London
UK

Competing interests: None declared.

TABLE 1   Diagnostic criteria for chronic fatigue syndrome (see text, p 48).

CDC 1994[1]	Oxford, UK[2]
Clinically evaluated, medically unexplained fatigue of at least 6 months' duration that is:	Severe, disabling fatigue of at least 6 months' duration that:
– of new onset	– affects both physical and mental functioning
– not a result of ongoing exertion	– was present for more than 50% of the time
– not substantially alleviated by rest	
– a substantial reduction in previous levels of activity	
The occurrence of four or more of the following symptoms:	Other symptoms, particularly myalgia, sleep, and mood disturbance, may be present.
– subjective memory impairment	
– tender lymph nodes	
– muscle pain	
– joint pain	
– headache	
– unrefreshing sleep	
– postexertional malaise (> 24 hours)	

Exclusion criteria

– Active, unresolved, or suspected disease likely to cause fatigue	– Active, unresolved, or suspect disease likely to cause fatigue
– Psychotic, melancholic, or bipolar depression (but not uncomplicated major depression)	– Psychotic, melancholic, or bipolar depression (but not uncomplicated major depression)
– Psychotic disorders	– Psychotic disorders
– Dementia	– Dementia
– Anorexia or bulimia nervosa	– Anorexia or bulimia nervosa
– Alcohol or other substance misuse	
– Severe obesity	

CDC, US Centers for Disease Control and Prevention.

Deliberate self harm

Search date April 2003

G Mustafa Soomro

Key Messages

- We found little RCT evidence for any intervention in people with deliberate self harm. Most RCTs and meta-analyses of small RCTs are likely to have been underpowered to detect clinically important outcomes of interventions.

- **Continuity of care** One systematic review of one RCT found limited evidence that follow up after hospital treatment with the same compared with a different therapist may increase repetition of deliberate self harm over 3 months, although this may be explained by a higher level of risk factors for repetition in the group receiving same therapist follow up, despite randomisation.

- **Dialectal behaviour therapy** One RCT found limited and equivocal evidence that dialectical behaviour therapy may reduce the proportion of people who repeat deliberate self harm over 12 months compared with usual care.

- **Emergency card** One systematic review found no significant difference in the proportion of people who repeated deliberate self harm over 12 months between emergency card (allowing emergency admission or contact with a doctor) and usual care.

- **Flupentixol depot injection** One small RCT found that flupentixol depot injection reduced the proportion of people who repeated deliberate self harm over 6 months compared with placebo. However, we were unable to draw reliable conclusions from this small study. Typical antipsychotics such as flupentixol are associated with a wide range of adverse effects.

- **Hospital admission** One RCT found no significant difference between hospital admission and immediate discharge in the proportion of people who repeated deliberate self harm over 16 weeks, but it is likely to have been too small to exclude a clinically important difference.

- **Intensive outpatient follow up plus outreach** One systematic review found no significant difference in the proportion of people who repeated deliberate self harm over 4–12 months between intensive intervention plus outreach and usual care.

- **Mianserin** RCTs provided insufficient evidence to assess mianserin.

- **Nurse led case management** One RCT found no significant difference between nurse led case management and usual care in the proportion of people who were admitted to emergency departments for episodes of deliberate self harm over 12 months.

- **Paroxetine** One RCT in people with deliberate self harm receiving psychotherapy found no significant difference between paroxetine and placebo in the proportion of people who repeated self harm over 12 months. It found that paroxetine increased diarrhoea and tremor compared with placebo.

- **Problem solving therapy** One systematic review of small RCTs found no significant difference between problem solving therapy and usual care in the proportion of people who repeated deliberate self harm over 6–12 months. Another systematic review found that problem solving therapy reduced depression, anxiety, and hopelessness, and improved problems compared with usual care.

- **Psychodynamic interpersonal therapy** One RCT found that psychodynamic interpersonal therapy for 4 weeks reduced repetition of deliberate self harm, depression, and suicidal ideation over 6 months compared with usual care. However, we were unable to draw reliable conclusions from one RCT.

- **Same number of therapy sessions given over long term versus over short term** One systematic review of one RCT found no significant difference in the proportion of people who repeated deliberate self harm at 12 months with therapy given over 3 months compared with 12 months.

- **Telephone contact** One RCT found no significant difference between telephone contact at 4 and 8 months and usual care in repetition of deliberate self harm, global functioning, and suicidal ideation over 12 months.

- **General practice based guidelines** One large cluster randomised trial comparing the use of general practitioner guidelines for management of deliberate self harm versus usual care found no significant difference in the proportion of people who repeated deliberate self harm over 12 months or in the time to repetition of self harm.

DEFINITION Deliberate self harm is an acute non-fatal act of self harm carried out deliberately in the form of an acute episode of behaviour by an individual with variable motivation.[1] The intention to end life may be absent or present to a variable degree. Other terms used to describe this phenomenon are "attempted suicide" and "parasuicide". The terms are not entirely satisfactory. Common methods of deliberate self harm include self cutting and self poisoning, such as overdosing on medicines. Some acts of deliberate self harm are characterised by high suicidal intent, meticulous planning (including precautions against being found out), and severe lethality. Other acts of deliberate self harm are characterised by no or low intention of suicide, lack of planning and concealing of the act, and low lethality of the method used. The related term of "suicide" is defined as an act with a fatal outcome that is deliberately initiated and performed by the person with the knowledge or expectation of its fatal outcome.[1] This review focuses on recent deliberate self harm as the main presenting problem and excludes RCTs in which deliberate self harm is assessed as an outcome associated with other disorders, such as depression or borderline personality disorder. Deliberate self harm is not defined in the *Diagnostic and statistical manual of mental disorders* (DSM IV)[2] or the *International classification of mental and behavioural disorders* (ICD-10).[3]

INCIDENCE/ PREVALENCE Based on data from 16 European countries between 1989–1992, the lifetime prevalence of deliberate self harm in people treated in hospital and other medical facilities, including general practice settings, is estimated at about 3% for women and 2% for men.[4] Over the last 50 years there has been a rise in the incidence of deliberate self harm in the UK.[4] A reasonable current estimate is about 400/100 000 population a year.[5] In two community studies in the USA, 3–5% of responders said that they had made an attempt at deliberate self harm at some time.[6] Self poisoning using organophosphates is particularly common in developing countries.[7] A large hospital (catering for 900 000 people) in Sri Lanka, reported 2559 adult hospital admissions and 41% occupancy of medical intensive care beds for deliberate self harm with organophosphates over 2 years.[8] An international survey using representative community samples of adults (aged 18–64 years) reported lifetime prevalence of self reported suicide attempts of 3.82% in Canada, 5.93% in Puerto Rico, 4.95% in France, 3.44% in West Germany, 0.72% in Lebanon, 0.75% in Taiwan, 3.2% in Korea, and 4.43% in New Zealand.[6]

AETIOLOGY/ RISK FACTORS Familial, biological, and psychosocial factors may contribute to deliberate self harm. Evidence for genetic factors includes a higher risk of familial suicide and greater concordance in monozygotic than dizygotic twins for deliberate self harm and suicide.[9] Evidence for biological factors includes reduced cerebrospinal fluid 5-hydroxyindole acetic acid (5-HIAA) levels and blunted prolactin response to fenfluramine challenge test, indicating a reduction in the function of serotonin in the central nervous system.[10] People who deliberately self harm also show traits of impulsiveness and aggression, inflexible and impulsive cognitive style, and impaired decision making and problem solving (see glossary, p 72).[11] Deliberate self harm is more likely in women, young adults, and people who are single or divorced, of low education level, unemployed, disabled, or suffering from a psychiatric disorder[12] particularly depression,[13] substance misuse,[14] borderline and antisocial personality disorders,[15] severe anxiety disorders,[16] and physical illness.[17]

PROGNOSIS Suicide is highest during the first year after deliberate self harm.[18] One systematic review found median rates of repetition of deliberate self harm of 16.0% (interquartile range [IQR] 12.0% to 25.0%) within the first year, 21.0% (IQR 12.0% to 30.0%) within 1–4 years, and 23% (IQR 11% to 32%) within 4 years or longer. It found median mortality from suicide after deliberate self harm of 1.8% (IQR 0.8% to 2.6%) within the first year, 3.0% (IQR 2.0% to 4.4%) within 1–4 years, 3.4% (IQR 2.5% to 6.0%) within 5–10 years, and 6.7% (IQR 5.0% to 11.0%) within 9 years or longer.[18] Repetition of deliberate self harm is more likely in people aged 25–49 years, who are unemployed, divorced, from lower social class, or who suffer from substance misuse, depression, hopelessness, powerlessness, personality disorders, have unstable living conditions or live alone, have a criminal record, previous psychiatric treatment, a history of stressful traumatic life events, or a history of coming from broken home or of family violence.[12] Factors associated with risk of suicide after deliberate self harm are age over 45 years, male sex, being unemployed, retired, separated, divorced, or widowed, living alone, poor physical health, psychiatric disorder (particularly depression, alcoholism, schizophrenia, and sociopathic personality disorder), high suicidal intent in current episode including leaving a written note, violent method used in current episode, and history of deliberate self harm.[19]

AIMS OF INTERVENTION	To reduce repetition of deliberate self harm, desire to self harm, to prevent suicide, and improve social functioning and quality of life, with minimal adverse effects.

OUTCOMES	Repetition of deliberate self harm, occurrence of suicide, admission to hospital, improvement in underlying psychiatric symptoms, improvement in coping, quality of life, and adverse effects. Some of the validated scales used for assessing psychiatric symptoms and deliberate self harm are: Symptom Checklist-90 (SCL-90), a self administered rating scale for assessing nine areas of psychopathology (somatisation, obsessive-compulsive, interpersonal sensitivity, depression, anxiety, hostility, phobic-anxiety, paranoid ideation, and psychoticism),[20–22] Beck Depression Inventory (a 21 item self administered Likert scale for measuring severity of depression),[23] Hospital Anxiety Depression Scale (a self administered 14 item Likert scale for measuring depression and anxiety),[24] Beck Scale for Suicidal Ideation (a 21-item self administered Likert scale covering thoughts and plans about suicide and aims at assessing the risk of a later suicide attempt),[25] Beck Hopelessness Scale (a 20 item true-false self administered items and aims at assessing hopelessness about the future),[26] and Global Severity Index (GSI; a mean of all items in SCL-90).[21]

METHODS	*Clinical Evidence* search and appraisal April 2003.

QUESTION **What are the effects of treatments for deliberate self harm in adults?**

OPTION **PAROXETINE**

One RCT in people with deliberate self harm receiving psychotherapy found no significant difference between paroxetine and placebo in the proportion of people who repeated self harm over 12 months. It found that paroxetine increased diarrhoea and tremor compared with placebo.

Benefits:	We found one systematic review (search date 1999),[27] which identified one RCT[28] (91 outpatients who had previously been admitted to hospital for deliberate self harm, without current depression, receiving psychotherapy) comparing paroxetine 40 mg daily versus placebo for 12 months. It found no significant difference between paroxetine and placebo in the proportion of people repeating deliberate self harm over 12 months (15/46 [33%] with paroxetine v 21/45 [47%] with placebo; RR 0.70, 95% CI 0.40 to 1.18).

Mental health

Harms: The RCT found that, compared with placebo, paroxetine significantly increased the proportion of people with diarrhoea (10/46 [22%] with paroxetine v 1/45 [2%] with placebo; P = 0.007), tremor (8/46 [17%] with paroxetine v 1/46 [2%] with control; P = 0.03), and delayed orgasm (9/46 [19%] with paroxetine v 0/45 [0%] with placebo; P = 0.003).[28] It also found that paroxetine was associated with large bruises in two people.

Comment: The review did not report any other outcomes.[27]

OPTION   MIANSERIN

RCTs provided insufficient evidence to assess mianserin.

Benefits: We found one systematic review (search date 1999),[27] which identified two RCTs.[29,30] The first RCT (38 people with borderline or histrionic personality disorder and a history of deliberate self harm, admitted to hospital after an episode of self harm) identified by the review found no significant difference between mianserin 30 mg daily and placebo in the proportion of people who repeated deliberate self harm over 6 months' treatment (8/17 [47%] with mianserin v 12/21 [57%] with placebo; RR 0.82, 95% CI 0.44 to 1.54), but it is likely to have been too small to detect a clinically important difference.[29] The second RCT (114 people admitted to hospital after deliberate self poisoning, history of deliberate self harm not stated) identified by the review compared mianserin 30–60 mg daily or nomifensine 75–150 mg daily versus placebo for 6 weeks' treatment (see comment below).[30] The RCT did not compare mianserin alone versus placebo. It found no significant difference between mianserin or nomifensine and placebo in the proportion of people who repeated deliberate self harm over 12 weeks (16/76 [21%] with mianserin or nomifensine v 5/38 [13%] with placebo; RR 1.60, 95% CI 0.63 to 4.04), but it is likely to have been too small to detect a clinically important difference.

Harms: The review[27] and RCTs[29,30] gave no information on adverse effects.

Comment: The review did not report any other outcomes.[27] Nomifensine was withdrawn worldwide in the 1980s because of association with immune haemolytic anaemia.[30]

OPTION   FLUPENTIXOL DEPOT INJECTION

One small RCT found that flupentixol depot injection reduced the proportion of people who repeated deliberate self harm over 6 months compared with placebo. However, we were unable to draw reliable conclusions from this small study. Typical antipsychotics such as flupentixol are associated with a wide range of adverse effects.

Benefits: We found one systematic review (search date 1999), which identified one RCT (30 people with a history of deliberate self harm) comparing flupentixol decanoate (20 mg im once every 4 weeks) versus placebo for 6 months.[27] It found that flupentixol significantly reduced the proportion of people who repeated deliberate self harm over 6 months compared with placebo (3/14 [21%] with flupentixol v 12/16 [75%] with placebo; RR 0.29, 95% CI 0.10 to 0.81).

Harms: The review gave no information on adverse effects (see comment below).[27]

Comment: We found insufficient evidence about the adverse effects of flupentixol in people with deliberate self harm. Typical antipsychotics such as flupentixol are associated with a wide range of adverse effects.[31] The review did not investigate other outcomes.[27]

OPTION   PROBLEM SOLVING THERAPY

One systematic review of small RCTs found no significant difference between problem solving therapy and usual care in the proportion of people who repeated deliberate self harm over 6–12 months. Another systematic review found that problem solving therapy reduced depression, anxiety, and hopelessness, and improved problems compared with usual care.

Benefits: We found one systematic review (search date 1999)[27] that assessed the effects of problem solving therapy (see glossary, p 72) on repetition of deliberate self harm and one systematic review (search date not stated)[32] that assessed the effects of problem solving therapy on depression, anxiety, and hopelessness. The first review identified five RCTs (571 people) comparing problem solving therapy versus usual care (standard care [from psychiatrist, community psychiatric nurse, or social worker], marital counselling, or general practitioner counselling).[27] Four of the RCTs were in people who had been admitted to hospital for deliberate self poisoning and included people with both a history of deliberate self harm and experiencing their first episode; one RCT was in people admitted to hospital after deliberate self harm who had self harmed at least once before in the previous year. The duration of interventions for four RCTs was 2–8 sessions, and for one RCT 3 months; follow up ranged from 6–12 months. The review found no significant difference between problem solving therapy and usual care in the proportion of people who repeated deliberate self harm over 6–12 months (45/290 [15%] with problem solving therapy v 54/281 [19%] with usual care; RR 0.77, 95% CI 0.55 to 1.08).[27] The second review (6 RCTs, including 5 identified by the first review) found that, compared with usual care, problem solving therapy significantly reduced depression (assessed by Beck Depression Inventory and Hospital Anxiety Depression Scale, 4 RCTs, 158 people, SMD −0.36 95% CI −0.61 to −0.11) and hopelessness (assessed by Beck Hopelessness Scale, 3 RCTs, 63 people; WMD −2.97 95% CI −4.81 to −1.13) and "improved problems" (2 RCTs, 211 people; OR 2.31, 95% CI 1.29 to 4.13; see comment below).[32]

Harms: The reviews gave no information on adverse effects.[27,32]

Comment: The second review did not state how improvement in problems was assessed.[32] The reviews did not assess other outcomes.[27,32]

OPTION   DIALECTICAL BEHAVIOUR THERAPY

One RCT found limited and equivocal evidence that dialectical behaviour therapy may reduce the proportion of people who repeat deliberate self harm over 12 months compared with usual care.

Benefits: We found one systematic review (search date 1999)[27] which identified one RCT (39 women with borderline personality disorder and a history of deliberate self harm who had self harmed in the previous 8 weeks) comparing dialectical behaviour therapy (see glossary, p 72) versus usual care (alternative therapy referrals). It found that dialectical behaviour therapy significantly reduced the proportion who repeated deliberate self harm over 1 year compared with usual care (5/19 [26%] with dialectical behaviour therapy v 12/20 [60%] with usual care; OR 0.24, 95% CI 0.06 to 0.93; see comment below).

Harms: The review gave no information on adverse effects.[27]

Comment: The results of the RCT are sensitive to the method of statistical calculation used; calculation of relative risk renders the difference between dialectical behaviour therapy and usual care non-significant (RR 0.44, 95% CI 0.19 to 1.01).[27] The review did not assess other outcomes.

OPTION   CONTINUITY OF CARE

One RCT found limited evidence that follow up after hospital treatment with the same compared with a different therapist may increase repetition of deliberate self harm over 3 months, although this may be explained by a higher level of risk factors for repetition in the group receiving same therapist follow up, despite randomisation.

Benefits: We found one systematic review (search date 1999), which identified one RCT (141 people with a history of deliberate self harm who had been admitted to hospital for 3 day crisis intervention [see glossary, p 72] after an episode of self harm) comparing follow up by the same therapist who assessed them in hospital versus different therapist follow up.[27] All participants also received a "motivational interview [see glossary, p 72], letter, and assessment of motivation towards therapy". It found that follow up by the same therapist significantly increased the proportion of people who repeated deliberate self harm over 3 months compared with different therapist follow up (12/68 [18%] with same therapist v 4/73 [5%] with different therapist; RR 3.22, 95% CI 1.09 to 9.51; see comment below).

Harms: The review gave no information on adverse effects.[27]

Comment: The authors commented that the increase in deliberate self harm in people who had continuity of care may have been because of a higher prevalence of risk factors (unspecified) for repetition in the same therapist group despite randomisation.[27] The review and RCTs did not assess other outcomes.

OPTION   SAME NUMBER OF SESSIONS OF THERAPY GIVEN OVER LONG TERM VERSUS OVER SHORT TERM

One systematic review of one RCT found no significant difference in the proportion of people who repeated deliberate self harm over 12 months with therapy given over 3 months compared with 12 months.

Benefits: We found one systematic review (search date 1999, 1 RCT, 80 people with deliberate self harm and a history of deliberate self harm) comparing 12 sessions of therapy given over 12 months versus the same number of session given over 3 months (see comment below).[27] It found no significant difference between longer and shorter duration of therapy in the proportion of people who repeated deliberate self harm over 12 months (9/40 [22%] with longer therapy v 9/40 [22%] with shorter therapy; RR 1.00, 95% 0.44 to 2.26).

Harms: The review gave no information on adverse effects.[27]

Comment: The RCT did not specify what type of therapy participants received.[27] The review did not assess other outcomes.

| OPTION | PSYCHODYNAMIC INTERPERSONAL THERAPY |

One RCT found that, compared with usual care, psychodynamic interpersonal therapy for 4 weeks reduced repetition of deliberate self harm, depression, and suicidal ideation over 6 months. However, we were unable to draw reliable conclusions from one RCT.

Benefits: We found no systematic review. We found one RCT (119 people admitted to hospital after deliberate self poisoning, 60% with a history of "deliberate self harm") that compared psychodynamic interpersonal therapy (see glossary, p 72) versus usual care (referral to usual services) for 4 weeks.[33] It found that, compared with usual care, brief psychodynamic interpersonal therapy significantly reduced repetition of deliberate self harm at 6 months (5/58 [9%] with psychodynamic interpersonal therapy v 17/61 [28%] with usual care; P = 0.009). It also found that brief psychodynamic interpersonal therapy significantly reduced depression (measured by Beck Depression Inventory, mean difference in score with interpersonal therapy v usual care –5.0, 95% CI –9.7 to –0.3) and suicidal ideation (measured by Beck Scale for Suicidal Ideation, mean difference in score –4.9, 95% CI –8.2 to –1.6).

Harms: The RCT gave no information on adverse effects.[33]

Comment: The RCT did not assess other outcomes.[33]

| OPTION | INTENSIVE OUTPATIENT FOLLOW UP PLUS OUTREACH |

One systematic review found no significant difference in the proportion of people who repeated deliberate self harm over 4–12 months between outreach plus intensive intervention and usual care.

Benefits: We found one systematic review (search date 1999, 6 RCTs, 1161 people admitted to hospital after deliberate self harm, 30–100% with a history of deliberate self harm) comparing intensive intervention plus outreach versus usual care over 3–12 months.[27] Intensive outpatient follow up plus outreach varied but usually involved in person or phone contact of the person in the community, including encouragement to attend health services. Usual care involved treatment by various professionals, not involving outreach. It found no significant difference between intensive intervention plus outreach and usual care in the proportion of people who repeated deliberate self harm over 4–12 months (92/580 [16%] with intensive intervention v 107/581 [18%] with usual care; RR 0.87, 95% CI 0.68 to 1.12).

Harms: The review gave no information on adverse effects.[27]

Comment: The review did not assess other outcomes.[27]

OPTION   EMERGENCY CARD

One systematic review found no significant difference in the proportion of people who repeated deliberate self harm over 12 months between emergency card (allowing emergency admission or contact with a doctor) and usual care.

Benefits: We found one systematic review (search date 1999, 2 RCTs, 1 RCT in 212 adults admitted to hospital after their first episode of deliberate self harm, 1 RCT in 105 children admitted to hospital after deliberate self harm, history of self harm not stated).[27] It compared emergency card (indicating that a doctor was available and how to contact them or allowing readmission to a paediatric hospital ward) versus usual care (referral to and treatment from usual inpatient, outpatient, or primary care services as appropriate). It found no significant difference in the proportion of people who repeated deliberate self harm over 12 months between emergency card and usual care (8/148 [5%] with emergency card v 19/169 [11%] with usual care; RR 0.48, 95% CI 0.22 to 1.07; see comment below).

Harms: The review gave no information on adverse effects.[27]

Comment: The review pooled results from RCTs of heterogeneous populations (adults and children) to try to increase the power of its meta-analysis but it may not be appropriate to pool results in such different groups.[27] The review did not assess other outcomes.

OPTION   HOSPITAL ADMISSION

One RCT found no significant difference between hospital admission and immediate discharge in the proportion of people who repeated deliberate self harm over 16 weeks, but it is likely to have been underpowered to detect a clinically important difference.

Benefits: We found one systematic review (search date 1999) which identified one RCT (77 people).[27] The RCT found no significant difference between hospital admission for a median of 17 hours and immediate discharge in the proportion of people who repeated deliberate self harm over 16 weeks (3/38 [8%] with hospital admission v 4/39 [10%] with immediate discharge; RR 0.77, 95% CI 0.18 to 3.21), but it is likely to have been underpowered to detect a clinically important difference.

Harms: The review gave no information on adverse effects.[27]

Comment: The review did not assess other outcomes.[27]

OPTION   GENERAL PRACTICE BASED GUIDELINES

One large cluster randomised trial comparing the use of general practitioner guidelines for management of deliberate self harm versus usual care found no significant difference in the proportion of people who repeated deliberate self harm over 12 months or in the time to repetition of self harm.

Benefits: We found no systematic review. We found one cluster randomised trial (98 general practices, 2084 people who had attended hospital emergency departments after deliberate self harm, 11–14 with a recent recorded history of deliberate self harm).[34] It compared inviting people for consultation with their general practitioner who followed guidelines for managing self harm versus usual care (provided by general practitioner or referral to mental health or other services as appropriate). It found no significant difference between use of guidelines and usual care in repetition of deliberate self harm (211/964 [22%] with guidelines v 189/968 [20%] with usual care; OR 1.17, 95% CI 0.94 to 1.47), mean repeat episodes per person (mean 0.48 with guidelines v 0.37 with usual care; incident rate ratio 1.24, 95% CI 0.92 to 1.68), and mean days to first episode of self harm (mean 105 with guidelines v 110 with usual care; HR 1.15, 95% CI 0.94 to 1.42).

Harms: The RCT gave no information on adverse effects.[34]

Comment: The RCT did not assess other outcomes.[34]

OPTION   NURSE LED CASE MANAGEMENT

One RCT found no significant difference between nurse led case management and usual care in the proportion of people who were admitted to emergency departments for episodes of deliberate self harm over 12 months.

Benefits: We found no systematic review. We found one RCT (467 people who had attended hospital emergency departments after deliberate self harm, 47% with a history of deliberate self harm) comparing nurse led case management (see glossary, p 72) versus usual care (triage, psychiatric assessment, and inpatient care if appropriate) for 12 months.[35] It found no significant difference between groups in rates of readmission to hospital as a result of deliberate self harm over 12 months (19/220 [9%] with nurse led case management v 25/247 [10%] with usual care; OR 0.84, 95% CI 0.45 to 1.57).

Harms: The RCT gave no information on adverse effects.[35]

Comment: The RCT did not assess other outcomes.[35]

OPTION   TELEPHONE CONTACT

One RCT found no significant difference between telephone contact at 4 and 8 months and usual care in repetition of deliberate self harm, global functioning, and suicidal ideation over 12 months.

Benefits: We found one RCT (216 people admitted to hospital after deliberate self harm, 51–54% with a history of deliberate self harm) that compared telephone contact at 4 and 8 months aimed at increasing motivation versus usual care (undefined).[36] It found no significant difference between telephone contact and usual care in the proportion of people repeating deliberate self harm over 12 months (14/83 [17%] with telephone contact v 15/89 [17%] with usual care; reported as non-significant, CI not reported; results not intention to treat, 19% lost to follow up). It found similar rates in overall functioning between telephone contact and usual care (assessed by Global Assessment of Functioning Scale: mean score 61.4 with telephone contact v 58.6 with usual care; CI not reported). It also found similar scores on the scale for suicidal ideation (mean score 5.8 with telephone contact group v 4.0 with usual care; CI not reported) and on the Symptom Checklist-90 scale at 12 months (mean score 0.82 with telephone contact group v 0.88 with usual care; CI not reported).

Harms: The RCT gave no information on adverse effects.[36]

Comment: None.

GLOSSARY

Case management Involves a case manager managing an individual's care including comprehensive assessment of their needs, development of individualised package of care, the arrangement of access to services, monitoring of quality of services provided, and long term flexible support.

Crisis intervention Involves short term help with current and acute difficult life events using variety of counselling, problem solving, and practical measures.

Dialectical behaviour therapy Is a multimodal cognitive behaviour therapy used particularly in the treatment of people with borderline personality disorder who repeatedly engage in deliberate self harm. It involves helping to replace extremes of emotions and behaviour with behaviour that is a moderate synthesis of extremes.

Motivational interviewing Uses principles of motivational psychology and is aimed at helping people to change and engage in demanding treatments.

Problem solving therapy Uses a set of sequential steps in solving problems and aims at minimising negative emotion and maximising identification, evaluation, and implementation of optimal solutions.

Psychodynamic interpersonal therapy Is a psychotherapeutic intervention aimed at improving interpersonal problems using the model developed by Hobson.

REFERENCES

1. Gelder M, Mayou R, Cowen P. Shorter oxford textbook of psychiatry. Oxford: Oxford University Press, 2001.

2. American Psychiatric Association. Diagnostic and statistical manual of mental disorders, 4th ed. Washington, DC: American Psychiatric Association, 1994.

3. World Health Organization. The ICD-10 classification of mental and behavioural disorders. Geneva: World Health Organization, 1992.

4. Schmidtke A, Bille-Brahe U, DeLeo D, et al. Attempted suicide Europe: rates, trends and sociodemographic characteristics of suicide attempters during the period 1989–1992. Results of the WHO/EURO Multicentre Study on Parasuicide. Acta Psychiatr Scand 1996;93:327–338.

5. The University of York. NHS Centre for Reviews and Dissemination. 1998. Deliberate self harm. Effective Health Care 4:1–12.

6. Weissman MM, Bland RC, Canino GJ, et al. Prevalence of suicide ideation and suicide attempts in nine countries. Psychol Med 1999;29:9–17.

7. Eddleston M. Patterns and problems of deliberate self-poisoning in the developing world. QJM 2000;93:715–731.

8. Eddleston M, Sheriff MH, Hawton K. Deliberate self harm in Sri Lanka: an overlooked tragedy in the developing world. BMJ 1998;317:133–135.

9. Roy A, Nielsen D, Rylander G, et al. Genetics of suicidal behaviour. In: Hawton K, van Heeringen K,

eds. *International handbook of suicide and attempted suicide*. Chichester: Wiley, 2000: 209–221.

10. Traskman-Bendz L, Mann JJ. Biological aspects of suicidal behaviour. In: Hawton K, van Heeringen K, eds. *International handbook of suicide and attempted suicide*. Chichester: Wiley, 2000: 65–78.

11. Williams JMG, Pollock LR. The psychology of suicidal behaviour. In: Hawton K, van Heeringen K, eds. *International handbook of suicide and attempted suicide*. Chichester: Wiley, 2000: 79–93.

12. Kerkhof AJFM. Attempted suicide: trends and patterns. In: Hawton K, van Heeringen K, eds. *International handbook of suicide and attempted suicide*. Chichester: Wiley, 2000: 49–64.

13. Lonnqvist JK. Psychiatric aspects of suicidal behaviour: depression. In: Hawton K, van Heeringen K, eds. *International handbook of suicide and attempted suicide*. Chichester: Wiley, 2000: 107–120.

14. Murphy GE. Psychiatric aspects of suicidal behaviour: substance abuse. In: Hawton K, van Heeringen K, eds. *International handbook of suicide and attempted suicide*. Chichester: Wiley, 2000: 135–146.

15. Linehan MM, Rizvi SL, Welch SS, et al. Psychiatric aspects of suicidal behaviour: personality disorder. In: Hawton K, van Heeringen K, eds. *International handbook of suicide and attempted suicide*. Chichester: Wiley, 2000: 147–178.

16. Allgulander C. Psychiatric aspects of suicidal behaviour: anxiety disorders. In: Hawton K, van Heeringen K, eds. *International handbook of suicide and attempted suicide*. Chichester: Wiley, 2000: 179–192.

17. Stenager EN, Stenager E. Physical illness and suicidal behaviour. In: Hawton K, van Heeringen K, eds. *International handbook of suicide and attempted suicide*. Chichester: Wiley, 2000: 405–420.

18. Owens D, Horrocks J, House A. Fatal and non-fatal repetition of self-harm. Systematic review. *Br J Psychiatry* 2002;181:193–199.

19. Hawton K. Treatment of suicide attempters and prevention of suicide and attempted suicide. In: Gelder MG, Lopez-Ibor JJ Jr, Andreasen NC, eds. *New Oxford textbook of psychiatry*. Oxford: Oxford University Press, 2000: 1050–1059.

20. Bridges K, Goldberg D. Self-administered scales of neurotic symptoms. In: Thompson C, ed. *The instruments of psychiatric research*. London: Wiley, 1989: 157–176.

21. Derogatis LR. Symptom Checklist-90-Revised (SCL-90-R). In: American Psychiatric Association, eds. *Handbook of psychiatric measures*. Washington, DC: American Psychiatric Association, 2000: 81–84.

22. Thompson C. Anxiety. In: Thompson C, ed. *The instruments of psychiatric research*. London: Wiley, 1989: 127–156.

23. Beck A, Steer A. Beck Depression Inventory (BDI). In: American Psychiatric Association, eds. *Handbook of psychiatric measures*. Washington, DC: American Psychiatric Association, 2000: 519–523.

24. Snaith RP, Zigmond AS. Hospital Anxiety and Depression Scale (HADS). In: American Psychiatric Association, eds. *Handbook of psychiatric measures*. Washington, DC: American Psychiatric Association, 2000:547–548.

25. Beck A, Kovacs M, Weissman A. Beck Scale for Suicidal Ideation (BSS). In: American Psychiatric Association, eds. *Handbook of psychiatric measures*. Washington, DC: American Psychiatric Association, 2000:264–266.

26. Beck A, Weissman A, Lester D, et al. Beck Hopelessness Scale (BHS). In: American Psychiatric Association, eds. *Handbook of psychiatric measures*. Washington, DC: American Psychiatric Association, 2000:268–270.

27. Hawton K, Townsend E, Arensman E, et al. Psychosocial and pharmacological treatments for deliberate self harm. In: The Cochrane Library, Issue 2, 2003. Oxford, Update Software. Search date 1999; primary sources Medline, PsychLit, Embase, Cochrane Controlled Trials Register, hand searches of 10 relevant journals, reference lists of relevant papers, and personal contact with trialists and other experts in the field.

28. Verkes RJ, Van der Mast RC, Hengeveld MW, et al. Reduction by paroxetine of suicidal behavior in patients with repeated suicide attempts but not major depression. *Am J Psychiatry* 1998;155:543–547.

29. Montgomery SA, Roy D, Montgomery DB. The prevention of recurrent suicidal acts. *Br J Clin Pharmacol* 1983;15:183S–188S.

30. Lasser KE, Alan PD, Woolhandler SJ, et al. Timing of new black box warnings and withdrawals for prescription medications. *JAMA* 2002;287:2215–2220.

31. British Medical Association and Royal Pharmaceutical Society of Great Britain. *British national formulary*. London: British Medical Association and Royal Pharmaceutical Society of Great Britain, 2002.

32. Townsend E, Hawton K, Altman DG, et al. The efficacy of problem-solving treatments after deliberate self-harm: meta-analysis of randomized controlled trials with respect to depression, hopelessness and improvement in problems. *Psychol Med* 2001;31:979–988. Search date not stated; primary sources Embase, PyschLit, Medline, Cochrane Controlled Trials Register, Cochrane Depression, Anxiety and Neurosis Review Group Trials Register, and hand searches of worldwide literature on deliberate self harm.

33. Guthrie E, Kapur N, Mackway-Jones K, et al. Randomised controlled trial of brief psychological intervention after deliberate self poisoning. *BMJ* 2001;323:135–138.

34. Bennewith O, Stocks N, Gunnell D, et al. General practice based intervention to prevent repeat episodes of deliberate self harm: cluster randomised controlled trial. *BMJ* 2002;324:1254–1257.

35. Clarke T, Baker P, Watts CJ, et al. Self-harm in adults: a randomised controlled trial of nurse-led case management versus routine care only. *J Mental Health* 2002;11:167–176.

36. Cedereke M, Monti K, Ojehagen A. Telephone contact with patients in the year after a suicide attempt: does it affect treatment attendance and outcome? A randomised controlled study. *Eur Psychiatry* 2002;17:82–91.

G Mustafa Soomro
Honorary Research Fellow
Section of Community Psychiatry
St George's Hospital Medical School, London, UK

Competing interests: None declared

Search date June 2003

James Warner, Rob Butler, and Pradeep Arya

Key Messages

- People in RCTs of treatments for dementia are often not representative of people with dementia. Few RCTs are conducted in primary care and few are conducted in people with types of dementia other than Alzheimer's disease.

Cognitive symptoms

- **Donepezil** One systematic review has found that donepezil improves cognitive function and global clinical state at up to 52 weeks compared with placebo in people with mild to moderate Alzheimer's disease. The review found no significant difference in patient rated quality of life at 12 or 24 weeks between donepezil and placebo. One large RCT identified by the review found that donepezil delayed the median time to "clinically evident functional decline" by 5 months compared with placebo. One open label RCT in people with mild to moderate Alzheimer's disease found no significant difference in cognitive function at 12 weeks between donepezil and rivastigmine, although fewer people taking donepezil withdrew from the trial for any cause.

- **Galantamine** RCTs have found that galantamine improves cognitive function and global clinical state over 6 months compared with placebo in people with Alzheimer's disease or vascular dementia.

- **Ginkgo biloba** RCTs found limited evidence that ginkgo biloba improved cognitive function over 24–26 weeks compared with placebo in people with Alzheimer's disease or vascular dementia.

- **Memantine** One systematic review has found that memantine improves cognitive function at 12–28 weeks compared with placebo in people with mild to moderate vascular dementia. Subsequent RCTs have found that memantine improves global clinical outcome and reduces care dependence at 12–28 weeks in people with more severe Alzheimer's disease or vascular dementia.

- **Reality orientation** One systematic review of small RCTs found that reality orientation improved cognitive function compared with no treatment in people with various types of dementia.

- **Oestrogen (in postmenopausal women)** One systematic review has found that, in postmenopausal women with mild to moderate Alzheimer's disease, oestrogen improves cognition over 7 weeks to 12 months' treatment compared with placebo or no treatment but there is concern that oestrogen treatment may increase the risk of developing breast cancer and cardiovascular events.

- **Physostigmine** One RCT in people with Alzheimer's disease found limited evidence that slow release physostigmine improved cognitive function over 12 weeks compared with placebo, but adverse effects, including nausea, vomiting, diarrhoea, dizziness, and stomach pain, were common.

- **Rivastigmine** One systematic review and one additional RCT have found that rivastigmine improves cognitive function compared with placebo in people with Alzheimer's disease or Lewy body dementia, but adverse effects such as nausea, vomiting, and anorexia are common. Subgroup analysis from one RCT in people with Alzheimer's disease suggests that people with vascular risk factors may respond better to rivastigmine than those without. One open label RCT in people with mild to moderate Alzheimer's disease found no significant difference in cognitive function at 12 weeks between rivastigmine and donepezil, although more people taking rivastigmine withdrew from the trial for any cause.

- **Tacrine** Two systematic reviews found limited evidence that tacrine improved cognitive function and global state at 3–36 weeks compared with placebo in people with Alzheimer's disease, but adverse effects, including nausea and vomiting, diarrhoea, anorexia, and abdominal pain, were common.

- **Lecithin** Small, poor RCTs identified by a systematic review provided insufficient evidence to assess lecithin in people with Alzheimer's disease.

- **Music therapy** Poor studies identified by a systematic review provided insufficient evidence to assess music therapy in people with dementia.

- **Nicotine** One systematic review found no RCTs of sufficient quality on the effects of nicotine in people with dementia.

- **Non-steroidal anti-inflammatory drugs** One RCT in people with Alzheimer's disease found no significant difference in cognitive function after 25 weeks' treatment with diclofenac plus misoprostol compared with placebo. Another RCT in people with Alzheimer's disease provided insufficient evidence to compare indometacin versus placebo in people with Alzheimer's disease.

- **Reminiscence therapy** One systematic review provided insufficient evidence to assess reminiscence therapy in people with dementia.

- **Selegiline** One systematic review found that, in people with mild to moderate Alzheimer's disease, selegiline for 2–4 months improved cognitive function compared with placebo. It found no significant difference in global clinical state or activities of daily living. RCTs assessing outcomes beyond 4 months found no significant difference between selegiline and placebo.

- **Vitamin E** One RCT in people with moderate to severe Alzheimer's disease found no significant difference in cognitive function after 2 years' treatment with vitamin E compared with placebo. However, it found that vitamin E reduced mortality, institutionalisation, loss of ability to perform activities of daily living, and the proportion of people who developed severe dementia.

Behavioural and psychological symptoms

- **Carbamazepine** One RCT found that carbamazepine reduced agitation and aggression over 6 weeks compared with placebo in people with various types of dementia and behavioural and psychological symptoms.

- **Reality orientation** One systematic review of small RCTs found that reality orientation improved behaviour compared with no treatment in people with various types of dementia.

- **Haloperidol** One systematic review in people with various types of dementia plus behavioural and psychological symptoms found no significant difference in agitation at 6–16 weeks between haloperidol and placebo. However, it found that haloperidol may reduce aggression. It found that haloperidol increased the frequency and severity of extrapyramidal symptoms compared with placebo. Another systematic review in people with various types of dementia plus behavioural and psychological symptoms found limited evidence that haloperidol and risperidone were similarly effective in reducing agitation over 12 weeks but that haloperidol caused more frequent and more severe extrapyramidal symptoms. Two RCTs in people with agitated behaviour associated with dementia found no significant difference in agitation between trazodone and haloperidol, but may have been too small to exclude a clinically important difference.

- **Olanzapine** One RCT identified by a systematic review in nursing home residents with Alzheimer's disease or Lewy body dementia plus behavioural and psychological symptoms found that olanzapine reduced agitation, hallucinations, and delusions over 6 weeks compared with placebo. Olanzapine has been associated with cerebrovascular adverse effects.

- **Risperidone** One systematic review and one subsequent RCT in people with various types of dementia, primarily Alzheimer's disease, all with behavioural and psychological symptoms, found that risperidone improved symptoms over 12 weeks compared with placebo. Another systematic review in people with various types of dementia plus aggressive behaviours found limited evidence that risperidone and haloperidol were similarly effective in reducing agitation over 12 weeks but that risperidone caused fewer and less severe extrapyramidal symptoms. Risperidone has been associated with cerebrovascular adverse events.

- **Sodium valproate** One RCT found that sodium valproate reduced agitation over 6 weeks compared with placebo in people with dementia plus behavioural and psychological problems. Another RCT found no significant difference in aggressive behaviour over 8 weeks between sodium valproate and placebo.

- **Trazodone** We found no RCTs comparing trazodone versus placebo. One small RCT in people with agitated behaviour associated with dementia found no significant difference in agitation over 9 weeks between trazodone and haloperidol. Another small RCT in people with Alzheimer's disease and agitated behaviour found no significant difference in outcomes over 16 weeks among trazodone, haloperidol, behaviour management techniques, and placebo. The RCTs may have been underpowered to detect a clinically important difference.

- **Donepezil; galantamine** RCTs provided inconclusive evidence about the effects of donepezil or galantamine compared with placebo on behavioural and psychiatric symptoms in people with mild to moderate Alzheimer's disease.

DEFINITION **Dementia** is characterised by chronic, global, non-reversible impairment of cerebral function. It usually results in loss of memory (initially of recent events), loss of executive function (such as the ability to make decisions or sequence complex tasks), and changes in personality. **Alzheimer's disease** is a type of dementia characterised by an insidious onset and slow deterioration, and involves speech, motor, personality, and executive function impairment. It should be diagnosed after other systemic, psychiatric, and neurological causes of dementia have been excluded clinically and by laboratory investigation. **Vascular dementia** is multi-infarct dementia involving a stepwise deterioration of executive function with or without language and motor dysfunction occurring as a result of cerebral arterial occlusion. It usually occurs in the presence of vascular risk factors (diabetes, hypertension, and smoking). Characteristically, it has a more sudden onset and stepwise progression than Alzheimer's disease. **Lewy body dementia** is a type of dementia involving insidious impairment of executive function with Parkinsonism, visual hallucinations, fluctuating cognitive abilities, and increased risk of falls or autonomic failure.[1,2] Careful clinical examination of people with mild to moderate dementia and the use of established diagnostic criteria accurately identifies 70–90% of cases confirmed at postmortem.[3,4]

INCIDENCE/ About 6% of people aged over 65 years and 30% of people aged
PREVALENCE over 90 years have some form of dementia.[5] Dementia is rare before the age of 60 years. Alzheimer's disease and vascular dementia (including mixed dementia) are each estimated to account for 35–50% of dementia, and Lewy body dementia is estimated to account for up to 20% of dementia in the elderly, varying with geographical, cultural, and racial factors.[1,5–10]

AETIOLOGY/ **Alzheimer's disease:** The cause of Alzheimer's disease is unclear.
RISK FACTORS A key pathological process is deposition of abnormal amyloid in the central nervous system.[11] Most people with the relatively rare condition of early onset Alzheimer's disease (before age 60 years) show an autosomal dominant inheritance owing to mutations on presenelin or amyloid precursor protein genes. Several genes (*APP*, *PS-1*, and *PS-2*) have been identified. Later onset dementia is sometimes clustered in families, but specific gene mutations have not been identified. Head injury, Down's syndrome, and lower premorbid intellect may be risk factors for Alzheimer's disease. **Vascular dementia** is related to cardiovascular risk factors, such as smoking, hypertension, and diabetes. **Lewy body dementia:** The cause of Lewy body dementia is unknown. Brain acetylcholine

activity is reduced in many forms of dementia, and the level of reduction correlates with cognitive impairment. Many treatments for Alzheimer's disease enhance cholinergic activity.[1,6]

PROGNOSIS **Alzheimer's disease:** Alzheimer's disease usually has an insidious onset with progressive reduction in cerebral function. Diagnosis is difficult in the early stages. Average life expectancy after diagnosis is 7–10 years.[10] **Lewy body dementia:** People with Lewy body dementia have an average life expectancy of about 6 years after diagnosis.[5] Behavioural problems, depression, and psychotic symptoms are common in all types of dementia.[12,13] Eventually, most people with dementia find it difficult to perform simple tasks without help.

AIMS OF INTERVENTION To improve cognitive function (memory, orientation, attention, and concentration); to reduce behavioural and psychological symptoms (wandering, aggression, anxiety, depression, and psychosis); to improve quality of life for both the individual and carer, with minimum adverse effects.

OUTCOMES Primary outcomes are quality of life, time to institutionalisation or death, functional scores, and scales of cognitive function, global assessment of function and behavioural and psychological symptoms. **Quality of life** of the person with dementia or their carer and **time to institutionalisation or death** are rarely reported because of the short duration of most trials.[14] Functional scores include the Disability Assessment for Dementia, a 40 item scale assessing 10 domains of function,[15] the Instrumental Activities of Daily Living Scale, maximum score 14 (lower scores indicate worse function).[16] **Cognitive symptoms and global assessment of function:** Quality of life of the person with dementia and their carer (rarely used in clinical trials). Comprehensive scales of cognitive function (e.g. Alzheimer's Disease Assessment Scale cognitive subscale [ADAS-cog], 70 point scale, lower scores indicate better function;[17] Mini Mental State Examination [MMSE], 30 point scale, lower scores indicate worse function;[18] Clinical Dementia Rating Scale [CDR], 3 point scale assessing six cognitive and functional parameters, higher scores indicate worse function;[14] Alzheimer's Disease Functional Assessment and Change Scale [ADFACS], 7 point scale, higher scores indicate worse function;[14] Severe Impairment Battery, 100 point scale used in people with severe Alzheimer's Disease, lower scores indicate worse function[19]). It has been suggested that ADAS-cog may be more sensitive than MMSE in assessing dementia, but neither scale directly reflects outcomes important to people with dementia or their carers. A 7 point change in the ADAS-cog has been regarded as clinically important. Measures of global state (e.g. Clinical Global Impression of Change [CGI-C] with caregiver input scale; Clinician's Interview Based Impression of Change-Plus [CIBIC-Plus], 7 point scale). **Behavioural and psychological symptoms:** Measures of psychiatric symptoms (e.g. Neuropsychiatric Inventory, 120 point scale, higher scores indicate greater difficulties; 12 item caregiver rated scale, maximum score 144, higher scores indicate greater difficulties; Dementia Mood Assessment Scale and Brief Psychiatric Rating Scale, higher scores indicate greater difficulties; Behave-AD scale, scores 0–75, higher scores indicate greater difficulties).

METHODS   *Clinical Evidence* search and appraisal June 2003. Dementia is often considered to have two domains of symptoms: cognitive impairment and non-cognitive symptoms (behavioural and psychological symptoms). We have separated the evidence into these two domains because they are often therapeutic targets at different stages of dementia and many RCTs focus on one or other domain of symptoms. In many RCTs, missing data were managed using "last observation carried forward", which does not account for the tendency of people with dementia to deteriorate with time. These RCTs may overestimate the benefit derived from interventions, especially when there are higher withdrawal rates in the intervention arm compared with controls. We found few RCTs in people with types of dementia other than Alzheimer's disease and most trials were placebo controlled rather than comparative.

QUESTION   **What are the effects of treatments on cognitive symptoms of dementia?**

OPTION   **DONEPEZIL**

One systematic review has found that donepezil improves cognitive function and global clinical state at up to 52 weeks compared with placebo in people with mild to moderate Alzheimer's disease. The review found no significant difference in patient rated quality of life at 12 or 24 weeks between donepezil and placebo. One large RCT identified by the review found that donepezil delayed the median time to "clinically evident functional decline" by 5 months compared with placebo. One open label RCT in people with mild to moderate Alzheimer's disease found no significant difference in cognitive function at 12 weeks between donepezil and rivastigmine, although fewer people taking donepezil withdrew from the trial for any cause.

Benefits: **Versus placebo:** We found one systematic review (search date 2003, 16 RCTs of 12, 24, and 52 weeks' duration, 4365 people, most with mild to moderate Alzheimer's disease) comparing donepezil versus placebo.[20] Nine RCTs identified by the review reported results using the Alzheimer's Disease Assessment Scale cognitive subscale (ADAS-cog) or the Clinician's Interview Based Impression of Change-Plus (CIBIC-Plus). The review found that donepezil 10 mg daily significantly improved cognitive function and global clinical state at 24 weeks compared with placebo (see table 1, p 101). It found no significant difference in patient rated quality of life at 12 or 24 weeks (at 24 weeks: WMD +2.79, 95% CI −2.56 to +8.14).[20] One RCT (24 weeks, 290 people with more severe Alzheimer's disease aged 48–92 years, Mini Mental State Examination [MMSE] score 5–17) identified by the review compared donepezil 5–10 mg daily versus placebo.[21] It found that donepezil significantly improved CIBIC-Plus scores at 24 weeks compared with placebo (mean difference 0.54, CI not reported, results presented graphically; NNT 5, 95% CI 4 to 10 for improved or no change on CIBIC-Plus).[21] Another RCT (431 people with mild to moderate Alzheimer's disease aged 49–94 years, MMSE score 12–20) identified by the review compared donepezil 10 mg daily versus placebo for 1 year.[22] It found that donepezil delayed the median time to "clinically evident functional decline" by 5 months compared with placebo (median: 357 days with donepezil v 208 days with placebo; CI not reported). It found that a significantly higher proportion of people had no "clinically evident functional decline" at 1 year with donepezil compared with placebo (no functional decline: 123/207 [59%] with donepezil v 92/208 [44%] with placebo; NNT 7, 95% CI 5 to 17). **Versus rivastigmine:** We found no systematic review. We found one open label RCT (111 people with mild to moderate Alzheimer's disease, MMSE score 10–26) comparing donepezil 5–10 mg daily versus rivastigmine (1.5–6.0 mg twice daily). It found no significant difference in cognitive function at 12 weeks between donepezil and rivastigmine (assessed by clinicians blind to intervention; mean difference in ADAS-cog –0.15, 95% CI –1.47 to +1.71).[23]

Harms: Adverse effects common to all cholinesterase inhibitors include anorexia, nausea, vomiting, and diarrhoea. **Versus placebo:** The RCTs identified by the review found that donepezil was associated with nausea, vomiting, and diarrhoea, which tended to be mild and transient.[20] The review found no difference between donepezil and placebo in the proportion of people who withdrew for any cause (see table 1, p 101).[20] Long term follow up of people taking donepezil (≤ 10 mg; open label extension) found that 86% experienced at least one adverse effect, often occurring later in the study. Common adverse events included agitation (24%), pain (20%), insomnia (11%), and diarrhoea (9%).[24] **Versus rivastigmine:** The RCT found that fewer people had at least one adverse event with donepezil than with rivastigmine, but the difference was not significant (24/56 [43%] with donepezil v 32/55 [58%] with rivastigmine; RR 0.74, 95% CI 0.51 to 1.07). It found that, compared with rivastigmine, donepezil significantly reduced the proportion of people who withdrew from the trial for any cause (6/56 [11%] with donepezil v 17/55 [31%] with rivastigmine; RR of withdrawal 0.35, 95% CI 0.15 to 0.81; NNH 5, 95% CI 3 to 20).[23]

Comment: In the RCT identified by the review in people with moderate to severe dementia, "clinically evident functional decline" was defined as a decline of at least 1 point on the Alzheimer's Disease Functional Assessment and Change Scale (ADFACS) or an increase of at least 1 point on the Clinical Dementia Rating Scale.[22] An unblinded extension of one of the RCTs identified by the review observed 133 people taking donepezil 3–10 mg daily for up to 240 weeks.[24] It found that improved cognitive function compared with baseline was present for 38 weeks in people taking donepezil, and throughout the period of observation cognitive function remained above the level estimated had people not been treated. Donepezil is taken once daily; this is a potential advantage over other cholinesterase inhibitors for people with dementia. Improvement usually starts within 2–4 months of starting donepezil. Open label studies should be interpreted with caution but do suggest that the effect of continued treatment is sustained in the long term.[23] We found no RCTs of donepezil in people with Lewy body or vascular dementia.

OPTION   GALANTAMINE

RCTs have found that galantamine improves cognitive function and global clinical state over 6 months compared with placebo in people with Alzheimer's disease or vascular dementia.

Benefits: **Versus placebo:** We found one systematic review (search date 2002, 7 RCTs)[25] in people with mild to moderate Alzheimer's disease and one additional RCT[26] in people with vascular dementia (see comment below). The review found that, compared with placebo, galantamine (12 or 16 mg twice daily) significantly improved cognitive function (measured by Alzheimer's Disease Assessment Scale cognitive subscale [ADAS-cog] score) and improved global status (measured by Clinician's Interview Based Impression of Change-Plus [CIBIC-Plus] score) over 6 months (see table 1, p 101). The additional RCT (592 people with vascular dementia or Alzheimer's disease plus cerebrovascular disease) compared galantamine 24 mg daily (396 people) versus placebo (196 people) for 6 months.[26] It found that galantamine significantly improved cognitive function from baseline at 6 months compared with placebo (4 point improvement in ADAS-cog: 35% with galantamine v 22% with placebo; NNT 8, 95% CI 5 to 17, absolute numbers not reported). It also found that galantamine significantly improved global clinical state at 6 months compared with placebo (CIBIC-Plus score "improved" or "no change": 74% with galantamine v 59% with placebo; NNT for "no change" 7, 95% CI 5 to 15).[26]

Harms: Adverse effects common to all cholinesterase inhibitors include anorexia, nausea, vomiting, and diarrhoea. **Versus placebo:** The review found that galantamine 12–16 mg daily significantly increased the proportion of people who withdrew for any cause over 6 months compared with placebo (see table 1, p 101). It also found that adverse effects were more frequent with higher doses of galantamine, including nausea (42% with galantamine 16 mg twice daily v 25% with placebo: OR 2.2, 95% CI 1.7 to 2.9) and vomiting (21% with galantamine 16 mg twice daily v 7% with placebo; OR 3.2, 95% CI 2.1 to 4.5). It also found that higher doses of galantamine increased the proportion of people who discontinued treatment because of adverse effects over 6 months (27% with galantamine 16 mg twice daily v 15% with galantamine 12 mg twice daily v 8% with placebo; 16 mg twice daily v placebo: OR 3.3, 95% CI 2.5 to 4.3).[25] The additional RCT comparing galantamine versus placebo in people with vascular dementia found that more people taking galantamine withdrew because of adverse effects (20% with galantamine v 8% with placebo; CI not reported).[26]

Comment: We found no RCTs of galantamine in people with Lewy body dementia.

OPTION   RIVASTIGMINE

One systematic review and one additional RCT have found that rivastigmine improves cognitive function in people with Alzheimer's disease or Lewy body dementia compared with placebo, but adverse

effects such as nausea, vomiting, and anorexia are common. Subgroup analysis from one RCT in people with Alzheimer's disease suggests that people with vascular risk factors may respond better to rivastigmine than those without. One open label RCT in people with mild to moderate Alzheimer's disease found no significant difference in cognitive function at 12 weeks between rivastigmine and donepezil, although more people taking rivastigmine withdrew from the trial for any cause.

Benefits: **Versus placebo:** We found one systematic review (search date 2000, 4 RCTs, 12 or 26 weeks' duration, 3370 people with mild to moderate Alzheimer's disease)[27] and one additional RCT[28] in people with Lewy body dementia (see comment below). The review found that rivastigmine (6–12 mg twice daily) produced small but significant improvements in cognitive function global clinical state over 26 weeks compared with placebo (see table 1, p 101). A subgroup analysis of an RCT[29] identified by the review[27] (699 people with Alzheimer's disease) comparing rivastigmine 1–4 mg daily or 6–12 mg daily versus placebo over 26 weeks found that people with vascular risk factors responded better than those without (mean Alzheimer's Disease Assessment Scale cognitive subscale difference −2.3). The additional RCT (120 people with Lewy body dementia) found that rivastigmine (dose titrated to 6 mg twice daily) significantly improved a computerised psychometric measure of cognitive function at 20 weeks compared with placebo (intention to treat analysis; P = 0.05; no further data reported) and improved a global measure of behavioural function (NNT for at least 30% improvement on Neuropsychiatric Inventory score 3, 95% CI 2 to 6).[28] **Versus donepezil:** See benefits of donepezil, p 79.

Harms: Adverse effects common to all cholinesterase inhibitors include anorexia, nausea, vomiting, and diarrhoea. **Versus placebo:** The systematic review in people with Alzheimer's disease found that rivastigmine increased the proportion of people who discontinued treatment for any cause compared with placebo (see table 1, p 101).[27] The RCT in people with Lewy body dementia found that rivastigmine increased the proportion of people who had nausea compared with placebo (37% with rivastigmine v 22% with placebo), vomiting (25% with rivastigmine v 15% with placebo), anorexia (19% with rivastigmine v 10% with placebo), and somnolence (9% with rivastigmine v 5% with placebo; no further data reported).[28] **Versus donepezil:** See harms of donepezil, p 80.

Comment: We found no RCTs of rivastigmine in people with vascular dementia.

OPTION   PHYSOSTIGMINE

One RCT in people with Alzheimer's disease found limited evidence that slow release physostigmine improved cognitive function over 12 weeks compared with placebo but adverse effects, including nausea, vomiting, diarrhoea, dizziness, and stomach pain, were common.

Benefits: **Versus placebo:** We found one systematic review (search date 2000, 15 RCTs) comparing physostigmine versus placebo in people mild to severe Alzheimer's disease (see comment below).[30] The RCTs differed widely in the preparations of physostigmine used, and most had weak reporting methods so the review could not perform a meta-analysis. Four were small trials of intravenous physostig-mine, which did not report quantitative results. Seven were small trials (131 people, 6 crossover design) of standard oral preparation. The crossover trials did not provide results before crossover. One RCT (16 people) found no significant difference in cognition between oral physostigmine and placebo but it is likely to have been too small to exclude a clinically important difference. Four RCTs (1456 people) used controlled release preparations, but three of these reported results only for people who responded to physostig-mine in a prestudy titration phase (see comment below). One RCT (170 people) found that slow release physostigmine 27 mg daily significantly improved cognition after 12 weeks compared with placebo (Alzheimer's Disease Assessment Scale cognitive sub-scale: WMD–2.0, 95% CI –3.6 to –0.5). It did not significantly improve activities of daily living or Clinician Based Impression of Change.

Harms: **Versus placebo:** Common adverse effects of physostigmine include nausea, vomiting, diarrhoea, dizziness, and stomach pain. In RCTs that randomised all people with Alzheimer's disease rather than selecting those who tolerated and responded to physostig-mine, withdrawals were more common with physostigmine (234/358 [65%] with physostigmine v 31/117 [26%] with placebo; OR 4.80, 95% CI 3.17 to 7.33).[30]

Comment: We found no RCTs of physostigmine in people with Lewy body or vascular dementia. Physostigmine is a sympathomimetic drug and has a short half life. Screening out non-responders to a drug before the trial is likely to overestimate its effectiveness.

OPTION   TACRINE

Two systematic reviews found limited evidence that tacrine improved cognitive function and global state at 3–36 weeks compared with placebo in people with Alzheimer's disease, but adverse effects, including nausea and vomiting, diarrhoea, anorexia, and abdominal pain, were common.

Benefits: **Versus placebo:** We found two systematic reviews comparing tacrine versus placebo in people with Alzheimer's disease (search date not reported, 12 RCTs, 1984 people;[31] search date 1997, 21 RCTs, including all 12 RCTs identified by the first review, 3555 people[32]). Various doses of tacrine were used in the RCTs, and the duration of treatment varied from 3–36 weeks. The first review found that, compared with placebo, tacrine significantly increased the proportion of people with overall clinical improvement (OR 1.58, 95% CI 1.18 to 2.11) and improved cognition (Mini Mental State Examination [MMSE] at 12 weeks: SMD 0.77, 95% CI 0.35 to 1.20; Alzheimer's Disease Assessment Scale cognitive subscale [ADAS-cog] at 12 weeks: SMD –2.7, 95% CI –1.36 to –2.78).[31] A subsequent subgroup analysis indicated that the five non-industry sponsored studies found no significant effect between tacrine and placebo, but most (6/7 [86%]) manufacturer supported studies found clinical benefit (1 RCT could not be located for inclusion in the subgroup analysis).[33] The second review assessed the methods and quality of tacrine RCTs and did not perform a meta-analysis.[32] It suggested that tacrine improved cognitive function in about 20% of people (improvement of 3–4 points in MMSE Scale score or ADAS-cog).

Harms: **Versus placebo:** The first review found that tacrine significantly increased the proportion of people who withdrew because of adverse effects, primarily elevated liver enzymes, compared with placebo (OR for withdrawal 3.6, 95% CI 2.8 to 4.7).[31] One RCT identified by the reviews found that tacrine 40–180 mg daily significantly increased withdrawals because of adverse events compared with placebo (265/479 [55%] with tacrine v 20/184 [11%] with placebo; RR 5.1, 95% CI 3.3 to 7.7; NNH 3, 95% CI 2 to 3), and that reversible elevation of liver enzymes was found in 133/265 (50%) of people taking tacrine.[34] Common adverse events included nausea and vomiting (35% with 160 mg daily), diarrhoea (18%), anorexia (12%), and abdominal pain (9%).

Comment: The reviews suggested that the quality of tacrine RCTs was generally poor.[31,32] We found no RCTs of tacrine in people with Lewy body or vascular dementia.

OPTION   LECITHIN

Small, poor RCTs identified by a systematic review provided insufficient evidence to assess lecithin in people with Alzheimer's disease.

Benefits: **Versus placebo:** We found one systematic review (search date 2002, 12 RCTs, 265 people with Alzheimer's disease, 21 with Parkinsonian dementia, 90 with subjective memory problems) comparing lecithin versus placebo (see comment below).[35] It found no significant difference between lecithin and placebo in cognition (1 RCT, 37 people, OR 0.91, 95% CI 0.25 to 3.34), functional performance (1 RCT, 30 people, WMD +0.76, 95% CI −0.91 to +2.43), or global impression (2 RCTs, 17/24 [71%] with lecithin v 12/28 [43%] with placebo; OR 3.01, 95% CI 0.92 to 9.81; see comment below).[35]

Harms: **Versus placebo:** The review found that adverse effects were more common with lecithin (14/34 [41%] with lecithin v 3/29 [10%] with placebo; OR 6.1, 95% CI 1.5 to 24.0).[35] The specific nature of the adverse effects was not stated.

Comment: One RCT (included in the systematic review) comparing lecithin versus placebo in people with minimal cognitive impairment found that some components of cognition were significantly better in the placebo group.[35] Most studies of lecithin were small and weak. Meta-analysis in the systematic review was hampered by diverse outcome criteria and it is likely that the meta-analyses were underpowered to detect a clinically important difference in outcomes. We found no RCTs of lecithin in people with Lewy body or vascular dementia.

OPTION   NICOTINE

One systematic review found no RCTs of sufficient quality on the effects of nicotine in people with dementia.

Benefits: One systematic review (search date 2001) found no RCTs of sufficient quality.[36]

Harms: We found no RCTs.

Comment: None.

OPTION   NON-STEROIDAL ANTI-INFLAMMATORY DRUGS

One RCT in people with Alzheimer's disease found no significant difference in cognitive function after 25 weeks' treatment with diclofenac plus misoprostol compared with placebo. Another RCT in people with Alzheimer's disease provided insufficient evidence to compare indometacin versus placebo in people with Alzheimer's disease.

Benefits: **Versus placebo:** We found two RCTs in people with Alzheimer's disease (see comment below).[37,38] The first RCT (41 people with Alzheimer's disease) found no significant difference in cognitive function after 25 weeks' treatment with diclofenac plus misoprostol compared with placebo (Alzheimer's Disease Assessment Scale cognitive subscale [ADAS-cog] score: mean difference +1.14, 95% CI –2.90 to +5.20) or global status (Clinician's Interview Based Impression of Change score: +0.24, 95% CI –0.26 to +0.74).[37] The second RCT (44 people with mild to moderate Alzheimer's disease) found that indometacin (indomethacin) ($\leq$150 mg daily) for 6 months significantly improved cognitive function compared with placebo (assessed by averaging percentage changes in scores on Mini Mental State Examination Scale, ADAS-cog, Boston Naming Test, and Token Test; mean increase 1.3% with indometacin v mean reduction 8.4% with placebo; results not intention to treat, 16/44 [36%] withdrew from the trial).[38]

Harms: In one RCT, more people withdrew by week 25 with diclofenac plus misoprostol than with placebo (12/24 [50%] with diclofenac plus misoprostol v 2/17 [12%] with placebo).[37] No serious drug related adverse events were reported.[37] In the RCT of indometacin, 21% of people on indometacin withdrew because of gastrointestinal symptoms.[38]

Comment: We found one systematic review of aspirin for vascular dementia (search date 2000), which identified no RCTs.[39] Earlier versions of a systematic review of aspirin in vascular dementia included one RCT (70 people), which was subsequently removed because of inadequate quality, including a lack of placebo control.[39] We found no RCTs of NSAIDs in people with Lewy body dementia.

OPTION   OESTROGEN

One systematic review has found that, in postmenopausal women with mild to moderate Alzheimer's disease, oestrogen improves cognition over 7 weeks to 12 months' treatment compared with placebo or no treatment but there is concern that oestrogen treatment may increase the risk of developing breast cancer and cardiovascular events.

Benefits: **Versus placebo:** We found one systematic review (search date 2000, 8 RCTs, 313 women with mild to moderate Alzheimer's disease aged over 56 years) comparing oestrogen 0.625–1.25 mg daily versus placebo or no treatment for 7 weeks to 12 months (see comment below).[40] The review found that oestrogen improved cognitive function compared with placebo or no treatment (5 RCTs, Mini Mental State Examination: WMD 2.3, 95% CI 1.7 to 3.4).

Harms: There is concern that oestrogen treatment may increase the risk of developing breast cancer and cardiovascular events.

Comment: Most RCTs in the review were small and heterogeneity may have distorted the results of the meta-analysis. We found no RCTs of oestrogen in people with Lewy body or vascular dementia. A meta-analysis of 14 observational studies (5990 people, length of follow up not stated) found that hormone replacement therapy is associated with a lower risk of developing dementia (dementia in 13% with hormone replacement therapy v 21% with controls; RR 0.56, 95% CI 0.46 to 0.68).[40] Observational studies provide only indirect evidence; the observed association may be explained by confounders (e.g. educational level, lifestyle factors).

OPTION   SELEGILINE

One systematic review found that, in people with mild to moderate Alzheimer's disease, selegiline for 2–4 months improved cognitive function compared with placebo. It found no significant difference in global clinical state or activities of daily living. RCTs assessing outcomes beyond 4 months found no significant difference between selegiline and placebo.

Benefits: **Versus placebo:** We found one systematic review (search date 2002, 17 RCTs) comparing selegiline versus placebo in people with mild to moderate Alzheimer's disease.[41] It found that, compared with placebo, selegiline 10 mg daily for 2–4 months significantly improved cognitive function (measured by various parameters: 11 RCTs, 866 people: WMD 2.40, 95% CI 0.06 to 4.74). It found no significant difference in global clinical state (5 RCTs, 275 people: WMD –0.03, 95% CI –0.13 to +0.07) or in activities of daily living (7 RCTs, 810 people: WMD –0.17, 95% CI –0.35 to 0). RCTs assessing outcomes beyond 4 months found no significant difference between selegiline and placebo.

Harms: **Versus placebo:** The RCTs identified by the first review found a similar proportion of adverse effects (anxiety, agitation, dizziness, nausea, dyspepsia) between selegiline and placebo.[41]

Comment: Many of the RCTs identified by the review were small and brief.[41] They used a variety of outcomes, making meta-analysis and comparison with other treatments difficult. Although selegiline may cause short term improvement, the improvement in cognition seems marginal and may not be of clinical importance. There is no evidence of long term benefit. We found no RCTs of selegiline in people with Lewy body or vascular dementia.

OPTION MEMANTINE

One systematic review has found that memantine improves cognitive function at 12–28 weeks compared with placebo in people with mild to moderate vascular dementia. Subsequent RCTs have found that memantine improves global clinical outcome and reduces care dependence at 12–28 weeks in people with more severe Alzheimer's disease or vascular dementia.

Benefits:

Versus placebo: We found one systematic review[42] and two subsequent RCTs[43,44] comparing memantine versus placebo. The review (search date 2002, 7 RCTs, 1532 people) did not meta-analyse many results because of differences in people included and in dose of memantine taken in the RCTs.[42] Two RCTs (154 people) included in the review were of poor quality and data are not reported here (see comment below). The review identified two RCTs (900 people with mild to moderate vascular dementia, Mini Mental State Examination [MMSE] score 10–22). They found that, compared with placebo, memantine significantly improved cognitive function at 28 weeks (measured by Alzheimer's Disease Assessment Scale cognitive subscale [ADAS-cog]: WMD –2.19, 95% CI –1.21 to –3.16; results not intention to treat). They found no significant difference in global clinical state (measured by Gottsfries-Brane-Steen scale: 2 RCTs, 595 people: WMD –1.81, 95% CI –4.21 to +0.58). Subgroup analysis in one of the RCTs identified by the review suggested that the largest treatment effect occurred in people with baseline MMSE scores of less than 15 (mean difference 3.17 points, P = 0.04) and in people without cerebrovascular macrolesions (mean difference 2.29 points; P = 0.002).[45] The first subsequent RCT (166 people with Alzheimer's disease [49%] or vascular dementia [51%], MMSE < 10, Global Deterioration Scale stages 5–7) found that memantine 10 mg daily significantly increased the proportion of people with improved global clinical outcome at 12 weeks compared with placebo (measured by Clinical Global Impression of Change; 60/82 [73%] with memantine v 38/84 [45%] with placebo; RR 1.62, 95% CI 1.24 to 2.12; NNT 4, 95% CI 3 to 7). It also found that memantine significantly reduced care dependence compared with placebo (measured by a Behavioural Rating Scale for Geriatric Patients [BGP] care dependence subscore: mean difference 2.0 points, CI not reported; P = 0.016).[43] The second subsequent RCT (252 people with moderate to severe Alzheimer's disease) found that memantine 20 mg daily for 28 weeks significantly improved cognitive function compared with placebo (measured by the Severe Impairment Battery [SIB]; WMD 6.10, 95% CI 2.99 to 9.21), and activities of daily living (measured by the Activities of Daily Living Scale: WMD 2.1, 95% CI 0.5 to 3.7; results not intention to treat; 71 [28%] people withdrew from the trial).[44] A resource utilisation analysis based on this RCT found that people taking memantine required significantly less caregiver time compared with people taking placebo (mean difference –52 hours/month, 95% CI –95 hours/month to –7 hours/month).[46]

Harms: The review found no significant difference between memantine and placebo in the proportion of people who had at least one adverse effect (2 RCTs, 351/460 [76%] with memantine v 327/440 [74%] with placebo; OR 1.11, 95% CI 0.82 to 1.51).[42] The subsequent RCTs also found that a similar proportion of people taking memantine and placebo had adverse effects.[44,46]

Comment: The methods of two memantine RCTs identified by the review were poor (follow up of 6 weeks, lack of blinding, unclear randomisation procedures, lack of intention to treat analysis, lack of ethics approval) and we have not reported the data here.[47,48] Memantine is a partial N-methyl-D-aspartate antagonist and has a different mechanism of action to cholinesterase inhibitors. Current evidence suggests it is well tolerated and may improve outcomes, especially in people with more severe dementia. However, it is difficult to compare memantine with cholinesterase inhibitors as most memantine RCTs are in people with more severe dementia and report different outcomes. Evidence for its use in mild to moderate dementia is inconclusive and more high quality trials are needed. We found no RCTs of memantine in people with Lewy body dementia.

OPTION   GINKGO BILOBA

RCTs found limited evidence that ginkgo biloba improved cognitive function over 24–26 weeks compared with placebo in people with Alzheimer's disease or vascular dementia.

Benefits: **Versus placebo:** We found one systematic review (search date 2002) comparing ginkgo biloba versus placebo in people with cognitive impairment, Alzheimer's disease, or vascular dementia (see comment below).[49] Trial duration ranged from 3–53 weeks, doses and preparations of ginkgo biloba varied widely, and diverse outcomes were assessed, making meta-analysis difficult.[49] The review included two large RCTs in people with Alzheimer's disease or vascular dementia. The first large RCT (216 people with mild to moderate Alzheimer's disease or vascular dementia) found that ginkgo biloba (≥ 200 mg daily) significantly increased the proportion of people who were rated as improved at 24 weeks (completer analysis: improvement in Clinician's Interview Based Impression of Change [criteria for improvement not defined] 57/79 [72%] with ginkgo biloba v 42/77 [55%] with placebo; RR 1.32, 95% CI 1.03 to 1.69).[49] The second large RCT (327 people, 236 people with Alzheimer's disease) had a high withdrawal rate; 137/309 (44%) people withdrew from the trial.[50] However, it provided an intention to treat analysis. It found that, in people with Alzheimer's disease, ginkgo biloba significantly improved cognition (intention to treat analysis for people with Alzheimer's disease, change in Alzheimer's Disease Assessment Scale cognitive subscale score [ADAS-cog]: −1.7, 95% CI −3.1 to −0.20; NNT for 4 point change in ADAS-cog: 8, 95% CI 5 to 50) and caregiver assessed improvement over 26 weeks compared with placebo (change in Geriatric Evaluation by Relative's Rating Instrument score: −0.16, 95% CI −0.25 to −0.06). It found no significant difference in mean Clinician's Global Impression of Change score (change in score: +0.1, 95% CI −0.1 to +0.2).[50]

Harms: The review found no significant difference between ginkgo biloba and placebo in the proportion of people who had at least one adverse effect (adverse effects not specified; 5 RCTs, 1070 people; 117/591 [19.7%] with ginkgo biloba v 59/471 [12.5%] with placebo; RR 0.95, 95% CI 0.72 to 1.26).[49]

Comment: Many of the RCTs in the review included people with memory and cognitive impairment other than dementia so the results of the meta-analysis may not be fully generalisable to people with Alzheimer's disease or vascular dementia. We found no RCTs of ginkgo biloba in people with Lewy body dementia. Preparations of ginkgo biloba available without prescription differ in terms of purity and concentration of active ingredients compared with high purity extract (EGb 761) used in most RCTs.

OPTION VITAMIN E

One RCT in people with moderate to severe Alzheimer's disease found no significant difference in cognitive function between vitamin E and placebo after 2 years' treatment. However, it found that vitamin E reduced mortality, institutionalisation, loss of ability to perform activities of daily living, and the proportion of people who developed severe dementia.

Benefits: **Versus placebo:** We found one systematic review (search date 2000, 1 multicentre RCT, 169 people with moderate to severe Alzheimer's disease; see comment below).[51] The RCT compared four treatments: vitamin E (α-tocopherol; 2000 IU daily); selegiline; vitamin E plus selegiline; or placebo.[52] It found no significant difference in cognitive function with high dose vitamin E alone for 2 years compared with placebo (measured by the cognitive portion of the Alzheimer's Disease Assessment Scale, lower scores indicate worse function: mean reduction in score 8.3 with vitamin E v 6.7 with placebo; reported as non-significant; no further details reported; see comment below). It found that vitamin E significantly increased event free survival compared with placebo (defined as death, survival until institutionalisation, loss of ability to perform activities of daily living, or severe dementia [clinical dementia rating of 3]; OR 0.49, 95% CI 0.25 to 0.96).[52]

Harms: **Versus placebo:** The RCT found no significant difference in adverse effects between placebo and vitamin E.[52] Other studies have found weak evidence of associations between high dose vitamin E and bowel irritation, headache, muscular weakness, visual complaints, vaginal bleeding, bruising, thrombophlebitis, deterioration of angina pectoris, worsening of diabetes, syncope, and dizziness.[53]

Comment: The groups in the RCT identified by the review were not matched evenly at baseline: the placebo group had a higher mean Mini Mental State Examination score, and these baseline scores were a significant predictor of outcome.[52] Attempts to correct for this imbalance suggested that vitamin E might increase mean survival, but the need for statistical adjustments weakens the strength of this conclusion. We found no RCTs of vitamin E in people with Lewy body or vascular dementia.

OPTION	MUSIC THERAPY

Poor studies identified by a systematic review provided insufficient evidence to assess music therapy in people with dementia.

Benefits: **Versus control:** We found one systematic review of music therapy (search date 1998, 21 studies, 336 people with various types of dementia).[54] It included studies with weak methods and found that music therapy significantly improved cognitive and behavioural outcomes compared with control interventions (mean effect size 0.79, 95% CI 0.62 to 0.95; see comment below). Significant effects were noted with different types of music therapy (active v passive, taped v live).

Harms: **Versus control:** The systematic review gave no information on harms.[54]

Comment: The primary studies lacked adequate controls, had potential for bias, used diverse interventions, and used inadequate outcome measures. Although one meta-analysis found significant benefits for music therapy on pooling the results of many studies, further high quality studies are needed to clarify whether the results are explained by a true effect or by bias. A previous Cochrane systematic review of music therapy has been withdrawn.[55]

OPTION	REALITY ORIENTATION

One systematic review of small RCTs found that reality orientation improved cognitive function compared with no treatment in people with various types of dementia.

Benefits: **Versus no treatment:** We found one systematic review (search date 2000, 6 RCTs, 125 people with various types of dementia).[56] The RCTs compared reality orientation (see glossary, p 97) versus no treatment and used different measures of cognition. The review found that reality orientation significantly improved cognitive function score compared with no treatment (SMD −0.59, 95% CI −0.95 to −0.22). No separate analysis was done for specific types of dementia.

Harms: **Versus no treatment:** The RCTs gave no information on adverse effects.[56]

Comment: The RCTs did not use standardised interventions or outcomes.[56]

OPTION	REMINISCENCE THERAPY

RCTs provided insufficient evidence to assess reminiscence therapy in people with dementia.

Benefits: We found one systematic review of reminiscence therapy (see glossary, p 97) (search date 2000, 2 RCTs, 42 people).[57] Analysis of pooled data was hindered by poor trial methods, diverse outcomes, and no separation of data for different types of dementia.

Harms: We found no RCTs.

Comment: None.

QUESTION What are the effects of treatments on behavioural and psychological symptoms of dementia?

OPTION HALOPERIDOL

One systematic review in people with various types of dementia plus behavioural and psychological symptoms found no significant difference in agitation at 6–16 weeks between haloperidol and placebo. However, it found that haloperidol may reduce aggression. It found that haloperidol increased the frequency and severity of extrapyramidal symptoms compared with placebo. Another systematic review in people with various types of dementia plus behavioural and psychological symptoms found limited evidence that haloperidol and risperidone were similarly effective in reducing agitation over 12 weeks but that haloperidol caused more frequent and more severe extrapyramidal symptoms. Two RCTs in people with agitated behaviour associated with dementia found no significant difference in agitation between trazodone and haloperidol, but may have been too small to exclude a clinically important difference.

Benefits: **Versus placebo:** We found one systematic review (search date 2000, 5 RCTs) comparing haloperidol versus placebo in people with various types of dementia, including Alzheimer's disease and vascular dementia, all with behavioural and psychological symptoms.[58] It found no significant difference in agitation at 6–16 weeks between haloperidol and placebo (4 RCTs, 369 people, change in symptoms from baseline measured by the Cohen-Mansfield Agitation Inventory or the psychomotor score of the Behavioural Symptoms Scale for Dementia [BSSD]; WMD –0.45, 95% CI –1.43 to +0.53). However, it found that haloperidol significantly reduced aggression from baseline at 3–6 weeks compared with placebo (4 RCTs, 489 people, change in symptoms from baseline measured by Multidimensional Observation Scale for Elderly Subjects aggression subscore, Behave-AD scale, aggression subscore, or the physical aggression score of the BSSD; WMD –0.92, 95% CI –1.75 to –0.09).[58] **Versus risperidone:** We found one systematic review (search date 2002, 2 RCTs, 402 people with Alzheimer's disease, vascular dementia, or mixed dementia, all with behavioural and psychological symptoms) comparing haloperidol versus risperidone for 12 weeks.[59] The reviewers could not perform a meta-analysis because of differences in outcomes assessed and people included in the trials (outpatients and people in hospital). The first RCT (58 people) identified by the review found no significant difference in agitation over 12 weeks between haloperidol and risperidone (measured by Cohen-Mansfield Agitation Inventory and Behave-AD scale; reported as non-significant; no further data reported). The second RCT (344 people) identified by the review compared three interventions: haloperidol, risperidone, and placebo. It found that a similar proportion of people taking haloperidol or risperidone had improvements in agitation (63% with haloperidol v 54% with risperidone; CI not reported). **Versus trazodone:** See benefits of trazodone, p 95.

Harms: **Versus placebo:** The review found that haloperidol (> 2 mg daily) significantly increased the proportion of people who had at least one extrapyramidal symptom or who withdrew because of adverse effects over 3–6 weeks (extrapyramidal symptom: OR 2.34, 95% CI 1.25 to 4.38; withdrawal: OR 2.99, 95% CI 1.26 to 7.10).[58] One study (2 year prospective, longitudinal, 71 people with dementia) found that the mean decline in cognitive scores in 16 people who took antipsychotics was twice that of people who did not (expanded Mini Mental State Examination: 21 with antipsychotics v 9 with no antipsychotics; P = 0.002).[60] **Versus risperidone:** The first RCT identified by the review did not compare adverse effects between haloperidol and risperidone directly. The second RCT found that haloperidol significantly increased frequency and severity of extrapyramidal symptoms compared with risperidone (frequency: 22% with risperidone v 15% with risperidone; P = 0.023; severity: measured by Extrapyramidal Symptoms Rating Scale score: mean +1.6 with haloperidol v –0.3 with risperidone; P < 0.05).[59] **Versus trazodone:** See harms of trazodone, p 95.

Comment: High response rates with placebo indicate that many behavioural problems resolve spontaneously in the short term. Most people with dementia are sensitive to adverse effects from antipsychotics, especially sedation and extrapyramidal symptoms. People with Lewy body dementia are particularly sensitive to these adverse effects,[61] suggesting that antipsychotics have a poor balance of benefits and harms in people with Lewy body dementia. More studies are needed to determine whether newer atypical antipsychotics have a better ratio of benefits to harms than older antipsychotics.

OPTION   OLANZAPINE

One RCT identified by a systematic review in nursing home residents with Alzheimer's disease or Lewy body dementia plus behavioural and psychological symptoms found that olanzapine reduced agitation, hallucinations, and delusions over 6 weeks compared with placebo. Olanzapine has been associated with cerebrovascular adverse effects.

Benefits: **Versus placebo:** We found one systematic review[59] (search date 2002), which identified one RCT[62] (double blind, 6 weeks' duration, 206 elderly US nursing home residents with Alzheimer's disease [177 people] or Lewy body dementia [29 people], all with psychotic or behavioural symptoms). The RCT compared olanzapine (given as a fixed dose of 5, 10, or 15 mg daily) versus placebo.[62] It found that agitation, hallucinations, and delusions were improved by the two lower doses but not by the highest dose of olanzapine compared with placebo (subscale of the Neuropsychiatric Inventory [nursing home version; higher scores indicate worse function]: –7.6 with olanzapine 5 mg v –6.1 with olanzapine 10 mg v –4.9 with olanzapine 15 mg v –3.7 with placebo).

Harms: **Versus placebo:** The RCT found that olanzapine increased sedation (25% with olanzapine 5 mg v 26% with olanzapine 10 mg v 36% with olanzapine 15 mg v 6% with placebo) and gait disturbance compared with placebo (20% with olanzapine 5 mg v 14% with olanzapine 10 mg v 17% with olanzapine 15 mg v 2% with placebo).[62]

Comment: See comment of haloperidol, p 92. Following the suggestion of an association between olanzapine and cerebrovascular adverse events, the Food and Drugs Administration in the USA and the Committee on Safety of Medicines in the UK have issued an alert that risperidone has not been shown to be safe in people with psychosis associated with dementia.[65,74]

OPTION RISPERIDONE

One systematic review and one subsequent RCT in people with various types of dementia, primarily Alzheimer's disease, all with behavioural and psychological symptoms, found that risperidone improved symptoms over 12 weeks compared with placebo. Another systematic review in people with various types of dementia plus aggressive behaviours found limited evidence that risperidone and haloperidol were similarly effective in reducing agitation over 12 weeks but that risperidone caused fewer and less severe extrapyramidal symptoms. Risperidone has been associated with cerebrovascular adverse events.

Benefits: **Versus placebo:** We found one systematic review[59] and one subsequent RCT.[63] The review (search date 2002, 2 RCTs, 969 people with Alzheimer's disease [67–73%], vascular dementia, or mixed dementia, all with behavioural symptoms, 56–68% women) compared risperidone versus placebo for 12 weeks.[59] It found that risperidone modestly but significantly improved behavioural and psychological symptoms over 12 weeks compared with placebo (measured by Behave-AD scale: mean difference with risperidone v placebo −1.80, 95% CI −3.22 to −0.38).[59] The subsequent RCT (167 people with Alzheimer's disease, vascular dementia, or mixed dementia, all with aggressive behaviours, mean age 83 years, 72% women) compared risperidone (mean 0.95 mg daily) versus placebo over 12 weeks.[63] It also found that risperidone significantly improved behavioural and psychological symptoms over 12 weeks compared with placebo (mean difference with risperidone v placebo measured by Behave-AD scale −4.50, 95% CI −6.45 to −2.46; measured by the Cohen-Mansfield Agitation Inventory aggression subscale −4.4, 95% CI −6.75 to −2.07). **Versus haloperidol:** See benefits of haloperidol, p 91.

Harms: **Versus placebo:** The review found that risperidone was associated with increases in extrapyramidal symptoms, somnolence, and mild peripheral oedema (no further data reported).[59] Adverse effects increased with higher doses. Data from four RCTs (1230 elderly people with dementia) of risperidone suggested that risperidone was associated with an increase in cerebrovascular adverse events (including strokes and transient ischaemic attacks, some of which were fatal) compared with placebo (29/764 [4%] with risperidone v 7/466 [2%] with placebo; CI not reported; see comment below).[64] **Versus haloperidol:** See harms of haloperidol, p 91.

Comment: See comment of haloperidol, p 92. Following the suggestion of an association between risperidone and cerebrovascular adverse events, the Food and Drugs Administration in the USA and the Committee on Safety of Medicines in the UK have issued an alert that risperidone has not been shown to be safe in people with psychosis associated with dementia.[65,74]

OPTION CARBAMAZEPINE

One RCT found that carbamazepine reduced agitation and aggression over 6 weeks compared with placebo in people with various types of dementia and behavioural and psychological symptoms.

Benefits: **Versus placebo:** We found no systematic review but found one RCT (single blind, 51 nursing home patients with agitation and Alzheimer's disease, vascular dementia, or mixed Alzheimer's disease and vascular dementia, 6 weeks' duration) comparing carbamazepine (individualised doses; modal dose 300 mg; mean serum level 5.3 µg/mL) versus placebo.[66] It found that carbamazepine significantly improved a measure of agitation and aggression (assessed by change in mean total Brief Psychiatric Rating Scale score: mean reduction 7.7 with carbamazepine v 0.9 with placebo; P = 0.03).

Harms: **Versus placebo:** The RCT found that adverse effects were significantly more common with carbamazepine than with placebo (16/27 [59%] with carbamazepine v 7/24 [29%] with placebo; P = 0.003). These were considered clinically important in two cases: one person with tics and one person with ataxia. Carbamazepine in the elderly may cause cardiac toxicity.

Comment: We found no RCTs of carbamazepine in people with Lewy body dementia.

OPTION SODIUM VALPROATE

One RCT found that sodium valproate reduced agitation over 6 weeks compared with placebo in people with dementia plus behavioural and psychological problems. Another RCT found no significant difference in aggressive behaviour over 8 weeks between sodium valproate and placebo.

Benefits: **Versus placebo:** We found no systematic review but found two RCTs.[67,68] The first RCT (single blind, 56 people in nursing homes with Alzheimer's disease or vascular dementia, all with agitation) compared sodium valproate versus placebo for 6 weeks.[67] It found that when several covariates were taken into account, sodium valproate significantly improved agitation and aggression compared with placebo (measured by Brief Psychiatric Rating Scale score; P = 0.05 only after adjustment) and a measure of global status (Clinical Global Impression rating: 68% with sodium valproate v 52% with placebo; P = 0.06). The second RCT (43 people with various types of dementia plus behavioural problems, crossover design) comparing sodium valproate 480 mg daily versus placebo for 3 weeks found no significant difference in aggressive behaviour over 8 weeks after crossover (mean change in Social Dysfunction and Aggression Scale-9 score −0.72 with sodium valproate v −0.72 with placebo; P = 0.99).[68] The RCT did not report results before crossover.

Harms: **Versus placebo:** The first RCT found that adverse effects, generally rated as mild, were significantly more common with sodium valproate than with placebo (68% with sodium valproate v 33% with placebo; P = 0.003).[67]

Comment: The need to perform adjustments for covariates in the first RCT weakens the findings.[67]

OPTION TRAZODONE

We found no RCTs comparing trazodone versus placebo. One small RCT in people with agitated behaviour associated with dementia found no significant difference in agitation over 9 weeks between trazodone and haloperidol. Another small RCT in people with Alzheimer's disease and agitated behaviour found no significant difference in outcomes over 16 weeks among trazodone, haloperidol, behaviour management techniques, and placebo. The RCTs may have been underpowered to detect a clinically important difference.

Benefits: **Versus placebo:** We found not RCTs. **Versus haloperidol:** We found no systematic review but found two RCTs.[69,70] The first RCT (double blind, 28 elderly people with agitated behaviour associated with Alzheimer's disease, vascular dementia, or mixed Alzheimer's disease and vascular dementia, 9 weeks' duration) compared trazodone 50–250 mg daily versus haloperidol 1–5 mg daily.[69] It found no significant difference in agitation between the groups, but the trial was too small to exclude a clinically important difference. The second RCT (double blind, 149 people with Alzheimer's disease and agitated behaviours, 16 weeks' duration) compared four treatments: haloperidol (mean dose 1.1 mg daily); trazodone (mean dose 200 mg daily); behaviour management techniques; or placebo.[70] It found no significant difference in outcome (Alzheimer's Disease Co-operative Study Clinical Global Impression of Change) between the four interventions, but it may have been too small to exclude a clinically important difference.

Harms: **Versus haloperidol:** In the first RCT, adverse effects were more common in the group treated with haloperidol than trazodone.[69] In the second RCT, no significant differences in adverse events were seen between the trazodone group and the placebo group.[70]

Comment: None.

OPTION DONEPEZIL

One RCT found that donepezil improved functional and behavioural symptoms at 24 weeks compared with placebo. Two RCTs found no significant difference in psychiatric symptoms at 6 months to 1 year between donepezil and placebo. Many of the people included in the RCTs did not have behavioural and psychological problems.

Benefits: **Versus placebo:** We found one systematic review (search date 2001)[71] and two additional RCTs.[21,72] The review did not report results for donepezil alone. It identified one RCT (286 people with mild to moderate Alzheimer's disease, Mini Mental State Examination [MMSE] score 10–26, at least 1 symptom on the Neuropsychiatric Inventory Score [NPI]) comparing donepezil (5 mg daily for 28 days, followed by 10 mg daily) versus placebo over 1 year.[73] It found no significant difference in psychiatric symptoms at 1 year (measured by NPI; reported as non-significant; no further data reported). The first additional RCT (208 people with mild to moderate Alzheimer's disease, at least 1 symptom on the Neuropsychiatric Inventory Score, Nursing Home version and living in a nursing home) found no significant difference in psychiatric symptoms after 24 weeks of treatment between donepezil and placebo (change in mean Neuropsychiatric Inventory Nursing Home version Q scores −4.9 with donepezil v −2.3 with placebo; reported as non-significant; no further data reported).[72] The second additional RCT (290 people with moderate to severe Alzheimer's disease aged 48–92 years, MMSE score 5–17, Disability Assessment for Dementia [DAD] score 2.5–100, at least 1 symptom on the NPI score) compared donepezil (5–10 mg daily) versus placebo.[21] It found that donepezil significantly improved functional and behavioural symptoms at 24 weeks compared with placebo (Disability Assessment for Dementia score; mean difference 8.23, $P < 0.001$; NPI score; mean difference 5.64; $P < 0.0001$).

Harms: See harms of donepezil, p 80.

Comment: Cholinesterase inhibitors improve cognitive function and are well tolerated in older people. Only one of the RCTs assessed behavioural and psychological problems as a primary outcome.[72] Many of the people included in the RCTs did not have behavioural and psychological problems.[21,72,73] Some people took sedatives, which may have affected the results.

OPTION | **GALANTAMINE**

RCTs provided inconclusive evidence about the effects of galantamine compared with placebo on behavioural and psychiatric symptoms in people with mild to moderate Alzheimer's disease.

Benefits: **Versus placebo:** We found one systematic review (search date 2002), which identified two RCTs that assessed the effects of galantamine on behavioural and psychological symptoms.[25] A meta-analysis was not performed because of differences in length of follow up between the trials. Both trials used the Neuropsychiatric Inventory (NPI) scale. The first RCT (386 people with mild to moderate Alzheimer's disease; Mini Mental State Examination score 10–22) found no significant difference in psychiatric symptoms at 3 months between galantamine (12–16 mg twice daily) and placebo (mean reduction in NPI score −0.30 with galantamine v +0.50 with placebo; WMD −0.80, 95% CI −2.67 to +1.07). The second RCT (978 people with mild to moderate Alzheimer's disease; Mini Mental State Examination score 12–24) found that galantamine 16 mg daily significantly reduced psychiatric symptoms at 6 months compared with placebo (mean reduction in NPI score −0.10 with galantamine v +2.00 with placebo; WMD −2.10, 95% CI −4.04 to −0.16). However, it found no significant difference with galantamine (8 or 24 mg daily).[25]

Harms: See harms of galantamine, p 81.

Comment: Neither RCT assessed behavioural and psychological problems as a primary outcome.[25] Many of the people included in the RCTs did not have behavioural and psychological problems. Some people took sedatives, which may have affected the results.

OPTION   REALITY ORIENTATION

One systematic review found that reality orientation improved behaviour compared with no treatment in people with various types of dementia.

Benefits: **Versus no treatment:** We found one systematic review (search date 2000, 6 RCTs, 125 people with various types of dementia).[56] It found that reality orientation (see glossary, p 97) significantly improved behavioural symptom score compared with no treatment (SMD −0.66, 95% CI −1.27 to −0.05). No separate analysis was done for specific types of dementia.

Harms: **Versus no treatment:** The RCTs gave no information on adverse effects.[56]

Comment: The RCTs did not use standardised interventions or outcomes.[56]

GLOSSARY

Reality orientation Involves presenting information that is designed to reorient a person in time, place, or person. It may range in intensity from a board giving details of the day, date, and season, to staff reorienting a patient at each contact.

Reminiscence therapy Involves encouraging people to talk about the past in order to enable past experiences to be brought into consciousness. It relies on remote memory, which is relatively well preserved in mild to moderate dementia.

REFERENCES

1. van Duijn CM. Epidemiology of the dementia: recent developments and new approaches. *J Neurol Neurosurg Psychiatry* 1996;60:478–488.
2. McKeith IG, Galasko D, Kosaka K, et al. Consensus guidelines for the clinical and pathological diagnosis of dementia with Lewy bodies (DLB): report of the consortium on DLB International workshop. *Neurology* 1996;47:1113–1124.
3. Rasmusson DX, Brandt J, Steele C, et al. Accuracy of clinical diagnosis of Alzheimer disease and clinical features of patients with non-Alzheimer's disease neuropathology. *Alzheimer Dis Assoc Disord* 1996;10:180–188.
4. Verghese J, Crystal HA, Dickson DW, et al. Validity of clinical criteria for the diagnosis of dementia with Lewy bodies. *Neurology* 1999;53:1974–1982.
5. Lobo A, Launer LJ, Fratiglioni L, et al. Prevalence of dementia and major subtypes in Europe: a collaborative study of population-based cohorts. *Neurology* 2000;54:S4–S9.
6. Farrer L. Intercontinental epidemiology of Alzheimer's disease: a global approach to bad gene hunting. *JAMA* 2001;285:796–798.

7. Skoog I. A population-based study of dementia in 85 year olds. *N Engl J Med* 1993;328:153–158.
8. McKeith IG. Clinical Lewy body syndromes. *Ann N Y Acad Sci* 2000;920:1–8.
9. Inkeda M, Hokoishi K, Maki N, et al. Increased prevalence of vascular dementia in Japan: a community-based epidemiological study. *Neurology* 2001;57:839–844.
10. McKeith I. The differential diagnosis of dementia. In: Burns A, Levy R, eds. *Dementia*. 1st ed. London: Chapman and Hall, 1994:39–57.
11. Hardy J. Molecular classification of Alzheimer's disease. *Lancet* 1991;1:1342–1343.
12. Eastwood R, Reisberg B. Mood and behaviour. In: Panisset M, Stern Y, Gauthier S, eds. *Clinical diagnosis and management of Alzheimer's disease*. 1st ed. London: Dunitz, 1996:175–189.
13. Absher JR, Cummings JL. Cognitive and noncognitive aspects of dementia syndromes. In: Burns A, Levy R, eds. *Dementia*. 1st ed. London: Chapman and Hall, 1994:59–76.
14. Burns A, Lawlor B, Craig S. Assessment scales in old age psychiatry. London: Martin Dunitz. 1998.
15. Gelinas I, Gauthier L, McIntyre M, et al. Development of a functional measure for persons

with Alzheimer's disease: the Disability Assessment for Dementia. *Am J Occup Ther* 1999;53:471–481.

16. Lawton MP, Brody EM. Assessment of older people: self-maintaining and instrumental activities of daily living. *Gerontologist* 1969;9:179–186.

17. Rosen WG, Mohs RC, Davis KL. A new rating scale for Alzheimer's disease. *Am J Psychiatry* 1984;141:1356–1364.

18. Folstein MF, Folstein SE, McHugh PR. Mini Mental State: a practical method for grading the cognitive state of patients for the clinician. *J Psychiatr Res* 1975;12:189–198.

19. Schmitt FA, Ashford W, Ernesto C, et al. The severe impairment battery: concurrent validity and the assessment of longitudinal change in Alzheimer's disease. *Alzheimer Dis Assoc Disord* 1997;11:S51–S56.

20. Birks JS, Melzer D, Beppu H. Donepezil for mild and moderate Alzheimer's disease. In: The Cochrane Library, Issue 3, 2003. Oxford: Update Software. Search date 2003; primary sources Cochrane Dementia and Cognitive Impairment Group Specialized Register of Clinical Trials, Medline, Psychlit, Embase, the Donepezil Study Group, and Eisai Inc.

21. Feldman H, Gauthier S, Hecker J, et al. A 24-week, randomized, double blind study of donepezil in moderate to severe Alzheimer's disease. *Neurology* 2001;57:613–620.

22. Mohs, RC, Doody, RS, Morris, JC, et al, and Study Group. A 1-year, placebo-controlled preservation of function survival study of donepezil in AD patients. *Neurology* 2001;57:481–488.

23. Wilkinson DG. Passmore AP. Bullock R. et al. A multinational, randomised, 12-week, comparative study of donepezil and rivastigmine in patients with mild to moderate Alzheimer's disease. *Int J Clin Pract* 2002;56:441–446.

24. Rogers SL, Doody RS, Pratt RD, et al. Long term efficacy and safety of donepezil in the treatment of Alzheimer's disease: final analysis of a US multicentre open-label study. *Eur Neuropsychopharmacol* 2000;10:195–203.

25. Olin J, Schneider L. Olin J, et al. Galantamine for Alzheimer's disease. In: The Cochrane Library, Issue 3, 2003. Oxford: Update Software. Search date 2002; primary sources Cochrane Dementia Group Specialized Register of Clinical Trials, Cochrane Controlled Trials Register, Embase, Medline, Psychlit, Combined Health Information Database, National Research Register, Alzheimer's Disease Education and Referral Centre Clinical Database, Biomed (Biomedicine and Health), GlaxoWellcome Clinical Trials Register, National Institutes of Health Clinical Trials Databases, Current Controlled Trials, Dissertation Abstracts, Index to UK Theses, hand searched reference lists, and additional information collected from an unpublished investigational brochure for galantamine.

26. Erkinjuntti T, Kurz A, Gauthier S, et al. Efficacy of galantamine in probable vascular dementia and Alzheimer's disease combined with cerebrovascular disease: a randomised trial. *Lancet* 2002;359:1283–1290.

27. Birks J, Iakovidou V, Tsolaki M, et al. Rivastigmine for Alzheimer's disease. In: The Cochrane Library, Issue 3, 2003. Oxford: Update Software. Search date 2000; primary sources Cochrane Controlled Trials Register, Cochrane Dementia Group Specialized Register of Clinical Trials, Medline, Embase, Psychlit, Cinahl, and hand searches of geriatric and dementia journals and conference abstracts.

28. McKeith I, Del Ser T, Spano P, et al. Efficacy of rivastigmine in dementia with Lewy bodies: a randomised, double-blind, placebo-controlled international study. *Lancet* 2000;356:2031–2036.

29. Kumar V, Anand R, Messina J, et al. An efficacy and safety analysis of Exelon in Alzheimer's disease patients with concurrent vascular risk factors. *Eur J Neurol* 2000;7:159–169.

30. Coelho F, Filho JM, Birks J. Physostigmine for Alzheimer's disease. In: The Cochrane Library, Issue 3, 2003. Oxford: Update Software. Search date 2000; primary sources the Cochrane Dementia Group Specialized Register of Clinical Trials and pharmaceutical companies.

31. Qizilbash N, Whitehead A, Higgins J, et al. Cholinesterase inhibition for Alzheimer disease. *JAMA* 1998;280:1777–1782. Search date not reported; primary sources Cochrane Dementia Group Registry of Clinical Trials, contact with trial investigators, and Parke-Davis Pharmaceuticals.

32. Arrieta JR, Artalejo FR. Methodology, results and quality of clinical trials of tacrine in the treatment of Alzheimer's disease: a systematic review of the literature. *Age Ageing* 1998;27:161–179. Search date 1997; primary sources Cochrane Library and Medline.

33. Koepp R, Miles SH. Meta-analysis of tacrine for Alzheimer's disease: the influence of industry sponsors. *JAMA* 1999;281:2287–2288.

34. Knapp MJ, Knopman DS, Solomon PR, et al. A 30-week randomized controlled trial of high-dose tacrine in patients with Alzheimer's disease. The Tacrine Study Group. *JAMA* 1994;271:985–991.

35. Higgins JPT, Flicker L. Lecithin for dementia and cognitive impairment. In: The Cochrane Library, Issue 3, 2003. Oxford: Update Software. Search date 2002; primary sources Cochrane Dementia and Cognitive Impairment Group Specialized Register of Clinical Trials, Medline, Embase, Psychlit, ISI, Current Contents, and hand searched reference lists and textbooks.

36. López-Arrieta JM, Rodríguez JL, Sanz F. Nicotine for Alzheimer's disease. In: The Cochrane Library, Issue 3, 2003. Oxford: Update Software. Search date 2001; primary source Cochrane Dementia Group Specialized Register of Clinical Trials.

37. Scharf S, Mander A, Ugoni A, et al. A double-blind, placebo-controlled trial of diclofenac/misoprostol in Alzheimer's disease. *Neurology* 1999;53:197–201.

38. Rogers J, Kirby LC, Hempleman SR, et al. Clinical trial of indomethacin in Alzheimer's disease. *Neurology* 1993;43:1609–1611.

39. Williams PS, Spector A, Orrell M, et al. Aspirin for vascular dementia. In: The Cochrane Library, Issue 3, 2003. Oxford: Update Software. Search date 2000; primary sources Medline, Cochrane Library Trials Register, Embase, Cinahl, Psychlit, Amed, Sigle, National Research Register, hand searched reference lists, and contact with specialists.

40. Hogervorst E, Williams J, Budge M, et al. The nature of the effect of female gonadal hormone replacement therapy on cognitive function in post-menopausal women: a meta-analysis. *Neuroscience* 2000;101:485–512. Search date 2000; primary sources Medline, Embase, Psychlit, and hand searches of reference lists.

41. Birks J, Flicker L. Selegiline for Alzheimer's disease. In: The Cochrane Library, Issue 3, 2003. Oxford: Update Software. Search date 2002; primary source Cochrane Dementia and Cognitive Impairment Group Register of Clinical Trials.

42. Areosa Sastre A, Sherriff F. Memantine for dementia. In: The Cochrane Library, Issue 3, 2003. Oxford: Update Software. Search date

2002; primary sources Cochrane Dementia and Cognitive Improvement Group Specialised Trials Register.

43. Winblad B, Poritis N. Memantine in severe dementia: results of the M-Best study (benefit and efficacy in severely demented patients during treatment with memantine). *Int J Geriatr Psychiatry* 1999;14:135–146.

44. Reisberg B, Doody R, Stoffler A, et al. Memantine in moderate to severe Alzheimer's disease. *New Engl J Med* 2003;348:1333–1341.

45. Wilcock G, Mobius HJ, Stoffler A. A double-blind, placebo-controlled multicentre study of memantine in mild to moderate vascular dementia (MMM500). *Int Clin Psychopharmacol* 2002;17:297–305.

46. Wimo A, Winblad B, Stoffler A, et al. Resource utilisation and cost analysis of memantine in patients with moderate to severe Alzheimer's disease. *Pharmacoeconomics* 2003;21:327–340.

47. Gortelmeyer R, Erbler H. Memantine in the treatment of mild to moderate dementia syndrome. A double-blind placebo-controlled study. *Arzneimittelforschung/Drug Research* 1992;42:904–913.

48. Ditzler K. Efficacy and tolerability of memantine in patients with dementia syndrome. A double-blind, placebo controlled trial. *Arzneimittelforschung/Drug Research* 1991;41:773–780.

49. Birks J, Grimley Evans J, Van Dongen M. Ginkgo biloba for cognitive impairment and dementia In: The Cochrane Library, Issue 3, 2003. Oxford, Update Software. Search date 2002; primary source Cochrane Dementia and Cognitive Impairment Group Specialised Register of Controlled Clinical Trials.

50. Le Bars P, Katz MM, Berman N, et al. A placebo-controlled, double-blind, randomised trial of an extract of Ginkgo biloba for dementia. *JAMA* 1997;278:1327–1332.

51. Tabet N, Birks J, Grimley Evans J. Vitamin E for Alzheimer's disease. In: The Cochrane Library, Issue 3, 2003. Oxford: Update Software. Search date 2000; primary sources Cochrane Dementia and Cognitive Impairment Group Specialized Register of Clinical Trials

52. Sano M, Ernesto C, Thomas RG, et al. A controlled trial of selegiline, α-tocopherol, or both as treatment for Alzheimer's disease. *N Engl J Med* 1997;336:1216–1222.

53. Myers DG, Maloley PA, Weeks D. Safety of antioxidant vitamins. *Arch Intern Med* 1996;156:925–935.

54. Koger SM, Chaplin K, Brotons M. Is music therapy an effective intervention for dementia? A meta-analytic review of the literature. *J Music Ther* 1999;36:2–15. Search date 1998; primary sources Medline, Psychlit, and hand searched reference lists.

55. Koger SM, Brotons M. Music therapy for dementia symptoms. In: Cochrane Library, Issue 3, 2003. Oxford: Update Software. Search date 2000; primary sources Medline, Cochrane Dementia and Cognitive Improvement Group Trials Register, Embase, Cinahl, and Psychlit.

56. Spector A, Orrell M, Davies S, et al. Reality orientation for dementia. In: The Cochrane Library, Issue 3, 2003. Oxford: Update Software. Search date 2000; primary sources Medline, Psychlit, Embase, Cochrane Database of Systematic Reviews, Omni, Bids, Dissertation Abstracts International, Sigle, plus internet searching of HealthWeb, Mental Health Infosources, American Psychiatric Association, Internet Mental Health, Mental Health Net, NHS Confederation, and hand searches of specialist journals.

57. Spector A, Orrell M. Reminiscence therapy for dementia. In: The Cochrane Library, Issue 3, 2003. Oxford: Update Software. Search date 2000; primary sources Cochrane Controlled Trials Register, Medline, Psychlit, Embase, Omni, Bids, Dissertation Abstracts International, Sigle, reference lists of relevant articles, internet sites, and hand searching of specialist journals.

58. Lonergan E, Luxenberg J, Colford J. Haloperidol for agitation in dementia. In: The Cochrane Library, Issue 3, 2003. Oxford: Update Software. Search date 2000; primary sources Cochrane Controlled Trials Register, Cochrane Dementia Group Specialized Register of Clinical Trials, Medline, Embase, Psychlit, Cinahl, and GlaxoWellcome Trials database.

59. Pwee KH, Shukla VK, Hermann N, et al. Novel antipsychotics for agitation in dementia: a systematic review. Ottawa: Canadian Coordinating Office for Health Technology Assessment; 2003. Technology report No 36. Search date 2002; primary sources Medline, Embase, Psychinfo, Ageline, Biosis Previews, Pascal, Toxfile, Health Technology Assessment website and other relevant websites, hand searches of bibliographies and conference proceedings, and contact with experts in the field.

60. McShane R, Keene J, Gedling K, et al. Do neuroleptic drugs hasten cognitive decline in dementia? Prospective study with necropsy follow up. *BMJ* 1997;314:266–269.

61. McKeith IG. Dementia with Lewy Bodies. *Br J Psychiatry* 2002;180:144–147.

62. Street JS, Clark WS, Gannon KS, et al. Olanzapine treatment of psychotic and behavioural symptoms in patients with Alzheimer's disease in nursing care facilities: a double-blind, randomised, placebo-controlled trial. *Arch Gen Psychiatry* 2000;57:968–976.

63. Brodaty H, Ames D, Snowdon J, et al. A randomized placebo-controlled trial of risperidone for the treatment of aggression, agitation, and psychosis of dementia. *J Clin Psychiatry* 2003;64:134–143.

64. Wooltorton E. Risperidone (Risperdal): increased rate of cerebrovascular events in dementia trials. *CMAJ* 2002;167:1269–1270.

65. Food and Drug Association. Medwatch. 2003 Safety Alert Risperidal (risperidone). Available online at http://www.fda.gov/medwatch/SAFETY/2003/risperdal.htm (last accessed 16 March 2004).

66. Tariot PN, Erb R, Podgorski CA, et al. Efficacy and tolerability of carbamazepine for agitation and aggression in dementia. *Am J Psychiatry* 1998;155:54–61.

67. Porsteinsson AOP, Tariot PN, Erb R, et al. Placebo-controlled study of divalproex sodium for agitation in dementia. *Am J Geriatr Psychiatry* 2001;9:58–66.

68. Sival RC, Haffmans PMJ, Jansen PAF, et al. Sodium valproate in the treatment of aggressive behaviour in patients with dementia — a randomised placebo controlled clinical trial. *Int J Geriatr Psychiatry* 2002;17:579–585.

69. Sultzer DL, Gray KF, Gunay I, et al. A double-blind comparison of trazodone and haloperidol for treatment of agitation in patients with dementia. *Am J Geriatr Psychiatry* 1997;5:60–69.

70. Teri L, Logsdon RG, Peskind E, et al. Treatment of agitation in AD: a randomised, placebofc-controlled clinical trial. *Neurology* 2000;55:1271–1278.

71. Trinh NH, Hoblyn J, Mohanty S, et al. Efficacy of cholinesterase inhibitors in the treatment of neuropsychiatric symptoms and functional impairment in Alzheimer disease: a meta-analysis.

JAMA 2003;289:210–216. Search date 2001; primary sources Medline, Dissertation Abstracts Online, Psychinfo, Biosis, Pubmed, Cochrane Controlled Trials Register, and hand searches of references of bibliographies and relevant articles.

72. Taroit PN, Cummings JL, Katz IR, et al. A randomized double blind placebo controlled study of the efficacy and safety of donepezil in patients with Alzheimer's disease in the nursing home setting. *J Am Geriatr Soc* 2001;49:1590–1599.

73. Winblad B, Engedal K, Sonininen H, et al. A 1-year, randomized, placebo-controlled study of donepezil in patients with mild to moderate AD. *Neurology* 2001;57:489–495.

74. Atypical antipsychotic drugs and stroke. Committee on Safety of Medicines. Available online at http://www.mca.gov.uk (last accessed 17 March 2004).

James Warner
Senior Lecturer/Consultant in Old Age
Psychiatry
Imperial College
London
UK

Rob Butler
Honorary Clinical Lecturer in Psychiatry
and Consultant in Old Age Psychiatry
University of Auckland and Waitemata
Health
Auckland
New Zealand

Pradeep Arya
Specialist Registrar
CNWL Mental Health Trust
London
UK

Competing interests: JW has been reimbursed by Novartis, the manufacturer of rivastigmine, for conference attendance and has received speaker fees from Janssen Pharmaceuticals for educational events. RB has been reimbursed by Novartis for conference attendance. PP, none declared.

TABLE 1 Effects on cognitive symptoms of donepezil, galantamine, and rivastigmine compared with placebo.

Drug	Dose (mg)	Duration (weeks)	Difference in ADAS-cog	NNT for at least 4 point change in ADAS-cog	OR for global improvement	OR for all cause withdrawal	Ref
Donepezil	10 od	24	−2.9 (−3.7 to −2.2)	N/A	2.1 (1.3 to 3.6)	1.4 (1.0 to 1.8)	20
Galantamine	12 bd	24	−3.3 (−3.9 to −2.7)	7 (4 to 10)	1.9 (1.4 to 2.5)	2.1 (1.5 to 2.9)	25
(observed case analysis)	16 bd	24	−3.3 (−4.1 to −2.4)	5 (5 to 12)	2.0 (1.6 to 2.5)	3.3 (2.5 to 4.3)	25
Rivastigmine	6–12 bd	28	−2.10 (−2.65 to −1.54)	17 (12 to 34)	1.5 (1.2 to 1.8)	2.4 (2.0 to 3.0)	28

Results are intention to treat unless stated. bd, twice daily; od, once daily; N/A, not applicable; Ref, reference.

Depression in children and adolescents

Search date May 2003

Philip Hazell

QUESTIONS

INTERVENTIONS

Key Messages

- **Cognitive behavioural therapy** One systematic review in children and adolescents with mild to moderate depression has found that cognitive behavioural therapy improves symptoms compared with non-specific support. One RCT in depressed adolescents with depressed parents found no significant difference in recovery from depression between cognitive behavioural therapy plus usual care and usual care alone over 2 years.

- **Interpersonal therapy** Two RCTs found that interpersonal therapy versus clinical monitoring or waiting list control increased recovery rate over 12 weeks in adolescents with mild to moderate depression.

- **Selective serotonin reuptake inhibitors** We found limited evidence that selective serotonin reuptake inhibitors improved symptoms of depression compared with placebo; one RCT found no significant difference, one RCT found significant results on some depression measures but not others, while one RCT found improvement in depressive symptoms with fluoxetine compared with placebo after 8–9 weeks. One RCT found that, in adolescents with major depression, paroxetine improved remission after 8 weeks compared with placebo. Another RCT found no significant difference in effects on outcomes between paroxetine and clomipramine, although it may have lacked power to detect clinically important effects. We found no RCTs on other selective serotonin reuptake inhibitors. Selective serotonin reuptake inhibitors are frequently associated with dizziness, light-headedness, drowsiness, poor concentration, nausea, headache, and fatigue if treatment is reduced or stopped.

- **Electroconvulsive therapy** We found no RCTs on electroconvulsive therapy in children and adolescents with depression.

- **Intravenous clomipramine** One small RCT found that, in non-suicidal adolescents, intravenous clomipramine improved depression scores at 6 days compared with placebo. However, the trial was too small and brief for us to draw reliable conclusions.

- **Lithium** One small RCT in children with depression and a family history of bipolar affective disorder found no significant difference between lithium and placebo in global assessment or depression scores after 6 weeks. However, the study may have lacked power to detect clinically important effects.

- **Monoamine oxidase inhibitors** One RCT found insufficient evidence to compare the reversible monoamine oxidase inhibitor moclobemide versus placebo in children aged 9–15 years with major depression, some of whom had a comorbid disorder. We found no RCTs on non-reversible monoamine oxidase inhibitors in children or adolescents.

- **St John's Wort** We found no RCTs on St John's Wort (*Hypericum perforatum*) in children or adolescents with depression.

- **Venlafaxine** One small RCT in children and adolescents with major depression receiving psychotheray found no significant difference between venlafaxine and placebo in improvement of depressive symptoms after 6 weeks. However, the study may have lacked power to detect clinically important effects.

- **Tricyclic antidepressants (in adolescents)** One systematic review in adolescents and children found no significant difference in depression scores between oral tricyclic antidepressants (amitriptyline, desipramine, imipramine, nortriptyline) and placebo after 4–10 weeks. However, subgroup analyses found that oral tricyclic antidepressants improved symptoms compared with placebo in adolescents but not children. There was no significant difference in rates of remission. The review also found that oral tricyclic antidepressants were associated with adverse effects. One RCT found no significant difference in improvement rates between oral clomipramine and paroxetine after 8 weeks.

- **Tricyclic antidepressants (in children)** Subgroup analyses in one systematic review found no significant difference between oral tricyclic antidepressants (amitriptyline, desipramine, imipramine, nortriptyline) and placebo in children with depression. The review also found that oral tricyclic antidepressants were associated with adverse effects.

- **Family therapy; specific psychological treatments other than cognitive behavioural therapy** We found insufficient evidence in children and adolescents about the effects of these interventions.

DEFINITION   Compared with adult depression (see depressive disorders, p 114), depression in children (6–12 years) and adolescents (13–18 years) may have a more insidious onset, may be characterised more by irritability than sadness, and occurs more often in association with other conditions such as anxiety, conduct disorder, hyperkinesis, and learning problems.[1] The term "major depression" is used to distinguish discrete episodes of depression from mild, chronic (1 year or longer) low mood or irritability, which is known as "dysthymia".[1] The severity of depression may be defined by the level of impairment and the presence or absence of psychomotor changes and somatic symptoms (see depressive disorders, p 114). In some studies, severity of depression is defined according to cut off scores on depression rating scales. A manic episode is defined by abnormally and persistently elevated, expansive, or irritable mood. Additional symptoms may include grandiosity, decreased need for sleep, pressured speech, flight of ideas, distractibility, psychomotor agitation, and impaired judgement.[2]

INCIDENCE/ PREVALENCE Estimates of prevalence of depression among children and adolescents in the community range from 2–6%.[3,4] Prevalence tends to increase with age, with a sharp rise at around the onset of puberty. Pre-adolescent boys and girls are affected equally by the condition, but depression is seen more frequently among adolescent girls than boys.[5]

AETIOLOGY/ RISK FACTORS The aetiology is uncertain, but may include genetic vulnerability,[6] childhood events, and current psychosocial adversity.[1]

PROGNOSIS In children and adolescents, the recurrence rate after a first depressive episode is 70% by 5 years, which is similar to the recurrence rate in adults. It is not clear whether this is related to the severity of depression.[1] Young people experiencing a moderate to severe depressive episode may be more likely than adults to have a manic episode within the following few years.[1,7] Trials of treatments for child and adolescent depression have found high rates of response to placebo (as much as two thirds of people in some inpatient studies).[8] A third of young people who experience a depressive episode will make a suicide attempt at some stage, and 3–4% will die from suicide.[1]

AIMS OF INTERVENTION To improve mood, social and occupational functioning, and quality of life; to reduce morbidity and mortality; to prevent recurrence of depressive disorder; and to minimise adverse effects of treatment.

OUTCOMES In children and adolescents, there are developmentally specific pseudo-continuous measures such as the Children's Depression Rating Scale and the Children's Depression Inventory, although some studies of adolescents use scales developed for use in adults such as the Hamilton Rating Scale for Depression. Pseudo-continuous measures reported by parents, such as the Children's Depression Inventory for Parents, are also used. Categorical outcomes are sometimes expressed as people no longer meeting specified criteria for depression on a structured psychiatric interview such as the Kiddie-SADS, which combines data from children and their parents. Global improvement in symptoms as judged by an investigator is sometimes reported using the Clinical Global Impressions Scale or the Clinical Global Assessment Scale.

METHODS *Clinical Evidence* search and appraisal May 2003, plus additional references identified by contributor.

QUESTION What are the effects of treatments?

OPTION TRICYCLIC ANTIDEPRESSANTS

One systematic review in adolescents and children found no significant difference in depression scores between oral tricyclic antidepressants (amitriptyline, desipramine, imipramine, nortriptyline) and placebo after 4–10 weeks. However, subgroup analyses found that oral tricyclic antidepressants improved symptoms compared with placebo in adolescents, but not in children. There was no significant difference in rates of remission. The review also found that oral tricyclic antidepressants were associated with adverse effects. One RCT found no significant difference in improvement rates between oral clomipramine and paroxetine after 8 weeks. One small RCT found that, in non-suicidal adolescents, intravenous clomipramine improved depression scores at 6 days compared with placebo.

Benefits:
Oral tricyclic antidepressants versus placebo: We found one systematic review (search date 2000, 13 RCTs, 506 children and adolescents aged 6–18 years, severity of depression not stated) comparing oral tricyclic antidepressants (amitriptyline, desipramine, imipramine, and nortriptyline) versus placebo.[8] It found no significant difference in overall improvement between tricyclic antidepressants and placebo after 4–10 weeks (OR 0.84, 95% CI 0.56 to 1.25). Subgroup analyses found a significant reduction in symptoms with tricyclic antidepressants versus placebo in adolescents (7 RCTs; 351 people; effect size SMD –0.47, 95% CI –0.92 to –0.02). However, there was no significant difference in children (3 RCTs; 65 people; effect size SMD +0.15, 95% CI –0.64 to +0.34). **Oral tricyclic antidepressants versus selective serotonin reuptake inhibitors:** See benefits of selective serotonin reuptake inhibitors (paroxetine with the predominantly serotonergic tricyclic antidepressant clomipramine), p 107. **Pulsed intravenous clomipramine:** We found one RCT (16 non-suicidal adolescent outpatients, aged 14–18 years, with major depression [21-item Hamilton Rating Scale for Depression score ≥ 18]), which compared pulse intravenous clomipramine (see glossary, p 112) 200 mg versus placebo.[9] It found that intravenous clomipramine significantly reduced Hamilton Rating Scale for Depression scores compared with placebo at 6 days (mean reduction in score: 15.0 with clomipramine v 9.0 with placebo, P < 0.05). However, it found no significant difference in remission rate (remission defined as ≥ 50% decrease in Hamilton Rating Scale for Depression scores; AR 7/8 [88%] with intravenous clomipramine v 3/8 [38%] with placebo; P = 0.06).[9] The study may have lacked power to detect a clinically important effect.

Harms:
Oral tricyclic antidepressants: The systematic review found that tricyclic antidepressants were more commonly associated with vertigo (OR 8.47, 95% CI 1.40 to 51.00), orthostatic hypotension (OR 4.77, 95% CI 1.11 to 20.50), tremor (OR 6.29, 95% CI 1.78 to 22.17), and dry mouth (OR 5.19, 95% CI 1.15 to 23.5) than placebo.[8] The review found no significant differences between tricyclic antidepressants and placebo in tiredness (OR 1.52, 95%

CI 0.63 to 3.67), sleep problems (OR 1.87, 95% CI 0.84 to 4.14), headache (OR 1.15, 95% CI 0.68 to 1.95), palpitations (OR 1.20, 95% CI 0.17 to 8.68), perspiration (OR 2.01, 95% CI 0.39 to 10.44), constipation (OR 1.94, 95% CI 0.72 to 5.24), or problems with micturition (OR 0.30, 95% CI 0.01 to 7.89). **Pulsed intravenous clomipramine:** The RCT did not report any adverse effects.[9]

Comment: We found single case reports and case series of toxicity and mortality from tricyclic antidepressants in overdose and therapeutic doses. Further research is needed to determine long term effects of intravenous clomipramine.

OPTION **MONOAMINE OXIDASE INHIBITORS**

One RCT found insufficient evidence to compare moclobemide versus placebo in children aged 9–15 years with major depression, some of whom had a comorbid disorder. We found no RCTs on non-reversible monoamine oxidase inhibitors in children or adolescents.

Benefits: We found no systematic review. **Reversible monoamine oxidase inhibitors:** We found one small RCT (20 Turkish children aged 9–15 years with major depression, including 13 children with a comorbid disorder) comparing moclobemide versus placebo for 5 weeks.[10] The RCT found that moclobemide significantly improved clinician rated scale scores (Clinical Global Impressions Scale — investigator assessment of severity of depression, adverse effects, and global recovery) compared with placebo after 5 weeks but not on parent rated (Children's Depression Inventory for Parents) and self reported measures (Children's Depression Inventory).[10] The small sample size limits the conclusions that may be drawn from this RCT.[10] **Non-reversible monoamine oxidase inhibitors:** We found no RCTs.

Harms: The RCT found no significant difference in adverse events assessed using Clinical Global Impression of adverse effects scale and self assessed adverse effects forms between moclobemide and placebo.[10] We found no information on the safety of moclobemide usage in children younger than 9 years.

Comment: None.

OPTION **SELECTIVE SEROTONIN REUPTAKE INHIBITORS**

We found limited evidence that selective serotonin reuptake inhibitors improved symptoms of depression compared with placebo; one RCT found no significant difference, one RCT found significant results on some depression measures but not others, and one RCT found improvement in depressive symptoms with fluoxetine compared with placebo after 8–9 weeks. One RCT found that, in adolescents with major depression, paroxetine improved remission after 8 weeks compared with placebo. Another RCT in people with major depression (aged 12–20 years) found no significant difference in effects on improvement rates between paroxetine and clomipramine, although it may have lacked power to detect clinically important effects. We found no RCTs on other selective

serotonin reuptake inhibitors. **Selective serotonin reuptake inhibitors are frequently associated with dizziness, light-headedness, drowsiness, poor concentration, nausea, headache, and fatigue if treatment is reduced or stopped.**

Benefits: **Fluoxetine:** We found one systematic review (search date 1998,[11] 2 RCTs[12,13]) and one subsequent RCT.[14] The systematic review did not pool results.[11] The first RCT identified by the review (40 adolescents, aged 13–18 years, of whom 30 completed the trial, severity of depression not stated) found no significant difference in the mean number of depression symptoms or psychosocial functioning (Clinical Global Impressions Scale) between fluoxetine 20–60 mg and placebo after 8 weeks (RR of failure to improve 1.00, 95% CI 0.36 to 2.75).[12] The second RCT identified by the review (96 children and adolescents aged 7–17 years with major depression) found that fluoxetine 20 mg significantly improved depression symptoms according to the self reported Children's Depression Scale compared with placebo after 8 weeks (proportion with improved Clinical Global Impressions Scale: 27/48 [56%] with fluoxetine v 16/48 [33%] with placebo; RR of failure to improve 0.66, 95% CI 0.45 to 0.96; proportion with improved self reported Children's Depression Rating Scale: 34% with fluoxetine v 18% with placebo; P < 0.01). The subsequent RCT (219 children and adolescents aged 8–17 years with major depression) found no significant difference between fluoxetine and placebo in response defined a priori on the Children's Depression Rating Scale at 8 weeks (response defined as ≥ 30% improvement in score: 71/109 [65%] with fluoxetine v 54/101 [54%] with placebo; P = 0.093).[14] The RCT found that fluoxetine significantly improved Children's Depression Rating Scale or Clinical Global Impressions Severity scale compared with placebo at 8 weeks (difference in mean improvement with fluoxetine v placebo; Children's Depression Rating Scale: 7.1, 95% CI 3.3 to 10.9; Clinical Global Impressions Severity Scale: 0.6, 95% CI 0.3 to 1.0). **Paroxetine:** We found two RCTs. The first RCT (180 adolescents, aged 12–18 years, of whom 133 completed the trial, severity of depression score of at least 12 on the Hamilton Rating Scale for Depression and < 60 on the Children's Global Assessment Scale) that compared effects of paroxetine 20–40 mg, imipramine (gradual upward titration to 200–300 mg), and placebo for 8 weeks with respect to end point response (Hamilton Rating Scale for Depression score ≤ 8 or a 50% reduction from baseline score) and change from baseline score (Hamilton Rating Scale for Depression).[15] The RCT did not include a direct statistical comparison of paroxetine with imipramine. The RCT found that paroxetine significantly improved response rate compared with placebo (AR for failure to respond 37% with paroxetine v 54% with placebo; ARI 17%, CI not reported; RR 0.68, 95% CI 0.49 to 0.95; P = 0.02). The second RCT (121 people aged 12–20 years with major depression) compared paroxetine versus clomipramine.[16] The RCT found no significant difference in rates of improvement after 8 weeks of treatment (achieving a score of 2 ["much" improved] or 1 ["very much" improved] on the Clinical Global Impressions Scale: 35/59 [59%] with paroxetine v 32/55 [58%] with clomipramine; P = 0.71). However, the trial may have lacked power to detect clinically important differences. **Other selective serotonin reuptake inhibitors:** We found no RCTs.

Harms: **Fluoxetine:** One of the RCTs included in the systematic review found significantly more weight loss with fluoxetine compared with placebo (data not reported).[12] The other included RCT did not report on adverse effects.[13] The subsequent RCT found that headache was reported significantly more often with fluoxetine versus placebo (P = 0.017).[14] **Paroxetine:** The first RCT reported more serious adverse events with paroxetine compared with placebo (12% with paroxetine v 2% with placebo).[15] The most common adverse events were somnolence (17% with paroxetine v 3% with placebo) and tremor (11% with paroxetine v 2% with placebo) but no statistical analyses were reported. A discontinuation syndrome after abrupt stopping or reduction in the dose of selective serotonin reuptake inhibitors has been described in a series of six cases.[17] The most frequent symptoms included dizziness, lightheadedness, drowsiness, poor concentration, nausea, headache, and fatigue.[17] The second RCT found significantly fewer adverse effects with paroxetine than with clomipramine (31/63 [49%] with paroxetine v 40/58 [69%] with clomipramine; P = 0.027).[16] The most common adverse events were dizziness (6.3% with paroxetine v 34.5% with clomipramine; P value not reported), headache (17.5% with paroxetine v 24.1% with clomipramine; P value not reported), and nausea (11.1% with paroxetine v 24.1% with clomipramine; P value not reported). There have been concerns about the safety of paroxetine in people under 18 years.

Comment: None.

OPTION   VENLAFAXINE

One small RCT in children and adolescents with major depression receiving psychotherapy found no significant difference between venlafaxine and placebo in improvement of depressive symptoms after 6 weeks. However, the study may have lacked power to detect clinically important effects.

Benefits: We found one systematic review (search date 1998,[11] 1 RCT[18]). The RCT (33 children and adolescents aged 8–17 years with major depression receiving psychotherapy) compared venlafaxine (37.5–75.0 mg/day in divided doses) and placebo for 6 weeks.[18] It found no significant difference in improvement of depressive symptoms with venlafaxine compared with placebo (Children's Depression Inventory: P = 0.37; Hamilton Rating Scale for Depression: P = 0.50; Children's Depression Rating Scale: P = 0.48).

Harms: The RCT reported nausea in a subgroup of participants aged ≥ 13 years.[18]

Comment: The RCT lacked power to rule out a clinically important difference.

OPTION   LITHIUM

One small RCT in children with depression and a family history of bipolar affective disorder found no significant difference between lithium and placebo in global assessment or depression scores after 6 weeks. However, the study may have lacked power to detect clinically important effects.

Benefits: We found no systematic review. We found one RCT (30 children, aged 6–12 years, with non-bipolar depression and family history of bipolar affective disorder) comparing lithium with placebo for 6 weeks.[19] The RCT found no significant difference between lithium and placebo (global assessment: P = 0.07; 9 depression items of the Kiddie-SADS interview: P = 0.91).

Harms: Of the 17 children randomised to lithium treatment, four were withdrawn because of adverse effects (3 had confusion, 1 had nausea and vomiting).[19]

Comment: The RCT lacked power to rule out a clinically important difference. It is not routine practice to give lithium alone to depressed children. Lithium is sometimes used to augment antidepressants and to prevent mania from developing with antidepressant use, but we found no RCTs of lithium for this indication.

OPTION   ST JOHN'S WORT (*HYPERICUM PERFORATUM*)

We found no RCTs on St John's Wort (*H perforatum*) in children or adolescents with depression.

Benefits: We found no systematic review and no RCTs.

Harms: We found no RCTs.

Comment: None.

OPTION   ELECTROCONVULSIVE THERAPY

We found no RCTs on electroconvulsive therapy in children and adolescents with depression.

Benefits: We found no systematic review and no RCTs.

Harms: We found no specific evidence on harms in children and adolescents. Known adverse effects in adults include memory impairment. See electroconvulsive therapy under depressive disorders, p 114.

Comment: None.

OPTION   SPECIFIC PSYCHOLOGICAL TREATMENTS

One systematic review has found that cognitive behavioural therapy increases resolution of symptoms compared with non-specific supportive therapies for children and adolescents with mild to moderate depression. One subsequent RCT in depressed adolescents with depressed parents found no significant difference in recovery from depression. We found limited evidence from two small RCTs that interpersonal therapy increases recovery in adolescents with mild to moderate depression

Mental health

compared with clinical monitoring alone or placement on a waiting list. We found insufficient evidence that family therapy or group treatments other than cognitive behavioural therapy are effective for depression in children and adolescents.

Benefits: **Cognitive behavioural therapy:** We found one systematic review (search date 1997, 6 RCTs, 376 children and adolescents with mild to moderate depression) of cognitive behavioural therapy (see glossary, p 111) versus other treatments ranging from waiting list control to supportive psychotherapy,[20] and one subsequent RCT.[21] The systematic review found that cognitive behavioural therapy significantly increased the rate of resolution of symptoms of depression compared with other treatments (OR 3.2, 95% CI 1.9 to 5.2; NNT 4, 95% CI 3 to 5).[20] The subsequent RCT (88 adolescents aged 13–18 years with major depression or dysthymia who had depressed parents) compared cognitive behavioural therapy (16 sessions) plus usual care with usual care alone.[21] The RCT found no significant difference in recovery rate between cognitive behavioural therapy plus usual care and usual care alone at 2 years (≥ 8 weeks with few or no depressive symptoms: 13/41 [31.7%] with cognitive behavioural therapy plus usual care v 14/47 [29.8%] with usual care alone; RR and P value not reported). A factor that could have contributed to the absence of a treatment effect was the higher level of impairment in the participants compared with other RCTs. **Interpersonal therapy:** We found two small RCTs comparing 12 weekly sessions of interpersonal therapy (see glossary, p 112) with clinical monitoring or waiting list control in adolescents with depression.[22,23] The first RCT (48 adolescents aged 12–18 years with major depressive disorder) found that interpersonal therapy significantly increased recovery rate compared with clinical monitoring (Hamilton Rating Scale for Depression < 6 or Beck Depressive Inventory score < 9: 18/24 [75%] with interpersonal therapy v 11/24 [46%] with clinical monitoring alone; RR 1.64, 95% CI 1.00 to 2.68; ARR 29%, 95% CI 3% to 56%).[22] The second RCT (46 adolescents with major depression) found no significant difference in the proportion of adolescents not manifesting severe depression between interpersonal therapy and being on a waiting list (defined by a cut off score on the Children's Depression Inventory: 17/19 [89%] with interpersonal therapy v 12/18 [67%] with waiting list; RR 1.33, 95% CI 0.94 to 1.93; ARR +22%, 95% CI −3% to +49%).[23] However, if the Children's Depression Inventory score was considered as a continuous measure, then the mean Children's Depression Inventory score was significantly lower after interpersonal therapy versus waiting list (P < 0.01). **Attachment based family therapy** We found one RCT (32 adolescents aged 13–17 years with major depression) comparing 6 weeks of attachment based family therapy (see glossary, p 112) versus 6 weeks of waiting list control.[24] It found no significant difference in remission rates between attachment based family therapy and waiting list control at 6 weeks (people no longer meeting criteria for major depression on the Kiddie-SADS interview: 13/16 [81%] with attachment based family therapy v 7/15 [47%] on the waiting list; RR 1.74, 95% CI 0.97 to 3.14). However, the study may have lacked the power to detect a clinically important difference between groups. **Systemic behavioural family therapy:** We found one RCT

(78 adolescents with major depressive disorder) comparing systemic behavioural family therapy (see glossary, p 112) versus non-specific supportive therapy.[25] The RCT found no significant difference in remission rates (combination of no longer meeting DSM-III-R criteria for major depression as determined by the Kiddie-SADS interview and Beck Depression Inventory score < 9: 29% with family therapy v 34% with non-specific supportive therapy). **Group administered cognitive behavioural therapy:** We found one RCT (123 adolescents aged 14–18 years with major depression or dysthymia) comparing group administered cognitive behavioural therapy versus waiting list control.[26] It found that cognitive behavioural therapy significantly increased the remission rate (as determined by Longitudinal Interval Follow-up Evaluation interview for DSM-III-R diagnoses: 46/69 [67%] with group cognitive behavioural therapy v 13/27 [48%] with waiting list control; P < 0.05). **Group therapeutic support versus group social skills training:** We found one RCT (66 adolescents aged 13–17 years, of whom 47 completed the protocol; 58 with major depression in the past year, 8 with dysthymia in the past year) comparing group therapeutic support versus group social skills training.[27] In 26 adolescents whose Kiddie-SADS scores were in the clinical range in the week before treatment, the RCT found no significant difference in remission rates (score of < 4 on Kiddie-SADS dysphoria and anhedonia symptoms: 8/16 [50%] with group therapeutic support v 4/10 [40%] with group social skills training; RR and P value not provided).

Harms: The RCTs did not report any adverse events.[21–30] We found no report of harms specifically for children and adolescents.

Comment: In the first RCT of interpersonal therapy, sessions were augmented by telephone contact.[22] No long term trials of pure treatment have been reported. However, we found one prospective study, in which 107 adolescents with depression had been randomised to cognitive behavioural therapy, systemic behavioural family therapy, or non-directive supportive therapy (see glossary, p 112).[31] After the initial trial phase of 16 weeks, they were allowed booster treatments and also had access to open treatment in any modality for the 2 years of follow up. They were assessed at 3 monthly intervals for the first 12 months and then again at 24 months. The study found no significant difference between groups in depressive symptoms (of 104 adolescents for whom there were sufficient follow up data, 38% experienced sustained recovery, 21% experienced persistent depression, and 41% had a relapsing course).[31]

GLOSSARY

Cognitive behavioural therapy A brief structured treatment (20 sessions over 12–16 weeks) aimed at changing the dysfunctional beliefs and negative automatic thoughts that characterise depressive disorders.[32] Cognitive behavioural therapy requires a high level of training for the therapist, and has been adapted for children and adolescents suffering from depression. A course of treatment is characterised by 8–12 weekly sessions, in which the therapist and the child collaborate to solve current difficulties. The treatment is structured and often directed by a manual. Treatment generally includes cognitive elements, such as the challenging of negative thoughts, and behavioural elements, such as structuring time to engage in pleasurable activity.

Interpersonal therapy A standardised form of brief psychotherapy (usually 12–16 weekly sessions) intended primarily for outpatients with unipolar non-psychotic depressive disorders. It focuses on improving the individual's interpersonal functioning and identifying the problems associated with the onset of the depressive episode.[33] In children and adolescents, interpersonal therapy has been adapted for adolescents to address common adolescent developmental issues, for example separation from parents, exploration of authority in relationship to parents, development of dyadic interpersonal relationships, initial experience with the death of a relative or friend, and peer pressure.

Non-directive supportive therapy Helping people to express feelings, and clarify thoughts and difficulties; therapists suggest alternative understandings and do not give direct advice but try to encourage people to solve their own problems.

Pulsed intravenous clomipramine An intravenous loading procedure for clomipramine.

Systemic behavioural family therapy A combination of two treatment approaches that have been used effectively for dysfunctional families. In the first phase of treatment, the therapist clarifies the concerns that brought the family into treatment, and provides a series of reframing statements designed to optimise engagement in therapy and identification of dysfunctional behaviour patterns (systemic therapy). In the second phase, the family members focus on communication and problem solving skills and the alteration of family interactional patterns (family behaviour therapy).

Attachment based family therapy A brief structured psychotherapy directed to adolescents and their parents or caregivers. It aims to repair attachment while promoting the autonomy of the adolescent. The treatment has five specific tasks; the focus of the family is shifted from "fixing" the individual to improving family relationships; an alliance is established with the individual; parental empathy for the individual is enhanced by exploring the parents' own stressors and history of attachment failure; the individual is encouraged to express previously unexpressed anger about core conflicts, and the individual is encouraged to make successful connections outside the home (e.g. at school, with peers, and at work).

REFERENCES

1. Birmaher B, Ryan ND, Williamson DE, et al. Childhood and adolescent depression: a review of the past 10 years, Part I. *J Am Acad Child Adolesc Psychiatry* 1996;35:1427–1439.

2. American Psychiatric Association. *Diagnostic and statistical manual of mental disorders, 4th ed.* Washington DC: American Psychiatric Association, 1994;328.

3. Costello EJ, Angold A, Burns BJ, et al. The Great Smoky Mountains Study of Youth. Goals, design, methods, and the prevalence of DSM-III-R disorders. *Arch Gen Psychiatry* 1996;53:1129–1136.

4. Costello EJ. Developments in child psychiatric epidemiology. *J Am Acad Child Adolesc Psychiatry* 1989;28:836–841.

5. Lewinsohn PM, Rohde P, Seely JR. Major depressive disorder in older adolescents: prevalence, risk factors, and clinical implications. *Clin Psychol Rev* 1998;18:765–794.

6. Rice F, Harold G, Thapar A. The genetic aetiology of childhood depression: a review. *J Child Psychol Psychiatry* 2002;43:65

7. Geller B, Fox LW, Fletcher M. Effect of tricyclic antidepressants on switching to mania and on the onset of bipolarity in depressed 6- to 12-year-olds. *J Am Acad Child Adolesc Psychiatry* 1993;32:43–50.

8. Hazell P, O'Connell D, Heathcote D, et al. Tricyclic drugs for depression in children and adolescents.

In: The Cochrane Library, Issue 3, 2002. Oxford: Update Software. Search date 2000; primary sources Medline, Excerpta Medica, and Cochrane trials database.

9. Sallee FR, Vrindavanam NS, Deas-Nesmith D, et al. Pulse intravenous clomipramine for depressed adolescents: double-blind, controlled trial. *Am J Psychiatry* 1997;154:668–673.

10. Avci A, Diler RS, Kibar M, et al. Comparison of moclobemide and placebo in young adolescents with major depressive disorder. *Ann Med Sci* 1999;8:31–40.

11. Williams JW, Mulrow CD, Chiquette E, et al. A systematic review of newer pharmacotherapies for depression in adults: evidence report summary. *Ann Intern Med* 2000;132:743–756. Search date 1998; primary sources Medline, Embase, Psychlit, Lilacs, Psyindex, Sigle, Cinahl, Biological Abstracts, Cochrane Controlled Trials, hand searches, and personal contacts.

12. Simeon JG, Dinicola VF, Ferguson HB, et al. Adolescent depression: a placebo-controlled fluoxetine treatment study and follow-up. *Prog Neuropsychopharmacol Biol Psychiatry* 1990;14:791–795.

13. Emslie GJ, Rush AJ, Weinberg WA, et al. A double-blind, randomized, placebo-controlled trial of fluoxetine in children and adolescents with depression. *Arch Gen Psychiatry* 1997;54:1031–1037.

14. Emslie GJ, Heiligenstein JH, Wagner KD, et al. Fluoxetine for acute treatment of depression in children and adolescents: a placebo-controlled, randomized clinical trial. *J Am Acad Child Adolesc Psychiatry* 2002;41:1205–1215.

15. Keller MB, Ryan ND, Strober M, et al. Efficacy of paroxetine in the treatment of adolescent major depression: a randomized, controlled trial. *J Am Acad Child Adolesc Psychiatry* 2001;40:762–772.

16. Braconnier A, Le Coent R, Cohen D. Paroxetine versus clomipramine in adolescents with severe major depression: a double-blind, randomized, multicenter trial. *J Am Acad Child Adolesc Psychiatry* 2003;42:22–29.

17. Diler RS, Avci A. Selective serotonin reuptake inhibitor discontinuation syndrome in children: six case reports. *Curr Ther Res Clin Exp* 2002;63:188–197.

18. Mandoki MW, Tapia MR, Tapia MA, et al. Venlafaxine in the treatment of children and adolescents with major depression. *Psychopharmacol Bull* 1997;33:149–154.

19. Geller B, Cooper TB, Zimerman B, et al. Lithium for prepubertal depressed children with family history predictors of future bipolarity: a double-blind, placebo-controlled study. *J Affect Disord* 1998;51:165–175.

20. Harrington R, Whittaker J, Shoebridge P, et al. Systematic review of efficacy of cognitive behavioural therapies in childhood and adolescent depressive disorder. *BMJ* 1998;316:1559–1563. Search date 1997; primary sources Medline, Psychlit, Cochrane, and hand searches of reference lists, book chapters, conference proceedings, and relevant journals in the field.

21. Clarke GN, Hornbrook M, Lynch F, et al. Group cognitive-behavioral treatment for depressed adolescent offspring of depressed patients in a Health Maintenance Organization. *J Am Acad Child Adolesc Psychiatry* 2002;41:305–313.

22. Mufson L, Weissman MM, Moreau D, et al. Efficacy of interpersonal psychotherapy for depressed adolescents. *Arch Gen Psychiatry* 1999;56:573–579.

23. Rossello J, Bernal G. The efficacy of cognitive-behavioral and interpersonal treatments for depression in Puerto Rican adolescents. *J Consult Clin Psychol* 1999;67:734–745.

24. Diamond GS, Reis BF, Diamond GM, et al. Attachment-based family therapy for depressed adolescents: a treatment development study. *J Am Acad Child Adolesc Psychiatry* 2002;41:1190–1196.

25. Brent DA, Holder D, Kolko D, et al. A clinical psychotherapy trial for adolescent depression comparing cognitive, family, and supportive therapy. *Arch Gen Psychiatry* 1997;54:877–885.

26. Clarke GN, Rohde P, Lewinsohn PM, et al. Cognitive-behavioral treatment of adolescent depression: efficacy of acute group treatment and booster sessions. *J Am Acad Child Adolesc Psychiatry* 1999;38:272–279.

27. Fine S, Forth A, Gilbert M, et al. Group therapy for adolescent depressive disorder: a comparison of social skills and therapeutic support. *J Am Acad Child Adolesc Psychiatry* 1991;30:79–85.

28. Lewinsohn PM, Clarke GN. Psychosocial treatments for adolescent depression. *Clin Psychol Rev* 1999;19:329–342.

29. Reinecke MA, Ryan NE, DuBois DL. Cognitive-behavioral treatment of depression and depressive symptoms during adolescence: a review and meta-analysis. *J Am Acad Child Adolesc Psychiatry* 1998;37:26–34.

30. Mendez Carrillo FX, Moreno PJ, Sanchez-Meca J, et al. Effectiveness of psychological treatment for child and adolescent depression: a qualitative review of two decades of research. *Psicol Conductual* 2000;8:487–510.

31. Birmaher B, Brent DA, Kolko D, et al. Clinical outcome after short-term psychotherapy for adolescents with major depressive disorder. *Arch Gen Psychiatry* 2000;57:29–36.

32. Haaga DAF, Beck AT. Cognitive therapy. In: Paykel ES, ed. *Handbook of affective disorders*. Edinburgh: Churchill Livingstone, 1992;511–523.

33. Klerman GL, Weissman H. Interpersonal psychotherapy. In: Paykel ES, ed. *Handbook of affective disorders*. Edinburgh: Churchill Livingstone, 1992;501–510.

Philip Hazell

Conjoint Professor of Child and Adolescent Psychiatry/Director Child and Youth Mental Health Service University of Newcastle Newcastle Australia

Competing interests: The author has been paid a fee by Pfizer, the manufacturer of sertraline, for speaking to general practitioners about the evidence for the treatment of depression in young people. The author's service has been in receipt of funding from Eli Lilly to participate in a relapse prevention trial of atomoxetine for attention deficit hyperactivity disorder.

Depressive disorders

Search date July 2002

John Geddes, Rob Butler, and Simon Hatcher

INTERVENTIONS

Key Messages

- We found no reliable direct evidence that one type of treatment (drug or non-drug) is superior to another in improving symptoms of depression. However, we found strong evidence that some treatments are effective, whereas the effectiveness of others remains uncertain. Of the interventions examined, prescription antidepressant drugs and electroconvulsive therapy are the only treatments for which there is good evidence of effectiveness in severe and psychotic depressive disorders. We found no RCTs comparing drug and non-drug treatments in severe depressive disorders.

- **Befriending (in mild to moderate depression)** One small RCT provided insufficient evidence to assess befriending.

- **Bibliotherapy (in mild to moderate depression)** One systematic review of RCTs in younger and older adults recruited by advertisement found limited evidence that bibliotherapy may reduce mild depressive symptoms compared with waiting list control or standard care. Another systematic review in people with combined anxiety and depression, anxiety, or chronic fatigue found that bibliotherapy may improve symptoms over 2–6 months compared with standard care. It is unclear whether people in the RCTs identified by the reviews are clinically representative of people with depressive disorders.

- **Care pathways (in mild to moderate depression)** Five RCTs in people aged over 18 years found that the effectiveness of antidepressant treatment may be improved by several approaches, including collaborative working between primary care clinicians and psychiatrists plus intensive patient education, case management, telephone support, and relapse prevention programmes. One RCT found that a clinical practice guideline and practice based education did not improve either detection or outcome of depression compared with usual care.

- **Care pathways versus usual care for long term outcomes (in mild to moderate depression)** One RCT found that a multifaceted "quality improvement programme" significantly improved symptoms and increased the proportion of people who returned to work over 1 year compared with usual care, but found no significant difference in outcomes at 2 years.

- **Cognitive therapy (in mild to moderate depression)** One systematic review in younger and older adults has found that cognitive therapy significantly improves the symptoms of depression compared with no treatment.

- **Cognitive therapy versus antidepressants for long term outcomes (in mild to moderate depression)** One systematic review and one additional RCT in younger and older adults found limited evidence by combining relapse rates across different RCTs that cognitive therapy may reduce the risk of relapse over 1–2 years compared with antidepressants.

- **Combining prescription antidepressant drugs and psychological treatment (in mild to moderate and severe depression)** One non-systematic review of RCTs in people aged 18–80 years has found that, in people with severe depression, adding drug treatment to interpersonal psychotherapy or to cognitive therapy compared with either psychological treatment alone improves symptoms, but found no significant difference in symptoms in people with mild to moderate depression. Subsequent RCTs in younger and older adults with mild to moderate depression have found that combining antidepressants plus psychotherapy improves symptoms significantly more than either antidepressants or psychotherapy alone. One RCT in older adults with mild to moderate depression found that cognitive behavioural therapy plus desipramine improved symptoms significantly more than desipramine alone.

- **Continuation drug treatment in mild to moderate depression (reduces risk of relapse in mild to moderate depression)** One systematic review and subsequent RCTs in younger and older adults have found that continuation treatment with antidepressant drugs compared with placebo for 4–6 months after recovery significantly reduces the risk of relapse. One RCT in people aged over 60 years has found that continuation treatment with dosulepin (dothiepin) significantly reduces the risk of relapse over 2 years compared with placebo.

Depressive disorders

- **Electroconvulsive therapy (in severe depression)** Two systematic reviews and additional RCTs in people aged over 16 years have found that electroconvulsive therapy significantly improves symptoms in severe depression compared with simulated electroconvulsive therapy.

- **Exercise (in mild to moderate depression)** One systematic review found limited evidence from poor RCTs that exercise may improve symptoms compared with placebo, and may be as effective as cognitive therapy or antidepressants.

- **Interpersonal psychotherapy (in mild to moderate depression)** One large RCT has found that interpersonal psychotherapy significantly improves rates of recovery from depression after 16 weeks compared with antidepressants or standard care.

- **Non-directive counselling (in mild to moderate depression)** One systematic review in people aged over 18 years with recent onset psychological problems, including depression, found that brief, non-directive counselling significantly reduced symptom scores in the short term (< 6 months) compared with usual care, but found no significant difference in scores in the long term (> 6 months).

- **Prescription antidepressant drugs (in mild to moderate and severe depression)** Systematic reviews in people aged 16 years or over have found that antidepressant drugs are effective in acute treatment of all grades of depressive disorders compared with placebo. Systematic reviews have found no significant difference in outcomes with different kinds of antidepressant drug. One systematic review in people aged 55 years or over with all grades of depressive disorder has found that tricyclic antidepressants, selective serotonin reuptake inhibitors, or monoamine oxidase inhibitors significantly reduce the proportion of people who fail to recover over 26–49 days compared with placebo. We found no specific evidence on adverse effects in older adults. However, the drugs differ in their adverse event profiles.

  - **Monoamine oxidase inhibitors** One systematic review found that monoamine oxidase inhibitors were less effective than tricyclic antidepressants in people with severe depressive disorders, but may be more effective in atypical depressive disorders with biological features such as increased sleep, increased appetite, mood reactivity, and rejection sensitivity.

  - **Selective serotonin reuptake inhibitors and related drugs** One systematic review found that selective serotonin reuptake inhibitors were associated with a lower rate of adverse effects compared with tricyclic antidepressants, but the difference was small. Another systematic review and one retrospective cohort study found no strong evidence that fluoxetine was associated with increased risk of suicide compared with tricyclic antidepressants or placebo. One RCT and observational data suggest that abrupt withdrawal of selective serotonin reuptake inhibitors is associated with symptoms including dizziness, nausea, paraesthesia, headache, and vertigo, and that these symptoms are more likely with drugs with a short half life, such as paroxetine.

  - **Tricyclic antidepressants** One systematic review found that tricyclic antidepressants were associated with higher rates of adverse effects compared with selective serotonin reuptake inhibitors, but the difference was small.

- **Problem solving treatment (in mild to moderate depression)** RCTs have found that problem solving treatment significantly improves symptoms over 3–6 months compared with placebo or control, and have found no significant difference in symptoms between problem solving treatment and drug treatment.

- **Psychological treatments (cognitive therapy, interpersonal psychotherapy, and problem solving treatment) in severe depression** RCTs found insufficient evidence to assess psychological treatments in severe depression.

- **St John's Wort (in mild to moderate depression)** Systematic reviews in people with mild to moderate depressive disorders have found that St John's Wort (*Hypericum perforatum*) significantly improves depressive symptoms over 4–12 weeks compared with placebo, and have found no significant difference in symptoms with St John's Wort versus prescription antidepressant drugs. The results of the reviews should be interpreted with caution because the RCTs did not use standardised preparations of St John's Wort, and doses of antidepressants varied. One subsequent RCT in people aged over 18 years with major depressive disorder found no significant difference in depressive symptoms at 8 weeks between a standardised preparation of St John's Wort and placebo or sertraline, but it is likely to have been underpowered to detect a clinically important difference between groups.

DEFINITION **Depressive disorders** are characterised by persistent low mood, loss of interest and enjoyment, and reduced energy. They often impair day to day functioning. Most of the RCTs assessed in this review classify depression using the *Diagnostic and statistical manual of mental disorders* (DSM IV)[1] or the *International classification of mental and behavioural disorders* (ICD-10).[2] DSM IV divides depression into major depressive disorder or dysthymic disorder. **Major depressive disorder** is characterised by one or more major depressive episodes (i.e. at least 2 wks of depressed mood or loss of interest accompanied by at least 4 additional symptoms of depression). **Dysthymic disorder** is characterised by at least 2 years of depressed mood for more days than not, accompanied by additional symptoms that do not reach the criteria for major depressive disorder.[1] ICD-10 divides depression into mild to moderate or severe depressive episodes.[2] **Mild to moderate depression** is characterised by depressive symptoms and some functional impairment. **Severe depression** is characterised by additional agitation or psychomotor retardation with marked somatic symptoms.[2] In this review, we use both DSM IV and ICD-10 classifications, but treatments are considered to have been assessed in severe depression if the RCT included inpatients. **Older adults:** Older adults are generally defined as people aged 65 years or older. However, some of the RCTs of older people in this review included people aged 55 years or over. The presentation of depression in older adults may be atypical: low mood may be masked and anxiety or memory impairment may be the principal presenting symptoms. Dementia should be considered in the differential diagnosis of depression in older adults.[3]

INCIDENCE/ PREVALENCE Depressive disorders are common, with a prevalence of major depression between 5% and 10% of people seen in primary care settings.[4] Two to three times as many people may have depressive symptoms but do not meet DSM IV criteria for major depression.

Women are affected twice as often as men. Depressive disorders are the fourth most important cause of disability worldwide and they are expected to become the second most important cause by the year 2020.[5,6] **Older adults:** Between 10% and 15% of older people have depressive symptoms, although major depression is relatively rare in older adults.[7]

AETIOLOGY/ RISK FACTORS The causes are uncertain but include both childhood events and current psychosocial adversity.

PROGNOSIS About half of people suffering a first episode of major depressive disorder experience further symptoms in the next 10 years.[8] **Older adults:** One systematic review (search date 1996, 12 prospective cohort studies, 1268 people, mean age 60 years) found that the prognosis may be especially poor in elderly people with a chronic or relapsing course of depression.[9] Another systematic review (search date 1999, 23 prospective cohort studies in people aged ≥ 65 years, including 5 identified by the first review) found that depression in older people was associated with increased mortality (15 studies; pooled OR 1.73, 95% CI 1.53 to 1.95).[10]

AIMS OF INTERVENTION To improve mood, social and occupational functioning, and quality of life; to reduce morbidity and mortality; to prevent recurrence of depressive disorder; and to minimise adverse effects of treatment.

OUTCOMES Depressive symptoms rated by the depressed person and clinician; social functioning; occupational functioning; quality of life; admission to hospital; rates of self harm; relapse of depressive symptoms; rates of adverse events. Trials often use continuous scales to measure depressive symptoms (such as the Hamilton Depression Rating Scale and the Beck Depression Inventory). **Older adults:** The Hamilton Depression Rating Scale is not ideal for older people because it includes several somatic items that may be positive in older people who are not depressed. It has been the most widely used scale, although specific scales for elderly people (such as the Geriatric Depression Scale) avoid somatic items.

METHODS The contributors conducted a validated search for systematic reviews and RCTs between May and September 1998 from the Cochrane Database of Systematic Reviews and the Database of Abstracts of Reviews of Effectiveness, *Best Evidence* and *Evidence-Based Mental Health*, Medline, Psychlit, and Embase. Studies were included by using epidemiological criteria and relevance to the clinical question. A *Clinical Evidence* search and appraisal was conducted in July 2002, including a search for data on depression in older adults. In this review, studies are included under the heading older adults if they specifically included people aged over 55 years.

QUESTION What are the effects of treatments?

OPTION PRESCRIPTION ANTIDEPRESSANT DRUGS

Systematic reviews in people aged 16 years or over have found that antidepressant drugs (monoamine oxidase inhibitors, selective serotonin reuptake inhibitors, or tricyclic antidepressants) improve symptoms in

acute treatment of all grades of depressive disorder compared with placebo. Two systematic reviews have found no significant difference in outcomes with different kinds of antidepressant drug, although one systematic review found that monoamine oxidase inhibitors were less effective than tricyclic antidepressants in people with severe depressive disorders, but may be more effective in atypical depressive disorders with reversed biological features such as increased sleep, increased appetite, mood reactivity, and rejection sensitivity. Systematic reviews have found that antidepressant drugs differ in their adverse event profiles. One systematic review has found that selective serotonin reuptake inhibitors were associated with fewer adverse effects compared with tricyclic antidepressants, but the difference was small. Another systematic review and one retrospective cohort study found no strong evidence that fluoxetine was associated with increased risk of suicide compared with tricyclic antidepressants or placebo. One RCT and observational data suggest that abrupt withdrawal of selective serotonin reuptake inhibitors is associated with symptoms including dizziness and rhinitis, and that these symptoms are more likely with drugs with a short half life, such as paroxetine. One systematic review in people aged 55 years or over with all grades of depressive disorder has found that tricyclic antidepressants, selective serotonin reuptake inhibitors, or monoamine oxidase inhibitors significantly reduce the proportion of people who fail to recover over 26–49 days compared with placebo. We found no specific evidence on adverse effects in older adults.

Benefits:
Antidepressants versus placebo: We found three systematic reviews.[11,12,13] The first review (search date 1995, 49 RCTs in people aged 18–70 years with mild to moderate or severe depressive disorders) included five RCTs in people admitted to hospital (probably with severe depressive disorders), 40 RCTs in a setting outside hospital, one in both settings, and three that did not specify the setting.[11] All RCTs identified by the review were of least 4 weeks' duration and included three way comparisons, including two antidepressant drugs (monoamine oxidase inhibitors [MAOIs], selective serotonin reuptake inhibitors [SSRIs], or tricyclic antidepressants [TCAs]) and placebo. The review only included RCTs that measured improvement in depressive symptoms using validated scales such as the Hamilton Depression Rating Scale and Montgomery-Asberg Depression Rating Scale. It found that the mean effect size (see glossary, p 133) for change in score with antidepressants versus placebo was 0.5, which means that 69% of people taking placebo had worse outcomes than the average person taking antidepressants (see comment below).[11] The second review (search date 1997, 15 RCTs, 1871 people aged ≥ 18 years) compared antidepressants (SSRIs, TCAs, MAOIs, amisulpride, amineptine, or ritanserin) versus placebo in people with dysthymia (chronic mild depressive disorders).[12] It found that antidepressants versus placebo significantly increased the proportion of people who responded to treatment at 4–12 weeks (response defined as a 50% decrease in Hamilton Depression Rating Scale score or scoring 1 or 2 on item 2 of the Clinical Global Impression Score; RR 1.9, 95% CI 1.6 to 2.3; NNT 4, 95% CI 3 to 5). The third systematic review (search date 1998, 18 RCTs, 838 people aged > 18 years with depression and a physical illness

[e.g. cancer, cardiovascular disorders, diabetes]) found that anti-depressants versus placebo significantly reduced the proportion of people who failed to recover over 4–12 weeks (177/366 [48%] with antidepressant v 229/325 [70%] with placebo; RR 0.68, 95% CI 0.60 to 0.77; NNT 4, 95% CI 3 to 7).[13] People allocated to antidepressants were more likely to withdraw from the study than were those on placebo (NNH 10, 95% CI 5 to 43). **In older adults; antidepressants versus placebo:** We found one systematic review (search date 2000, 17 RCTs, 1326 people aged ≥ 55 years with mild to moderate or severe depression) comparing antidepressants versus placebo.[14] It found that TCAs, SSRIs, or MAOIs versus placebo significantly reduced the proportion of people who failed to recover over 26–49 days (125/245 [51%] with TCAs v 167/223 [75%] with placebo: RR 0.68, 95% CI 0.59 to 0.68, NNT 4, 95% CI 4 to 5; 261/365 [72%] with SSRIs v 310/372 [83%] with placebo: RR 0.86, 95% CI 0.79 to 0.93, NNT 9, 95% CI 9 to 10; 34/58 [59%] with MAOIs v 57/63 [90%] with placebo: RR 0.64, 95% CI 0.50 to 0.81, NNT 4, 95% CI 3 to 4).[14] **TCAs versus SSRIs:** We found three systematic reviews (search dates 1999,[15] 1997,[16] and 1998[17]) and one subsequent RCT[18] in people with mild to moderate or severe depression comparing SSRIs versus TCAs. The reviews found no significant difference in overall effectiveness between TCAs and SSRIs.[15,16] The second review (search date 1997, 95 RCTs, 10 533 people aged 18–80 years) found that SSRIs may be slightly more acceptable overall than TCAs, as measured by the number of people who withdrew from clinical trials for any cause (RR of withdrawal 0.88, 95% CI 0.83 to 0.93; NNH 26, 95% CI 18 to 46).[16] The third systematic review (search date 1998, 28 RCTs, 5940 people aged ≥ 18 years) compared the efficacy of newer antidepressants versus placebo or versus older antidepressants in primary care.[17] The average response rate was 63% for newer agents, 35% for placebo, and 60% for TCAs (RR for SSRIs versus placebo 1.6, 95% CI 1.2 to 2.1). The subsequent RCT (152 people with major depression) compared adherence on dosulepin (dothiepin) versus fluoxetine over 12 weeks and found no significant difference between the drugs.[18] However, the RCT was probably underpowered to detect a clinically important difference. **MAOIs versus TCAs:** We found one systematic review (search date not stated, 55 RCTs) comparing MAOIs versus TCAs in several subgroups of people with depression aged 18–80 years.[19] It found that MAOIs were less effective than TCAs in people with severe depressive disorders but may be more effective in atypical depressive disorders (depressive disorders with reversed biological features, e.g. increased sleep, increased appetite, mood reactivity, and rejection sensitivity). **Antidepressants plus benzodiazepines:** We found one systematic review (search date 1999, 8 RCTs, 679 people aged 18–65 years, 1 RCT in people aged 20–73 years with major depression) comparing combination treatment with antidepressants plus benzodiazepines versus antidepressants alone.[20] It found that combination treatment versus antidepressants alone was significantly more likely to produce a response within 1 week (RR of > 50% reduction on symptom rating scale 1.64, 95% CI 1.19 to 2.27), although this difference was not apparent at 6 weeks.

Harms: **Common adverse events with TCAs versus SSRIs:** One systematic review (search date 1996) compared adverse events with TCAs versus SSRIs in people aged 18 years or over with all severities of depression (see table 1, p 136).[21] **Adverse effects with different SSRIs:** One large cohort study of people receiving four different SSRIs (fluvoxamine [983 people], fluoxetine [692 people], sertraline [734 people], and paroxetine [13 741 people]) in UK primary care found that reports of common adverse events (nausea/vomiting, malaise/lassitude, dizziness, and headache/migraine) varied between SSRIs (fluvoxamine 78/1000 participant months; fluoxetine 23/1000 participant months; RR v fluvoxamine 0.29, 95% CI 0.27 to 0.32; paroxetine 28/1000 participant months; RR 0.35, 95% CI 0.33 to 0.37; sertraline 21/1000 participant months; RR 0.26, 95% CI 0.25 to 0.28).[22] Only 52% of people responded to the questionnaire, although this response rate was similar for all four drugs. A study of spontaneous reports to the UK Committee on Safety of Medicines found no difference in safety profiles between the same four SSRIs.[23] **Suicide with TCAs versus SSRIs:** One systematic review (search date not stated, which included RCTs completed by December 1989) pooled data from 17 double blind RCTs in people with depressive disorders aged 12–90 years comparing a TCA (731 people) versus fluoxetine (1765 people) or versus placebo (569 people).[24] It found no significant difference in the rate of suicidal acts between the groups (TCAs 0.4%, fluoxetine 0.3%, and placebo 0.2%), but development of suicidal ideation was less frequent in the fluoxetine group (1% fluoxetine v 3% placebo, P = 0.04; and v 4% TCAs, P = 0.001). One historical cohort study followed 172 598 people who had at least one prescription for 1/10 antidepressants during the study period in general practice in the UK.[25] The risk of suicide was higher in people who received fluoxetine (19/10 000 person years, 95% CI 9 to 34) than in those receiving dosulepin (RR of suicide v dosulepin 2.1, 95% CI 1.1 to 4.1). In a nested case controlled subanalysis in people with no history of suicidal behaviour or previous antidepressant prescription, the risk remained the same, although the confidence interval broadened to make the result non-significant (RR 2.1, 95% CI 0.6 to 7.9). Although the apparent association may be because of residual confounding, there remains uncertainty about the possible association between fluoxetine and suicide. However, any absolute increase in risk is unlikely to be large. **Withdrawal effects with SSRIs:** We found one RCT in people aged 18 years or over (average age 30–40 years) comparing abrupt discontinuation of fluoxetine (96 people) versus continued treatment (299 people) in people who had been taking the drug for 12 weeks.[26] Abrupt discontinuation was associated with increased dizziness (7% v 1%), dysmenorrhoea (3% v 0%), rhinitis (10% v 3%), and somnolence (4% v 0%). However, there was a high withdrawal rate in this study because of the return of symptoms of depression (39%), so these may be underestimates of the true rate of withdrawal symptoms. Between 1987 and 1995 the rate of spontaneous reports of suspected withdrawal reactions per million defined daily doses to the World Health Organization Collaborating Centre for International Drug Monitoring was higher for paroxetine than for sertraline and fluoxetine.[27] The most common withdrawal effects were dizziness, nausea, paraesthesia, headache, and vertigo. **MAOIs versus TCAs:** The systematic review found that MAOIs were associated with a similar level of overall adverse effects as were TCAs.[19] Adverse effects associated with MAOIs included hypotension, dizziness, mydriasis, piloerection, oedema, tremor, anorgasmia, and insomnia. **During pregnancy:** One systematic review (search date 1999) assessing the risk of fetal harm of antidepressants in pregnancy found four small prospective studies published since 1993.[28] No evidence of increased risk was found, although the risk of adverse effects cannot be excluded. Decreased birth weights of infants exposed to fluoxetine during the third trimester were identified in one study, and direct drug effects and withdrawal syndromes were identified in some neonates. **In older adults:** We found no specific evidence on adverse effects in older adults.

Comment: **Antidepressants versus placebo:** The first review found that results were sensitive to the diagnostic criteria used; the mean effect size for antidepressants was 0.5 in those RCTs in which depressive disorders were diagnosed according to standard criteria (mainly *Diagnostic and statistical manual of mental disorders*, 3rd edition, revised) and 0.4 in those RCTs that did not use objective diagnostic criteria.[11] **In older adults:** The systematic review of antidepressants versus placebo in older people was limited by the diversity of populations included and by the brevity of the studies.[13] The reviewers recommended at least 6 weeks of antidepressant treatment in elderly people to achieve optimal effect. A systematic review is under way to examine adverse effects in elderly people. Metabolic and physical changes with age mean that older people may be more prone to adverse effects such as falls. Because older people often take more medications, they may be at greater risk of drug interactions.

OPTION   CARE PATHWAYS

Five RCTs in people aged over 18 years found that the effectiveness of antidepressant treatment may be improved by several approaches, including collaborative working between primary care clinicians and psychiatrists plus intensive patient education, case management, telephone support, and relapse prevention programmes. One RCT found that a clinical practice guideline and practice based education did not improve either detection or outcome of depression compared with usual care.

Benefits: We found no systematic review but found six RCTs.[29–34] **Collaborative working between primary care clinicians and psychiatrists plus intensive patient education:** The first RCT (217 people aged 19–76 years with mild to moderate or major depression in primary care in the USA) found that, compared with standard treatment (including antidepressants), the addition of a multifaceted programme, including collaborative working between primary care physician and psychiatrist plus intensive patient education, improved outcomes over 12 months.[29] Improvement in depressive symptoms assessed using the Symptom Checklist-90 was significant only in the subgroup of people with major depressive disorder (91 people; AR of clinical response of > 50% reduction in symptom checklist 74% v 44% with standard treatment; NNT 4, 95% CI 3 to 10).[29] **Care management:** The second RCT (613 people, mean age 46 years) in a Health Maintenance Organization in Seattle (USA) compared three interventions: usual care (antidepressants), usual care plus feedback (in which doctors received a detailed report on each person at 8 and 16 wks after randomisation), or usual care plus feedback plus care management (in which the care manager assessed people with depression by telephone at 8 and 16 wks, doctors received a detailed report, and care managers facilitated the follow up).[30] It found that feedback plus care management versus usual care significantly increased the proportion of people with a clinically important reduction in depressive symptoms at 6 months after randomisation (about 56% of people with care management v 40% with usual care [results presented graphically]; OR 2.22, 95% CI 1.31 to 3.75). **Clinical practice guideline and practice based education:** The third RCT (cluster randomised, based in UK primary care, people aged over 16 years) compared the effects of a clinical practice guideline and practice based education versus usual care.[31] It found that the intervention did not improve either detection or outcome of depression. **Telephone support:** The fourth RCT (302 people with major depressive disorder or dysthymia aged 19–90 years) compared usual physician care (selective serotonin reuptake inhibitor [SSRI]; 117 people), usual care plus nurse telehealth (SSRI plus 12–14 telephone support calls during 16 wks of treatment; 62 people), or usual care plus telehealth plus peer support (123 people).[32] Nurse telehealth versus usual clinician care significantly increased the proportion of people with a 50% reduction in symptoms at 6 months (57% with nurse telehealth v 38% with usual care; NNT 6, 95% CI 4 to 18). **Relapse prevention programme:** The fifth RCT (386 people aged > 18 with recurrent major depression or dysthymia who had largely recovered after 8 wks of antidepressant treatment) compared a relapse prevention programme (2 primary care visits and 3 telephone calls) versus usual care for 1 year.[33] It found that relapse prevention versus usual care significantly improved depressive symptoms over 1 year (results presented graphically; P = 0.04) but found no significant difference in relapse rates (35% in both groups). **Multifaceted quality improvement programme:** The sixth RCT compared a multifaceted "quality improvement programme" including antidepressants plus psychotherapy or plus cognitive behavioural therapy (see glossary, p 132) versus usual care and assessed outcomes at 1 and 2 years (see which treatments are most effective at improving long term outcome, p 131).[34] **Older adults:** We found no systematic review or RCTs specifically in older adults.

Harms: The RCTs gave no information about adverse effects.[29–34]

Comment: None.

OPTION **ST JOHN'S WORT (HYPERICUM PERFORATUM)**

Two systematic reviews in people with mild to moderate depressive disorders have found that St John's Wort (H perforatum) significantly improves depressive symptoms over 4–12 weeks compared with placebo,

Depressive disorders

and have found no significant difference in symptoms between St John's Wort and prescription antidepressant drugs. The results of the reviews should be interpreted with caution because the RCTs did not use standardised preparations of St John's Wort, and doses of antidepressants varied. One subsequent RCT in people aged over 18 years major depressive disorder found no significant difference in depressive symptoms at 8 weeks between a standardised preparation of St John's Wort and placebo or sertraline, but it is likely to have been underpowered to detect a clinically important difference between groups.

Benefits: We found two systematic reviews[35,36] and one subsequent RCT.[37] The first review (search date 1998) identified 17 RCTs (1168 people aged > 18 years with mild to moderate depression) comparing St John's Wort versus placebo (16 RCTs using single preparations of hypericum, and 1 RCT using combinations of hypericum and 4 other plant extracts; see comment below).[35] It also identified 10 RCTs (1123 people) comparing St John's Wort versus other antidepressants or sedative drugs (8 RCTs using single preparations of hypericum, and 2 RCTs using combinations of hypericum and valeriana). It found that H perforatum preparations versus placebo significantly increased the proportion of people who responded over 4–12 weeks (response defined as a Hamilton Depression Rating Scale score of < 10 or < 50% of baseline score; 267/465 [57%] with hypericum v 122/485 [25%] with placebo; RR 2.47, 95% CI 1.69 to 3.61), and found no significant difference in the proportion of people who responded with St John's Wort versus antidepressants or sedatives (177/352 [50%] with single preparations of hypericum v 176/339 [52%] with placebo; 88/130 [68%] v 66/132 [50%]; RR 1.01, 95% CI 0.87 to 1.16; combinations RR 1.52, 95% CI 0.78 to 2.94). The second review (search date 2000, 23 RCTs, 2776 people with mild to moderate depression) included 14 RCTs identified by the first review, but applied different inclusion criteria for RCTs and excluded 13 of the RCTs included in the first review.[36] It identified 14 RCTs (1336 people) comparing St John's Wort versus placebo and nine RCTs (1394 people) comparing St John's Wort versus other antidepressants. It found that St John's Wort versus placebo significantly increased the proportion of people who responded over 4–8 weeks (390/690 [57%] v 184/646 [28%]; RR 1.98, 95% CI 1.49 to 2.62), but found no significant difference in depressive symptoms over 4–6 weeks with St John's Wort versus other antidepressants (422/694 [61%] v 423/700 [60%]; RR 1.00, 95% CI 0.91 to 1.11). These results did not change when only RCTs that met stricter methodological treatment were combined (6 RCTs; St John's Wort v placebo: 153/257 [60%] v 79/232 [34%]; RR 1.77, 95% CI 1.16 to 2.70; St John's Wort v other antidepressants: 260/440 [59%] v 261/468 [56%]; RR 1.04, 95% CI 0.94 to 1.15). The subsequent RCT (340 people aged over 18 years with major depressive disorder defined as a total score of ≥ 20 on the Hamilton Depression Rating Scale) compared St. John's Wort (standardised extract, hypericin 0.12%–0.28%, 900–1500 mg/day) versus placebo or sertraline (50–100 mg/day).[37] It found no significant difference in the proportion of people who responded at 8 weeks with St John's Wort compared with placebo (response defined as Clinical Global Impression Score of 1 [very much improved] or 2 [much improved] or a Hamilton Depression Rating Scale score of < 8: 24% with St John's Wort v 32% with placebo v 25% with sertraline; P = 0.21 for St John's Wort v placebo; P for St John's Wort v sertraline not stated). The RCT is likely to have been underpowered to detect a clinically important difference between groups.[37] **Older adults:** We found no systematic review or RCTs specifically in older adults.

Harms: We found three systematic reviews that assessed adverse effects associated with St John's Wort.[35,36,38] The first review (search date 1998) found that adverse events were poorly reported in the trials.[35] Adverse effects were reported by 26% of people taking St John's Wort versus 45% of people taking standard antidepressants (RR 0.57, 95% CI 0.47 to 0.69), and by 15% of people taking combinations of hypericum and valeriana versus 27% taking amitriptyline or desipramine (RR 0.49, 95% CI 0.23 to 1.04). The second systematic review (search date 2000) found no significant difference in the proportion of people who had adverse effects (including gastrointestinal effects, headaches, restlessness, and fatigue) with St John's Wort versus placebo (43/236 [18%] v 29/177 [16%]; RR 1.04, 95% CI 0.68 to 1.58), and found that St John's Wort versus antidepressants significantly reduced the proportion of people with adverse effects (260/440 [59%] v 261/448 [58%]; RR 0.59, 95% CI 0.52 to 0.71).[36] The third systematic review (search date 1997) included RCTs and observational surveillance studies after marketing of St John's Wort.[38] It found that the most common adverse effects of St John's Wort in the included studies were gastrointestinal symptoms, dizziness/confusion, tiredness/sedation, and dry mouth, although all occurred less frequently than on conventional drugs. Findings from observational studies were consistent with these results. Photosensitivity is theoretically possible; however, only two cases have been reported.

Comment: The results of the systematic reviews must be interpreted with caution because the preparations and doses of H perforatum and types and doses of antidepressants varied widely.[35,36] More RCTs are needed using standardised preparations. Interactions with other drugs are possible and should be considered.

OPTION **ELECTROCONVULSIVE THERAPY**

Two systematic reviews and additional RCTs in people aged over 16 years have found that electroconvulsive therapy significantly improves symptoms in severe depression compared with simulated electroconvulsive therapy.

Benefits: We found two systematic reviews,[39,40] three additional RCTs,[41–43] and two subsequent RCTs.[44,45] The first review (search date not stated, 6 RCTs published between 1960 and 1978, 205 people with severe depressive disorder, age range not stated) compared electroconvulsive therapy (ECT) versus simulated ECT (in which people received everything but electric stimulation; see comment below).[39] It found that people given real versus simulated ECT were significantly more likely to respond to treatment (response defined as global clinical state or a "clinically significant" difference in scores on depressive scales such as the Hamilton Depression Rating Scale: 73/109 [67%] v 33/96 [34%]; pooled RR 1.95, 95% CI 1.43 to 2.65; NNT 3, 95% CI 2 to 5; calculated by the author from data in the article). The second review (search date 1998, which included 11 additional RCTs published between 1987 and 1998) also found good evidence for the beneficial effects of ECT, but did not quantify its conclusions.[40] The results of the additional and subsequent RCTs are consistent with the findings of the review.[41–45] **Older adults:** We found no systematic review or RCTs specifically in older adults.

Harms: The systematic reviews gave no information on adverse effects,[39,40] and we found no good evidence about possible adverse cognitive effects of ECT. However, people often complain of memory impairment after ECT. One of the main difficulties in studying the association between memory impairment and ECT is that depressive disorders also lead to cognitive impairment that usually improves during the course of treatment. For this reason, most of the small studies in this area find an average improvement in memory in people treated with ECT. This does not rule out the possibility of more subtle, subjective memory impairment secondary to ECT. Adverse memory effects may vary according to the dose and electrode location.

Comment: Because ECT may be unacceptable to some people and because it is a short term treatment, there is consensus that it should normally be reserved for people who cannot tolerate or have not responded to drug treatment, although it may be useful when a rapid response is required.

OPTION PSYCHOLOGICAL TREATMENTS

One systematic review in younger and older adults with mild to moderate depression has found that cognitive therapy significantly improves symptoms compared with no treatment. One systematic review in people aged over 18 years with recent onset psychological problems, including depression, found that brief, non-directive counselling significantly reduced symptom scores in the short term (< 6 months) compared with usual care, but found no significant difference in scores in the long term (> 6 months). RCTs in younger and older adults with mild to moderate depression found that problem solving treatment or interpersonal psychotherapy significantly improved depressive symptoms in the short term compared with placebo, and found no significant difference in symptoms with problem solving treatment or interpersonal psychotherapy compared with antidepressant treatment. RCTs found insufficient evidence to assess the relative efficacy of drug and non-drug treatment in severe depression. One systematic review in people aged over 55 years with mild to moderate depression found no significant difference in symptoms between psychological treatments (such as cognitive therapy or cognitive behaviour therapy) and no treatment. However, it also found no significant difference in symptoms between psychological treatments and similar but non-specific attention. This review was based on a small number of RCTs, the populations varied (although most were community samples), and many of the studies were short term. RCTs found limited evidence about the effects of psychological treatments in severe depression.

Benefits: The evidence comparing psychological treatments versus drug or no treatment is summarised in table 2 (see table 2, p 137).[46–50] RCTs found insufficient evidence to assess the relative efficacy of drug and non-drug treatment in severe depression (see comment below). **Older adults:** We found one systematic review (search date 1995, 14 small RCTs, < 24 people, age > 55 years in an outpatient or community setting) of pharmacological and psychological treatments.[51] It found four RCTs in older adults that compared psychological treatments versus no treatment. None of the RCTs found a significant difference between treatment and no treatment, measured on the Hamilton Depression Rating Scale. It also found six RCTs comparing different psychological treatments. Five of six comparisons of "rational" treatments (such as cognitive therapy or cognitive behavioural therapy [see glossary, p 133]) versus no treatment in older adults found significant benefit with treatment. Combined, the "rational" treatments performed significantly better than no treatment (mean difference in the Hamilton Depression Rating Scale score −7.3, 95% CI −10.1 to −4.4), but were not significantly different from the "non-specific attention" control. None of the RCTs found significant differences in effectiveness between psychological treatments.

Harms: The systematic review and RCTs gave no information on adverse effects.[46–50]

Comment: Large RCTs are needed in more representative people in a range of clinical settings, including primary care. Because of varying exclusion criteria, the generalisability of the studies is questionable (see table 2, p 137). Other factors to be considered when psychological treatments are compared with drug treatment include whether serum concentrations of drugs reach therapeutic concentrations, whether changes in medication are allowed (reflecting standard clinical practice), and whether studies reflect the natural course of depressive disorders. It is difficult to conduct studies of psychological treatments for severe depression because of the ethics surrounding withholding a proved treatment (antidepressant drugs) in a group of people at risk of self harm or neglect.[52]

| OPTION | PSYCHOLOGICAL TREATMENTS PLUS PRESCRIPTION ANTIDEPRESSANT DRUGS |

One non-systematic review of RCTs in people aged 18–80 years has found that, in people with severe depression, adding drug treatment to interpersonal psychotherapy or to cognitive therapy compared with either psychological treatment alone improves symptoms, but found no significant difference in symptoms in people with mild to moderate depression. Subsequent RCTs in younger and older adults with mild to moderate depression have found that combining antidepressants plus psychotherapy improves symptoms significantly more than either antidepressants or psychotherapy alone. One RCT in older adults with mild to moderate depression found that cognitive behavioural therapy plus desipramine improved symptoms significantly more than desipramine alone.

Benefits: We found no systematic review, but found one non-systematic review[52] and two subsequent RCTs.[53,54] The non-systematic review (6 RCTs, 595 people aged 18–80 years with major depression) found that, in more severe depressive disorders, antidepressants plus interpersonal psychotherapy (see glossary, p 133) or plus cognitive therapy (see glossary, p 133) significantly increased the proportion of people who responded after 16 weeks of treatment compared with interpersonal psychotherapy or cognitive therapy alone (response defined as 4 wks with Hamilton Depression Rating Scale score < 7; P = 0.001).[52] It found no advantage in combining antidepressants and specific psychological treatments in mild to moderate depressive disorders (P = 0.10). The first subsequent RCT (681 adults with chronic depressive disorder, mean age 43 years) compared three interventions: nefazodone alone, cognitive behavioural therapy (see glossary, p 132) alone, or nefazodone plus cognitive behavioural therapy.[53] It found that combined treatment significantly improved the proportion of people with a clinical response compared with either treatment alone (defined as at least 50% reduction in Hamilton Depression Rating Scale score and a score of ≤ 15; 152/226 [67%] with combined treatment v 92/220 [42%] with nefazodone alone v 90/226 [40%] with psychotherapy alone; combined treatment v either single intervention; P < 0.001; NNT 5, 95% CI 3 to 6). The second subsequent RCT (167 people with a major depressive episode) compared antidepressants (fluoxetine, amitriptyline, or moclobemide) plus short term psychodynamic supportive psychotherapy (see glossary, p 133) versus antidepressants alone (see comment below).[54] It found that combined treatment versus antidepressants significantly increased the proportion of people who had improved after 24 weeks (improvement defined as Hamilton Depression Rating Scale score of ≤ 7, Clinical Global Impression score of 1 or 2, Symptom Checklist-90 or Quality of Life Depression Scale score of at least 1 standard deviation from baseline; mean success rate 41% v 59%; NNT 5, 95% CI 3 to 11). **Older adults:** We found one RCT (102 people aged > 60 years with major depressive disorder) that compared three interventions: desipramine plus cognitive behavioural therapy; desipramine alone; or cognitive behavioural therapy alone.[55] It found that all three groups showed a significant reduction in symptoms from baseline as assessed using the Hamilton Depression Rating Scale after 16–20 weeks of treatment (reduction of 0.20 with desipramine, 0.36 with cognitive behavioural therapy, and 0.41 with combined treatments; P < 0.05 for all comparisons). It found that combined treatments versus desipramine alone significantly improved symptoms over 16–20 weeks (P < 0.05). It found no significant difference among the three groups in the proportion of people who withdrew for any cause (desipramine 34%, cognitive behavioural therapy 23%, and combined treatments 33%; P = 0.52).

Harms: The non-systematic review and RCTs gave no information on adverse effects.[52–55]

Comment: A systematic review is needed to address this question. In the second subsequent RCT, 38/167 people initially randomised refused the proposed treatment: 27/84 (32%) of people offered antidepressants and 11/83 (13%) of people offered combined treatment.[54] This makes the results of the RCT very difficult to interpret.

One systematic review found limited evidence from poor RCTs that exercise may improve symptoms compared with placebo, and may be as effective as cognitive therapy. One poor RCT in older adults identified by the review found limited evidence that exercise may be as effective as antidepressants in improving symptoms and may reduce relapse over 10 months.

Benefits: We found one systematic review (search date 1999, 14 RCTs, 851 people).[56] It found limited evidence that exercise versus no treatment may improve symptoms and found that exercise may be as effective as cognitive therapy (see glossary, p 133). However, it suggested that these results were inconclusive because of methodological problems in all of the RCTs; randomisation was adequately concealed in only three of the RCTs, intention to treat analysis was undertaken in only two, and assessment of outcome was blinded in only one of the RCTs. **Older adults:** The systematic review[56] identified one RCT (156 people with major depression, mean age 57 years) comparing aerobic exercise, sertraline hydrochloride (a selective serotonin reuptake inhibitor), and combined treatment for 16 weeks.[57] It found that the proportion of people who recovered (those no longer meeting criteria for depression or with a Hamilton Depression Rating Scale score < 8) was not significantly different across the treatment groups (60% with exercise v 69% with sertraline v 66% with combined treatments). A 10 month follow up of this RCT found lower rates of relapse with exercise versus medication (30% with exercise v 52% with sertraline v 55% with combined treatment).[58] However, about half of the people in the medication group engaged in exercise during follow up, making it difficult to draw firm conclusions about effects of exercise. The clinical importance of the observed difference at 10 months remains unclear.

Harms: The review gave no information about adverse effects.[56]

Comment: There is a need for a well designed RCT of the effects of exercise in people with all grades of depression assessing clinical outcomes over an adequate time period.

One systematic review of RCTs in younger and older adults recruited by advertisement found limited evidence that bibliotherapy may reduce mild depressive symptoms compared with waiting list control or standard care. Another systematic review in people with combined anxiety and depression, anxiety, or chronic fatigue found that bibliotherapy may improve symptoms over 2–6 months compared with standard care. It is unclear whether people in the RCTs identified by the reviews are clinically representative of people with depressive disorders.

Benefits: **Younger and older adults:** We found two systematic reviews (search date not stated[59] and search date 1999[60]). The first review identified six small short term RCTs of bibliotherapy (see glossary, p 132) versus waiting list control in 273 people (described as adults in 4 RCTs and elderly in 2 RCTs; no age range provided) recruited by advertisement through the media and probably with only mild depression (see comment below).[59] The mean effect size (see glossary, p 133) of bibliotherapy was 0.82 (95% CI 0.50 to 1.15). This means that 79% of people in the waiting list control group had a worse outcome than the average person in the bibliotherapy group. The second systematic review identified eight randomised and non-randomised trials in younger and older people, but only one of them included people with depression.[60] It found that, in people with combined anxiety and depression, anxiety, or chronic fatigue, bibliotherapy may improve symptoms over 2–6 months compared with standard care. The RCT identified by the second review that included people with depression found that bibliotherapy versus standard care significantly improved symptoms of anxiety over 4 weeks as assessed using the Hamilton Depression Rating Scale, but found no significant difference in symptoms of depression at 4 or 12 weeks. **Older adults:** We found no systematic review or RCTs specifically in older adults.

Harms: None reported.

Comment: The review did not clearly describe the characteristics of the people in the RCTs it identified, and it is unclear whether people were receiving interventions in addition to bibliotherapy.[59] Further RCTs are needed in clinically representative groups.

OPTION   BEFRIENDING

One small RCT provided insufficient evidence to assess befriending.

Benefits: We found one small RCT (86 women with chronic depression, aged > 18 years, primarily aged 25–40 years, based in London, UK) of befriending (see glossary, p 132) versus waiting list control.[61] Initial identification was by postal screening of women registered with, but not attending, primary care. It found that befriending versus waiting list control significantly increased the proportion of women with remission of symptoms at 13 months (65% with befriending v 39% with control; P < 0.05; NNT 4, 95% CI 2 to 18). **Older adults:** We found no systematic review or RCTs specifically in older adults.

Harms: The RCT gave no information on harms.[61]

Comment: In the RCT, 14% of women in the befriending group were taking antidepressants and 12% of women in the waiting list control group.[61] Fewer than half of the women screened by post were interested in befriending as a treatment option.

What are the effects of continuation treatment with antidepressant drugs?

OPTION CONTINUATION TREATMENT WITH ANTIDEPRESSANT DRUGS

One systematic review and subsequent RCTs in younger and older adults have found that continuation treatment with antidepressant drugs compared with placebo for 4–6 months after recovery significantly reduces the risk of relapse. One RCT in people aged over 60 years has found that continuation treatment with dosulepin significantly reduces the risk of relapse over 2 years compared with placebo.

Benefits: We found one systematic review (search date not stated, 6 RCTs, 312 people, age range not stated).[62] It found that continuation of antidepressant medication versus placebo for 4–6 months after acute treatment reduced the relapse rate by nearly half (RR 0.6, 95% CI 0.4 to 0.7). Several more recent RCTs confirmed this reduction in risk of early relapse with continuing antidepressant treatment for 6–12 months after acute treatment. **Older adults:** We found one RCT (69 people aged > 60 years with mild to moderate or severe depression who had recovered sufficiently and consented to enter a 2 year trial of continuation treatment [see glossary, p 133]), which compared dosulepin (dothiepin) versus placebo.[63] It found that dosulepin versus placebo reduced the risk of relapse over 2 years by 55% (RR 0.45, 95% CI 0.22 to 0.96).

Harms: Adverse effects seem to be similar to those reported in trials of acute treatment.

Comment: We found no adequate systematic review of maintenance treatment (see glossary, p 133), but several RCTs have found that maintenance treatment reduced recurrence compared with placebo in recurrent depressive disorder. However, they all have problems with their methods (e.g. high withdrawal rates)[64] and will be considered in future *Clinical Evidence* updates. A systematic review of antidepressant treatment duration is in progress.[65]

QUESTION Which treatments are most effective at improving long term outcome (≥ 1 year)?

OPTION IMPROVING LONG TERM OUTCOMES

One systematic review and one additional RCT in younger and older adults found limited evidence by combining relapse rates across different RCTs that cognitive therapy may reduce the risk of relapse over 1–2 years compared with antidepressants. One RCT found that a multifaceted "quality improvement programme" significantly improved symptoms and increased the proportion of people who returned to work over 1 year compared with usual care, but found no significant difference in outcomes at 2 years.

Benefits: **Cognitive therapy versus antidepressants:** We found one systematic review (search date not stated) comparing cognitive therapy (see glossary, p 133) versus antidepressants in people with mainly mild to moderate depressive disorders.[46] The review identified eight small RCTs (261 people, mean age 39.3 years) that assessed long term (1–2 year) relapse rates after treatment had stopped. Relapse was defined as a return of depressive symptoms (Beck Depression Inventory Score > 16) at 6–9 months after a 2 month remission. It found limited evidence by combining relapse rates across different RCTs that, overall, 30% of people treated with cognitive therapy relapsed compared with 60% of those treated with either antidepressants or antidepressants plus cognitive therapy. We found one small additional RCT (40 people) comparing cognitive therapy versus normal clinical management (antidepressants) for residual depressive symptoms in people who had responded to antidepressants. It also found that, at 2 years, fewer people relapsed with cognitive therapy than with antidepressants.[66]

Care pathways versus usual care: One RCT (1356 people aged > 18 years with mild to moderate or major depression in 46 primary care clinics in US Health Maintenance Organizations) compared a multifaceted "quality improvement programme" (including antidepressants plus psychotherapy or plus cognitive behavioural therapy [see glossary, p 132]) versus usual care (including mailed practice guidelines).[34] It found that the quality improvement programme versus usual care significantly increased the proportion of people who improved on continuous depression rating scales over 1 year. It found that, among people initially employed, 90% of people in the quality improvement programme worked at 1 year versus 85% of the people receiving usual care ($P = 0.05$). For people initially not working, there was no difference in employment rates at 12 months with quality improvement versus usual care (17% v 18%). A 2 year follow up of this RCT found no significant difference in outcomes with quality improvement versus usual care.[67] **Older adults:** We found no systematic review or RCTs specifically in older adults.

Harms: See harms of prescription antidepressant drugs, p 121.

Comment: The review did not present information on the proportion of people who recovered and continued to remain well after 2 years.[46] The largest RCT identified by the review found that only a fifth of people remained well over 18 months' follow up, and that there were no significant differences between interpersonal psychotherapy (see glossary, p 133), cognitive therapy, or drug treatment.[46] It is possible that different people respond to different treatments. Further large scale comparative studies are needed of the long term effectiveness of treatments in people with all severities of depressive disorders.

GLOSSARY

Befriending Consists of a befriender meeting the person to talk and socialise for at least 1 hour a week, acting as a friend.

Bibliotherapy Advising people to read written material such as *Feeling good: the new mood therapy* by David Burns (New York: New American Library, 1980).

Brief, non-directive counselling Helping people to express feelings and clarify thoughts and difficulties; therapists suggest alternative understandings and do not give direct advice but try to encourage people to solve their own problems.

Cognitive behavioural therapy Brief (20 sessions over 12–16 wks) structured treatment, incorporating elements of cognitive therapy and behavioural therapy. Behavioural therapy is based on learning theory and concentrates on changing behaviour.

Cognitive therapy Brief (20 sessions over 12–16 wks) structured treatment aimed at changing the dysfunctional beliefs and negative automatic thoughts that characterise depressive disorders. It requires a highly trained therapist.[68]

Continuation treatment Continuation of treatment after successful resolution of a depressive episode to prevent relapse.

Effect size This expresses the degree of overlap between the range of scores in the control and experimental groups. The effect size can be used to estimate the proportion of people in the control group who had a poorer outcome than the average person in the experimental group; a proportion of 50% indicates that the treatment has no effect.

Interpersonal psychotherapy Standardised form of brief psychotherapy (usually 12–16 weekly sessions) primarily intended for outpatients with unipolar non-psychotic depressive disorders. It focuses on improving the person's interpersonal functioning and identifying the problems associated with the onset of the depressive episode.[69]

Maintenance treatment Long term treatment of recurrent depressive disorder to prevent the recurrence of further depressive episodes.

Problem solving treatment Consists of three stages: (1) identifying the main problems for the person; (2) generating solutions; and (3) trying out the solutions. Potentially briefer and simpler than cognitive therapy and may be feasible in primary care.[48]

Psychodynamic supportive psychotherapy Aims to facilitate change by detecting and resolving underlying psychological conflicts. The treatment aims to be less challenging by incorporating supportive elements.

REFERENCES

1. American Psychiatric Association. *Diagnostic and statistical manual of mental disorders*, 4th ed. Washington, DC: American Psychiatric Association, 1994.
2. World Health Organization. *The ICD-10 classification of mental and behavioural disorders*. Geneva: World Health Organization, 1992.
3. Rosenstein, Leslie D. Differential diagnosis of the major progressive dementias and depression in middle and late adulthood: a summary of the literature of the early 1990s. *Neuropsychol Rev* 1998;8:109–167.
4. Katon W, Schulberg H. Epidemiology of depression in primary care. *Gen Hosp Psychiatry* 1992;14:237–247.
5. Murray CJ, Lopez AD. Regional patterns of disability-free life expectancy and disability-adjusted life expectancy: global burden of disease study. *Lancet* 1997;349:1347–1352.
6. Murray CJ, Lopez AD. Alternative projections of mortality and disability by cause 1990–2020: global burden of disease study. *Lancet* 1997;349:1498–1504.
7. Beekman ATF, Copeland JRM, Prince MJ. Review of community prevalence of depression in later life. *Br J Psychiatry* 1999;174:307–311.
8. Judd LL, Akiskal HS, Maser JD, et al. A prospective 12 year study of subsyndromal and syndromal depressive symptoms in unipolar major depressive disorders. *Arch Gen Psychiatry* 1988;55:694–700.
9. Cole MG, Bellavance F, Mansour A. Prognosis of depression in elderly community and primary care populations: a systematic review and meta-analysis. *Am J Psychiatry* 1999;156:1182–1189. Search date 1996;

primary sources Medline 1981–1996, Psychinfo 1984–1996, and hand searches of the bibliographies of relevant articles.

10. Saz P, Dewey ME. Depression, depressive symptoms and mortality in persons aged 65 and older living in the community: a systematic review of the literature. *Int J Geriatr Psychiatry* 2001;16:622–630. Search date 1999; primary sources Embase, Medline, personal files, and hand searches of reference lists.
11. Joffe R, Sokolov S, Streiner D. Antidepressant treatment of depression: a meta-analysis. *Can J Psychiatry* 1996;41:613–616. Search date 1995; primary source Medline.
12. Lima MS, Moncrieff J. Drugs versus placebo for dysthymia. In: Cochrane Library, Issue 2, 2002. Oxford: Update Software. Search date 1997; primary sources Biological Abstracts, Medline, Psychlit, Embase, Lilacs, Cochrane Library, personal communication, conference abstracts, unpublished trials from the pharmaceutical industry, and book chapters on the treatment of depression.
13. Gill D, Hatcher S. Antidepressants for depression in medical illness. In: The Cochrane Library, Issue 2, 2002. Oxford: Update Software. Search date 1998; primary sources Medline, Cochrane Library Trials Register, Cochrane Depression and Neurosis Group Trials Register, and hand searches of two journals and reference lists.
14. Wilson K, Mottram P, Sivanranthan A, et al. Antidepressant versus placebo for the depressed elderly. In: The Cochrane Library, Issue 2, 2002. Oxford: Update Software. Search date 2000;

primary sources Psychlit, Medline, Embase, Cinahl, Cochrane Controlled Trials register, CCDAN trials register, and hand searches.

15. Geddes JR, Freemantle N, Mason J, et al. Selective serotonin reuptake inhibitors (SSRIs) for depression. In: The Cochrane Library, Issue 2, 2002. Oxford: Update Software. Search date 1999; primary sources Medline, Embase, Cochrane Group Register of Controlled Trials, hand searches of reference lists of all located studies, and contact with manufacturers.

16. Anderson IM. Selective serotonin reuptake inhibitors versus tricyclic antidepressants: a meta-analysis of efficacy and tolerability. J Affect Disord 2000;58:19–36. Search date 1997; primary sources Medline, and hand searches of reference lists of meta-analyses and reviews.

17. Mulrow CD, Williams JW, Chiqueete E, et al. Efficacy of newer medications for treating depression in primary care people. Am Med J 2000;108:54–64. Search date 1998; primary sources Cochrane Depression Anxiety and Neurosis Group Specialised Register of Clinical Trials, hand searches of trials and 46 pertinent meta-analyses, and consultation with experts.

18. Thompson C, Peveler RC, Stephenson D, et al. Compliance with antidepressant medication in the treatment of major depressive disorder in primary care: a randomized comparison of fluoxetine and a tricyclic antidepressant. Am J Psychiatry 2000;157:338–343.

19. Thase ME, Trivedi MH, Rush AJ. MAOIs in the contemporary treatment of depression. Neuropsychopharmacology 1995;12:185–219. Search date not stated; primary sources Medline and Psychological Abstracts.

20. Furukawa TA, Streiner DL, Young LT. Antidepressant and benzodiazepine for major depression. In: The Cochrane Library, Issue 2, 2002. Oxford: Update Software. Search date 1999; primary sources Medline, Embase, International Pharmaceutical Abstracts, Biological Abstracts, LILACS, Psychlit, Cochrane Library, Cochrane Depression, Anxiety and Neurosis Group Trial Register, SciSearch, hand searches of reference lists, and personal contacts.

21. Trindade E, Menon D. Selective serotonin reuptake inhibitors (SSRIs) for major depression. Part I. Evaluation of the clinical literature. Ottawa: Canadian Coordinating Office for Health Technology Assessment, 1997 August Report 3E. Evidence-Based Mental Health 1998;1:50. Search date 1996; primary sources Medline, Embase, Psychinfo, International Pharmaceutical Abstracts, Pascal, Health Planning and Administration, Mental Health Abstracts, Pharmacoeconomics and Outcomes News, Current Contents databases, scanning bibliographies of retrieved articles, hand searching of journals, and consulting researchers.

22. Mackay FJ, Dunn NR, Wilton LV, et al. A comparison of fluvoxamine, fluoxetine, sertraline and paroxetine examined by observational cohort studies. Pharmacoepidemiol Drug Safety 1997;6:235–246.

23. Price JS, Waller PC, Wood SM, et al. A comparison of the post marketing safety of four selective serotonin reuptake inhibitors including the investigation of symptoms occurring on withdrawal. Br J Clin Pharmacol 1996;42:757–763.

24. Beasley CM Jr, Dornseif BE, Bosomworth JC, et al. Fluoxetine and suicide: a meta-analysis of controlled trials of treatment for depression. BMJ 1991;303:685–692. Search date not stated, but included trials that had been completed/analysed by December 1989; primary sources not given in

detail but based on clinical report form data from trials and data from the Drug Experience Network Database.

25. Jick SS, Dean AD, Jick H. Antidepressants and suicide. BMJ 1995;310:215–218.

26. Zajecka J, Fawcett J, Amsterdam J, et al. Safety of abrupt discontinuation of fluoxetine: a randomised, placebo controlled study. J Clin Psychopharmacol 1998;18:193–197.

27. Stahl MM, Lindquist M, Pettersson M, et al. Withdrawal reactions with selective serotonin reuptake inhibitors as reported to the WHO system. Eur J Clin Pharmacol 1997;53:163–169.

28. Wisner KL, Gelenberg AJ, Leonard H, et al. Pharmacologic treatment of depression during pregnancy. JAMA 1999;282:1264–1269. Search date 1999; primary sources Medline, Healthstar, hand searches of bibliographies of review articles, and discussions with investigators in the field.

29. Katon W, Von Korff M, Lin E, et al. Collaborative management to achieve treatment guidelines: impact on depression in primary care. JAMA 1995;273:1026–1031.

30. Simon GE, Vonkorff M, Rutter C, et al. Randomised trial of monitoring, feedback, and management of care by telephone to improve treatment of depression in primary care. BMJ 2000;320:550–554.

31. Thompson C, Kinmonth AL, Stevens L, et al. Effects of a clinical-practice guideline and practice-based education on detection and outcome of depression in primary care: Hampshire Depression Project randomised controlled trial. Lancet 2000;355:185–191.

32. Hunkeler EM, Meresman JF, Hargreaves WA, et al. Efficacy of nurse telehealth care and peer support in augmenting treatment of depression in primary care. Arch Fam Med 2000;9:700–708.

33. Katon W, Rutter C, Ludman EJ, et al. A randomized trial of relapse prevention of depression in primary care. Arch Gen Psychiatry 2001;58:241–247.

34. Wells KB, Sherbourne C, Schoenbaum M, et al. Impact of disseminating quality improvement programs for depression in managed primary care: a randomized controlled trial. JAMA 2000;283:212–220.

35. Linde K, Mulrow CD. St John's Wort for depression. In: The Cochrane Library, Issue 2, 2002. Oxford: Update Software. Search date 1998; primary sources Medline, Embase, Psychlit, Psychindex, specialised databases: Cochrane Complementary Medicine Field, Cochrane Depression and Neurosis CRG, Phytodok, hand searches of references of pertinent articles, and contact with manufacturers, and researchers.

36. Whiskey A, Werneke U, Taylor D. A systematic review and meta-analysis of Hypericum perforatum in depression: a comprehensive clinical review. Int Clin Psychopharmacol 2001;16:239–252. Search date 2000; primary sources (in English or German) Medline, Embase, and hand searched references of primary studies.

37. Davidson JRT, Gadde KM, Fairbank JA. Effect of Hypericum perforatum (St John's wort) in major depressive disorder: a randomized controlled trial. JAMA 2002;287:1807–1814.

38. Ernst E, Rand JI, Barnes J, et al. Adverse effects profile of the herbal antidepressant St John Wort (Hypericum perforatum L). Eur J Clin Pharmacol 1998;54:589–594. Search date 1997; primary sources AMED, Cochrane Library 1997 Issue 2, Embase, Medline, hand searched reference lists, contacted WHO Collaborating Centre for International Drug Monitoring, UK Committee on Safety of Medicines, and German Bundesinstitut

für Arzneimittel und Medizinproducte plus 12 German manufacturers of hypericum products.

39. Janicak PG, Davis JM, Gibbons RD, et al. Efficacy of ECT: a meta-analysis. *Am J Psychiatry* 1985;142:297–302. Search date not stated; primary source Medline.

40. Wijeratne C, Halliday GS, Lyndon RW. The present status of electroconvulsive therapy: a systematic review. *Med J Austr* 1999;171:250–254. Search date 1998; primary source Medline.

41. Johnstone EC, Deakin JF, Lawler P, et al. The Northwick Park electroconvulsive therapy trial. *Lancet* 1980;1:1317–1320.

42. Brandon S, Cowley P, McDonald C, et al. Electroconvulsive therapy: results in depressive illness from the Leicestershire trial. *BMJ* 1984;288:22–25.

43. Gregory S, Shawcross CR, Gill D. The Nottingham ECT study. A double-blind comparison of bilateral, unilateral and simulated ECT in depressive illness. *Br J Psychiatry* 1985;146:520–524.

44. Vaughan McCall W, Reboussin DM, Weiner RD, et al. Titrated moderately suprathreshold vs fixed high-dose right unilateral electroconvulsive therapy. *Arch Gen Psychiatry* 2000;57:438–444.

45. Sackeim HA, Prudic J, Devanand DP, et al. A prospective, randomized, double-blind comparison of bilateral and right unilateral electroconvulsive therapy at different stimulus intensities. *Arch Gen Psychiatry* 2000;57:425–434.

46. Gloaguen V, Cottraux J, Cucherat M, et al. A meta-analysis of the effects of cognitive therapy in depressed people 1998. *J Affect Disord* 1998;49:59–72. Search date not stated; primary sources Medline, Embase, references in books and papers, previous reviews and meta-analyses, abstracts from congress presentations, and preprints sent by authors.

47. Elkin I, Shea MT, Watkins JT, et al. National Institute of Mental Health treatment of depression collaborative research program: general effectiveness of treatments. *Arch Gen Psychiatry* 1989;46:971–982.

48. Mynors-Wallis LM, Gath DH, Lloyd-Thomas AR, et al. Randomised controlled trial comparing problem solving treatment with amitriptyline and placebo for major depression in primary care. *BMJ* 1995;310:441–445.

49. Dowrick C, Dunn G, Ayuso-Mateos JL, et al. Problem solving treatment and group psychoeducation for depression: multicentre randomised controlled trial. *BMJ* 2000;321:1450–1454.

50. Bower P, Rowland N, Mellor Clark J, et al. Effectiveness and cost effectiveness of counselling in primary care. In: The Cochrane Library, Issue 2, 2002. Oxford: Update Software. Search date 2001; primary sources Medline, Embase, Psychlit, Cinahl, Cochrane Controlled Trials Register, CCDAN trials register, personal contact with experts and CCDAN members, search of unpublished sources (clinical trials, books, dissertations, agency reports, etc.), and hand searches of one journal and reference lists.

51. McCusker J, Cole M, Keller E, et al. Effectiveness of treatments of depression in older ambulatory people. *Arch Intern Med* 1998;158:705–712. Search date 1995; primary sources Medline, Psychinfo, and hand searches of references.

52. Thase ME, Greenhouse JB, Frank E, et al. Treatment of major depression with psychotherapy or psychotherapy — pharmacotherapy combinations. *Arch Gen Psychiatry* 1997;54:1009–1015. Pooled results of six research protocols conducted 1982–1992 at the Mental Health Clinical Research Center, University of Pittsburgh School of Medicine.

53. Keller MB, McCullough JP, Klein DN, et al. A comparison of nefazodone, the cognitive behavioral-analysis system of psychotherapy, and their combination for the treatment of chronic depression. *N Engl J Med* 2000;342:1462–1470.

54. De Jonghe F, Kool S, van Aalst G, Dekker J, Peen J. Combining psychotherapy and antidepressants in the treatment of depression. *J Affect Disord* 2001;64:217–229.

55. Thompson LW, Coon DW, Gallagher-Thompson D, Sommer BR, Koin D. Comparison of desipramine and cognitive behavioural therapy in the treatment of elderly outpatients with mild-to-moderate depression. *Am J Geriatr Psychiatry* 2001;9:225–240.

56. Lawlor DA, Hopker SW. The effectiveness of exercise as an intervention in the management of depression: systematic review and meta-regression analysis of randomised controlled trials. *BMJ* 2001;322:763–767. Search date 1999; primary sources Medline, Embase, Sports Discus, Psychlit, Cochrane Library, and hand searches of reference lists and nine journals.

57. Blumenthal JA, Babyak MA, Moore KA, et al. Effects of exercise training on older people with major depression. *Arch Intern Med* 1999;159:2349–2356.

58. Babyak M, Blumenthal JA, Herman S, et al. Exercise treatment for major depression: maintenance of therapeutic benefit at 10 months. *Psychosom Med* 2000;62:633–638.

59. Cuijpers P. Bibliotherapy in unipolar depression: a meta-analysis. *J Behav Ther Exp Psychiatry* 1997;28:139–147. Search date not stated; primary sources Psychlit, Psychinfo, and Medline.

60. Bower P, Richards D, Lovell K. The clinical and cost-effectiveness of self-help treatments for anxiety and depressive disorders in primary care: a systematic review. *Br J Gen Pract* 2001;51:838–845. Search date 1999; primary sources Psychinfo, Medline, Embase, Cinahl, Cochrane Library, Counselling in Primary Care Counsel.lit database, National Research Register, personal contact with researchers, hand searches of reference lists and two journals.

61. Harris T, Brown GW, Robinson R. Befriending as an intervention for chronic depression among women in an inner city: randomised controlled trial. *Br J Psychiatry* 1999;174:219–224.

62. Loonen AJ, Peer PG, Zwanikken GJ. Continuation and maintenance therapy with antidepressive agents: meta-analysis of research. *Pharm Week Sci* 1991;13:167–175. Search date not stated; primary sources references of textbooks and review articles, Medline, Embase, and review of reference lists of primary studies.

63. Old age depression interest group. How long should the elderly take antidepressants? A double-blind placebo-controlled study of continuation/prophylaxis therapy with dothiepin. *Br J Psychiatry* 1993;162:175–182.

64. Keller MB, Kocsis JH, Thase ME, et al. Maintenance phase efficacy of sertraline for chronic depression: a randomized controlled trial. *JAMA* 1998;280:1665–1672.

65. Carney S, Geddes J, Davies D, et al. Antidepressants treatment duration for depressive disorder (protocol). In: The Cochrane Library, Issue 4, 2001. Oxford: Update Software.

66. Fava GA, Rafanelli C, Grandi S, et al. Prevention of recurrent depression with cognitive behavioral therapy: preliminary findings. *Arch Gen Psychiatry* 1998;55:816–820.

67. Sherbourne CD, Wells KB, Duan N, et al. Long term effectiveness of disseminating quality improvement for depression in primary care. *Arch Gen Psychiatry* 2001;58:696–703.

68. Haaga DAF, Beck AT. Cognitive therapy. In: Paykel ES, ed. *Handbook of affective disorders*. Edinburgh: Churchill Livingstone, 1992:511–523.

69. Klerman GL, Weissman H. Interpersonal psychotherapy. In: Paykel ES, ed. *Handbook of affective disorders*. Edinburgh: Churchill Livingstone, 1992:501–510.

John Geddes
Professor of Epidemiological Psychiatry
University of Oxford
Oxford
UK

Rob Butler
Honorary Senior Lecturer in
Psychiatry/Consultant in Old Age
Psychiatry
University of Auckland and Waitemata
Health

Simon Hatcher
Senior Lecturer in Psychiatry/Honorary
Consultant in Liaison Psychiatry
University of Auckland
Auckland
New Zealand

Competing interests: RB has been reimbursed by Novartis for attending a conference. JG and SH none declared.

We would like to acknowledge the previous contributors of this chapter, including James Warner.

TABLE 1 Adverse events (% of people) with selective serotonin reuptake inhibitors versus tricyclic antidepressants (see text, p 121).[21]

Adverse effects	SSRI event rates (%)	TCA event rates (%)
Dry mouth	21	55
Constipation	10	22
Dizziness	13	23
Nausea	22	12
Diarrhoea	13	5
Anxiety	13	7
Agitation	14	8
Insomnia	12	7
Nervousness	15	11
Headache	17	14

SSRI, selective serotonin reuptake inhibitors; TCA, tricyclic antidepressants.

TABLE 2 Effects of specific psychological treatments for depressive disorders (see text, p 127).

Intervention	Evidence	Benefits	Harms	Disadvantages
Cognitive therapy	1 SR (48 RCTs of psychological therapies [2765 people, mean age 39.3 y] mainly outpatients in secondary care; therefore, probably with mild to moderate depression; people with psychotic or bipolar symptoms were excluded); 20 RCTs compared CT with waiting list or placebo and 17 compared it with drug treatment[46]	79% of people receiving placebo were more symptomatic than the average person receiving CT (P < 0.0001).[43] 65% of people receiving CT were less symptomatic than the average person treated with antidepressant drugs (P < 0.0001)[46]	No harms reported	Requires extensive training. Limited availability. RCTs in primary care suggest limited acceptability to some people
Interpersonal psychotherapy	No SR. 1 large RCT (people with mild to moderate depression, mean age 35 y) compared interpersonal psychotherapy v either drug treatment, CT, or placebo plus clinical management for 16 wks[47]	Rates of recovery from depression: interpersonal psychotherapy (43%; NNT 5, 95% CI 3 to 19), imipramine (42%; NNT 5, 95% CI 3 to 22), placebo clinical management (21%)[47]	No harms reported	Requires extensive training. Limited availability
Problem solving therapy	No SR. 1 large RCT (452 people aged 18–65 y with mild to moderate depression or adjustment disorders) compared PS, group treatment, and control.[49] 1 RCT (91 people aged 18–65 y with mild to moderate depression) compared problem solving, placebo, and amitriptyline[48]	PS v control significantly increased the proportion of people who were not depressed at 6 mo, but no significant difference at 1 y.[49] PS v placebo significantly improved symptoms at 12 wks, and no significant difference in symptoms with PS v amitriptyline[48]	No harms reported	Requires some training. Limited availability
Non-directive counselling	1 SR (7 RCTs, 772 people aged over 18 y with recent onset psychological problems, including depression in UK primary care) compared counselling v standard physician care[50]	Counselling v standard care significantly improved symptoms in the short term (1–6 mo; WMD −2.03, 95% CI −3.82 to −0.24), but no significant difference in the long term (> 6 mo; WMD −0.03, 95% CI −0.39 to +0.32)[50]	No harms reported	Requires some training. Limited availability

CT, cognitive therapy; mo, month; PS, problem solving; SR, systematic review; y, year.

Domestic violence towards women

Search date July 2003

Joanne Klevens and Laura Sadowski

QUESTIONS

Effects of interventions initiated by healthcare professionals, aimed at female victims of domestic violence 141

INTERVENTIONS

Likely to be beneficial
Advocacy 143
Safety planning. 145

Unknown effectiveness
Cognitive behaviour orientated
   counselling 141
Couple counselling 141
Grief resolution orientated
   counselling 141

Peer support groups 145
Shelters 144

Unlikely to be beneficial
Non-specific counselling 141

See glossary, p 147

Key Messages

- **Advocacy** One RCT and one non-randomised controlled trial found that advocacy reduced reabuse compared with no treatment. The RCT also found an improvement in women's quality of life with advocacy compared with no treatment. One controlled trial in pregnant Hispanic women found no significant difference in rates of reabuse between combined counselling plus mentoring (similar to advocacy) and a resource card, but found that counselling plus mentoring slightly reduced rates of reabuse compared with unlimited counselling.

- **Safety planning** One RCT found that providing telephone sessions on safe behaviour in addition to usual care increased safe behaviour at 6 months compared with usual care alone. We found limited evidence from one non-randomised controlled trial in pregnant women that helping participants to make a safety plan reduced spouse abuse and increased safe behaviour at 12 months.

- **Cognitive behaviour orientated counselling** One controlled trial found that cognitive behaviour orientated therapy improved women's assertiveness and reduced their exposure to abuse compared with baseline levels, whereas non-specific support did not. However, the study did not directly compare effects of interventions.

- **Couple counselling** Controlled trials found that both gender specific counselling and couple counselling reduced physical aggression, psychological aggression and depression in wives from baseline levels, but they found no significant differences between treatments. One controlled trial found no significant difference between group and individual couple counselling on reduction in physical violence or on psychological wellbeing.

- **Grief resolution orientated counselling** One controlled trial found that grief resolution orientated counselling improved self esteem and self efficacy from baseline, whereas feminist orientated counselling did not. However, the study did not directly compare effects of interventions.

- **Peer support groups** We found no systematic reviews or controlled trials on the effect of peer support groups.

- **Shelters** We found no reliable controlled trials. One cohort study found a reduced incidence of violence in the weeks following shelter stay for women choosing to use the shelter when they were also engaged in other types of help seeking behaviour compared with women not choosing to stay at the shelter. Women choosing to stay at the shelter who had not sought help elsewhere experienced an increase in violence.

- **Non-specific counselling** Two controlled trials and one comparative cohort study found no effect of counselling compared with no treatment on medical care utilisation rates, reported exposure to violence and threats of violence, or depression, anxiety, and self esteem.

DEFINITION Domestic violence, also called intimate partner violence, is actual or threatened physical or sexual violence, or emotional or psychological abuse (including coercive tactics) by a current or former spouse or dating partner (including same sex partners).[1] Other terms commonly used to describe domestic violence include domestic abuse, spouse abuse, marital violence, and battering.

INCIDENCE/ PREVALENCE Between 10–69% of women participating in population based surveys in 48 countries from around the world reported being physically assaulted by a partner during their lifetime.[2] Rates of assault by a partner are 4.3 times higher among women than men.[3] Nearly 25% of surveyed women in the USA reported being physically and/or sexually assaulted by a current or former partner at some time during their lives, and 1.5% were victimised during the previous 12 months.[3] Rates of violence against pregnant women range from 0.9–20%.[4] Between 11.7–24.5% of women in prenatal clinics[5–8] and 5.5–17% of women in primary or ambulatory care reported being abused by a partner in the past year.[9–12]

AETIOLOGY/ RISK FACTORS A recent systematic review found that physical domestic violence toward women is associated with lower levels of education and unemployment, low family income, marital discord, and with the partner's lower level of occupation, childhood experiences of abuse, witnessing interparental violence, higher levels of anger, depression, heavy or problem drinking, drug use, jealousy, and lack of assertiveness with spouse.[13] A similar review of research on psychological aggression found that the few demographic and psychological variables assessed were either inconsistently associated with psychological domestic violence or were found to be associated with psychological domestic violence in studies with serious methodological limitations.[14]

PROGNOSIS There are few prospective studies documenting the course of domestic violence and its outcomes. Cross sectional surveys suggest that domestic violence persists for at least two thirds of women.[15,16] Among black and Hispanic people, persistence of domestic violence seems to be dependent on initial severity.[17] For all ethnic groups, half of those reporting moderate domestic violence did not report occurrences of domestic violence at the 5 year follow up, but for people of black or Hispanic origin reporting severe domestic violence only a third did not report occurrences of domestic violence at the 5 year follow up. A case control study conducted in middle class working women found that, compared with non-abused women, women abused by their partners during the previous 9 years were significantly more likely to have or report headaches (48% v 35%), back pain (40% v 25%), sexually transmitted diseases (6% v 2%), vaginal bleeding (17% v 6%), vaginal infections (30% v 21%), pelvic pain (17% v 9%), painful intercourse (13% v 7%), urinary tract infections (22% v 12%), appetite loss (9% v 3%), digestive problems (35% v 19%), abdominal pain (22% v 11%), and facial injuries (8% v 1%).[18] After adjusting for age, race, insurance status, and cigarette smoking, a cross sectional survey found that women experiencing psychological abuse are also more likely to report poor physical and mental health, disability preventing work, arthritis, chronic pain, migraine and other frequent headaches, sexually transmitted infections, chronic pelvic pain, stomach ulcers, spastic colon, frequent indigestion, diarrhoea, or constipation (see table 1, p 149).[19]

AIMS OF INTERVENTION

To improve quality of life and psychological and physical wellbeing; to reduce risk of physical and mental illness, injury, or death.

OUTCOMES

Self reported rates of domestic violence, mortality, non-fatal injuries, gynaecological and reproductive/obstetrical complications (e.g. chronic pelvic pain, miscarriage, recurrent vaginal infections), chronic disorders that may have a psychosomatic component (e.g. chronic pain, sleep or eating disorders, or hypertension), and psychological conditions (e.g. depression, suicide, substance abuse, anxiety, low self esteem, low self efficacy, or poor assertiveness) associated with intimate partner violence, as well as quality of life, physical and functional status, and adverse effects of treatment. Utilisation of domestic violence services was also considered as an intermediate outcome. Scales frequently used were the Severity of Violence Against Women Scale, Spielberger's 20 item State-Trait Anxiety Inventory, Hudson's Index of Self-esteem, Self-efficacy Scale, Modified Conflict Tactics Scale, Beck Depression Inventory, and Index of Spouse Abuse Scale (see glossary, p 147).

METHODS

Clinical Evidence search and appraisal July 2003. *Clinical Evidence* searched Medline from 1966, Embase from 1980, PsycINFO from 1985, ASSIA from 1987, Cinahl from 1982, MIDIRS from 1990; Cochrane Library 2002 issue 4 and TRIP database; and identified systematic reviews, RCTs, other controlled trials, and observational studies using the following search terms: intimate partner violence, domestic violence, battered women, woman abuse, woman battering, family violence, husband to wife violence, marital violence, battered wives, conjugal violence, spouse abuse, violence against women, and abused women; and prevention, treatment, or intervention. We excluded public education, system level interventions, civil protection orders, screening for domestic violence or protocols focusing on identification of domestic violence victims, as well as interventions targeting only men (e.g. batterer treatment). Couple interventions were included only if women participated regularly in the intervention and reoccurrence of violence or other outcomes among women were measured. Given the paucity of studies, none were excluded because of methodological limitations; however, when high non-participation, attrition, or high rates of loss to follow up were found, these are mentioned in the comment sections.

| QUESTION | What are the effects of interventions initiated by health care professionals, aimed at female victims of domestic violence? |

| OPTION | INDIVIDUAL, COUPLE, OR GROUP COUNSELLING |

Two controlled trials and one cohort study found no effect of counselling compared with no treatment on medical care utilisation rates, reported exposure to violence and threats of violence, or depression, state anxiety, and self esteem. One controlled trial found that grief resolution orientated counselling improved self esteem and self efficacy from baseline, whereas feminist orientated counselling did not. Similarly, one controlled trial found that cognitive behaviour orientated therapy improved women's assertiveness and reduced exposure to abuse from baseline, whereas non-specific support did not. One RCT and one controlled trial reported that gender specific or couple therapy reduced subsequent exposure to violence among couples from baseline, but found no significant differences between these two types of counselling.

Benefits:
Versus no treatment: We found three systematic reviews (search dates 1997[20] and 2001[21,22]), which between them identified one cohort study[23] and one controlled trial.[24] We found one additional controlled trial.[25] The cohort study (117 women), conducted in Sweden, evaluated an intervention comprising emergency room counselling (see glossary, p 147) by a social worker and psychiatrist, overnight hospital stay even if not warranted by injuries, counselling after release, and referrals to social and legal services offered to women self identified as battered.[23] Women receiving counselling had similar rates of utilisation of somatic and psychiatric care during the 5 year period after treatment compared with those who declined treatment or withdrew. No numbers or description of types of services were reported. The controlled trial identified by the systematic reviews (290 pregnant Hispanic women) compared three interventions: unlimited counselling, unlimited counselling plus a mentor, or a wallet sized resource card.[24] Clinics were assigned randomly (see comment). Women in all three groups reported a decrease in levels of violence and threats of violence at follow up 2 months postpartum, which was sustained through follow up at 6, 12, and 18 months. The trial found no significant difference in severity of violence between either type of counselling group and resource card intervention (mean on the Severity of Violence Against Women Scale [see glossary, p 147]: 34.7 for counselling plus mentor v 39.5 for unlimited counselling only v 38.2 for resource card; see note below for explanation of this score). Physical violence and threats of violence scores remained consistently lower at each follow up for the counselling plus mentor group (but not reaching statistical significance), whereas scores for women in the counselling only group were consistently higher than those in the resource card group. The additional controlled trial (33 women in two shelters in South Korea) compared a problem solving/empowerment group intervention versus no intervention.[25] Anxiety proneness scores (measured using Spielberger's 20 item State Trait Anxiety Inventory [see glossary, p 148]) decreased significantly in the intervention group compared with the control

group (size of change from pre-test to post-test: −11.81 v −0.35; P < 0.01), but there were no significant differences between groups in current levels of anxiety (−9.88 v −9.35; P = 0.91), self esteem (measured using Rosenberg's Self-esteem Scale [see glossary, p 147]: 1.56 v 1.29; P = 0.84), or depression (measured using the CES-D [see glossary, p 147]: −13.31 v −5.76; P = 0.13). **Grief resolution orientated counselling versus feminist orientated counselling:** We found one systematic review[22] (search date 2001, 1 quasi-randomised trial, 20 women). In the trial included in the review,[26] women requesting counselling at a battered women's programme were alternately allocated to grief resolution or feminist orientated individual counselling for 8 weeks. Women in both groups improved based on pre–post evaluation with Hudson's Index of Self-esteem (see glossary, p 147) and a Self-efficacy Scale (see glossary, p 147). Pre–post score differences were statistically significant only for women in the grief resolution orientated group for both self esteem (66.9 v 53.5; P < 0.01) and self efficacy (63.3 v 74.7; P < 0.01), whereas women in the feminist orientated group showed no significant changes between pre- and post-intervention scores (self esteem: 45.7 v 39.5; self efficacy: 68.4 v 77.7). Differences between treatments were not reported. **Cognitive behaviour orientated counselling** We found one controlled trial (20 women in Colombia, aged 19–50 years) that compared 20 twice weekly 3 hour sessions of cognitive behavioural treatment versus non-structured support group.[27] Two women in the cognitive behavioural therapy group and four in the non-structured support group reported new episodes of domestic violence after the intervention began. Levels of assertiveness improved significantly in the intervention group (from pre- to post-intervention; P < 0.05), whereas in the control group they did not. Differences between treatments were not reported. **Group counselling versus individual couple counselling:** One systematic review (search date 1997) identified one controlled trial (68 couples).[20] It found no difference between group and individual couple intervention in reduction in physical violence or in psychological wellbeing. Withdrawal rates were higher in the group programme. **Gender specific versus couple counselling:** We identified one RCT[28] and one non-randomised controlled trial (124 couples) comparing gender specific counselling versus couple counselling.[29] In the RCT, 49 couples who indicated a desire to remain in their current relationship were randomly assigned to gender specific counselling or couple counselling.[28] There were no differences in victims' reports of subsequent physical violence at 6 month follow up for 26 (62%) of the couples (reports: 8.3% among couple therapy participants v 7.1% for gender specific therapy; P = 0.91). In the non-randomised controlled trial, volunteer married and intact couples who reported at least two acts of husband to wife physical aggression (75 couples), excluding couples with alcohol dependence, mental disease, and who reported severe injuries, or women who feared their partner, were alternately assigned to couple therapy or gender specific therapy.[29] The past year prevalence of husband to wife physical aggression was reduced from 100% before treatment to 74% after treatment (P < 0.01) in both groups, based on the Modified Conflict Tactics Scale (see glossary, p 147). With both treatments, there were significant decreases from pre-treatment scores to 1 year follow up in husband to wife psychological aggression (93.37 to 44.79; $P < 0.005$) and mild (19.31 to 8.63; $P < 0.001$) and severe physical aggression (3.34 to 1.71; $P < 0.05$), as well as wives' depression on the Beck Depression Inventory (see glossary, p 147) (12.39 to 8.79; $P < 0.005$), with no differences between treatments. Women in couples group therapy reported that physical aggression resulted from content discussed in 2% of the sessions, with no differences between treatments.

Harms: No harms were reported for individual or group counselling. However, a potential harm of any intervention targeting victims of domestic violence is escalation of violence as a result of reprisal. Qualitative assessment of weekly reports did not support the belief that women who received couple counselling were placed in any further danger than those who attended individual therapy.[28]

Comment: It is unclear whether the controlled trial comparing counselling versus no intervention was an RCT because the allocation method was not described.[24] Rotating assignment to groups may have increased the possibility of contamination across groups. In the quasi-randomised trial comparing grief orientated versus feminist orientated counselling, the scoring range was unclear, and the authors did not indicate whether the original 14 point Lickert scale was used.[26] The trial conducted in South Korea, comparing a group problem solving/empowering intervention versus no intervention, had high withdrawal rates (47% in group intervention v 43% in the no intervention group).[25] In the second trial comparing gender specific interventions versus couple intervention, two thirds of eligible couples declined to participate.[29] In addition, 67% of the participants withdrew at the start or dropped out during treatment or before follow up.

OPTION   ADVOCACY

One RCT and one non-randomised controlled trial found that advocacy reduced reabuse compared with no treatment. The RCT also found an improvement in women's quality of life with advocacy compared with no treatment. One controlled trial in pregnant Hispanic women found no significant difference in rates of reabuse between combined counselling plus mentoring (similar to advocacy) and a resource card, but found that counselling plus mentoring slightly reduced rates of reabuse compared with unlimited counselling.

Benefits: **Versus no treatment:** We found one systematic review[30] (search date 2002, 1 RCT,[31] 278 women) and one additional non-randomised controlled trial.[32] The RCT included in the review allocated 278 battered women leaving shelter stay either to a trainee advocate or to a control group.[31] Advocates worked with participants for about 6.4 hours each week over a 10 week period. It found significant reductions in psychological abuse and increases in quality of life at 6, 12, 18, and 24 months of follow up, but it found no significant change from baseline for depression. The RCT reported no significant differences between groups for psychological abuse or depression, but found that advocacy significantly improved quality of life ($P = 0.01$) and reduced reabuse at 24 months compared with control (reabuse rate: 76% with advocacy v

89% with control; $P < 0.01$). The additional non-randomised controlled trial (81 women seeking temporary restraining orders with incomes below the poverty line and access to a telephone, who had no obvious mental disorder, were not already represented by an attorney, or receiving extensive violence related resources) allocated 22 women to law school advocates and 59 to standard court services without an advocate.[32] Women assisted by advocates reported less physical reabuse (5% v 25%) and psychological reabuse (10% v 47%) compared with women receiving standard court services at 6 months of follow up. **Versus counselling:** We found one systematic review (search date 2001, 1 controlled trial,[24] 290 pregnant Hispanic women).[22] The controlled trial compared unlimited counselling plus a mentor (who might be considered to have acted as an advocate) versus unlimited counselling only versus a resource card.[24] Participants in all three groups reported a reduction in levels of violence and threats of violence at follow up 2 months postpartum. Although women receiving unlimited counselling plus mentoring reported less physical violence than women receiving unlimited counselling only (mean on the Severity of Violence Against Women Scale [see glossary, p 147] adjusted for entry scores: 34.7 v 39.5; $P < 0.05$), neither of these interventions had significantly different results compared with women receiving only a resource card. There were no differences at 6, 12, or 18 month follow up assessments.

Harms: No harms were reported. However, a potential harm for any intervention targeting victims of domestic violence is escalation of violence as a result of reprisal.

Comment: In the additional controlled trial (81 women below the poverty line), 41% of those approached did not consent to participate.[32] An additional 13% did not appear for their first appointment. Assignment to the intervention group was based on women's acceptance of free legal representation from a law student. The RCT[31] evaluated the effect of advocacy for women exiting shelters, and the controlled trial involving women below the poverty line utilised law school advocates in a legal setting (interventions not available in a healthcare setting).[32] Although referral to an advocate (usually available at community based intimate partner violence services) at any time was considered an intervention to which a healthcare professional could potentially refer a victim; the extent to which the effectiveness of these interventions for women exiting shelter or women seeking restraining orders can be generalised to women in other conditions is unknown.

| OPTION | SHELTERS |

We found no reliable controlled trials. One cohort study found a reduced incidence of violence in the weeks after shelter stay for women choosing to use the shelter when they were also engaged in other types of help seeking behaviour compared with women not choosing to stay at the shelter. Women choosing to stay at the shelter who had not sought help elsewhere experienced an increase in violence.

Benefits: We found one systematic review (search date 1997), which found no reliable studies.[20]

Harms: The systematic review identified one cohort study (243 women), which found that violence increased among women staying at shelters who had not sought other types of help.[33] However, women choosing shelters had previously experienced twice as much violence as those not choosing shelters.

Comment: The systematic review identified one cohort study (243 women) in women who spontaneously went to a shelter (see glossary, p 147) and women sent by the prosecutors' offices compared those who voluntarily chose to stay at the shelter compared with those who chose not to stay. [33] Stay ranged from 1–30 days. The study found that women choosing shelter and not seeking any other help were more likely to experience new episodes of violence during the 6 weeks after leaving the shelter compared with those who did not choose to stay at the shelter (OR 1.8; P = 0.13, after adjusting for initial risk of violence, days outside the shelter, and attrition). However, in women who engaged in at least one other type of help seeking behaviour, shelter use reduced the risk of new violence compared with shelter non-use (OR 0.6; P < 0.05), suggesting that shelter stay is only effective when women use other resources. Conclusions must be drawn carefully from this study because losses to follow up were 36%, and results were based on subgroup analyses.[33] In the study, help seeking behaviour was defined as the number of distinct kinds of help seeking actions taken during the 6 months before the baseline interview and included previous shelter stay, calling the police, trying to get a restraining order, seeking criminal justice prosecution, seeking counselling, and trying to get help from legal aid or a private attorney.[20]

OPTION   PEER SUPPORT GROUPS

We found no systematic reviews, RCTs, non-randomised controlled trials, or cohort studies of peer support groups in women experiencing domestic violence.

Benefits: We found no RCTs, non-randomised controlled trials, or cohort studies of peer support groups (see glossary, p 147) in women experiencing domestic violence.

Harms: We found no RCTs, non-randomised controlled trials, or cohort studies.

Comment: None.

OPTION   SAFETY PLANNING

One RCT found that providing telephone sessions on safe behaviour in addition to usual care increased safe behaviour at 6 months compared with usual care alone. We found limited evidence from one non-randomised controlled trial in pregnant women that helping participants to make a safety plan reduced spouse abuse and increased safe behaviour at 12 months.

Benefits: We found one systematic review (search date 2002, 1 RCT, and 1 non-randomised trial).[30] The RCT (150 English and Spanish speaking women recruited from a family violence unit in an urban District

Attorney's office) compared standard services offered by the District Attorney's office versus standard services plus six telephone sessions on safety behaviours.[34] The RCT found that additional sessions on safety behaviours improved safety behaviour compared with standard treatment at 3 and 6 months (safety behaviours were assessed using the Safety Behaviour Checklist of 15 behaviours, adjusted for relevance [e.g. if no firearms in the home, adopting the safety behaviour of removing the firearm was not applicable]; mean increase of two safety behaviours for sessions v standard care; effect size 0.91 at 3 months and 0.64 at 6 months). In the non-randomised trial included in the review, 199 pregnant women attending public prenatal clinics who had been physically or sexually assaulted in the past year by their partner were recruited consecutively first into the control group to receive standard prenatal care (67 women) and then into the safety planning group (132 women).[35] Women in the control group received a wallet sized resource card with information on community resources. In the safety planning group, trained nurses helped participants to prepare a safety plan and provided them with information on applying for legal protection orders and filing for criminal charges, as well as community resource phone numbers. This information was provided during three evenly spaced sessions throughout pregnancy and was reinforced with a brochure at the end of each session. After adjusting for entry levels of violence, women in the safety planning group reported less ongoing physical and non-physical abuse on the Index of Spouse Abuse Scale (see glossary, p 147) at 12 months (37.6 v 56.9; P = 0.007), and fewer threats and instances of actual violence on the Severity of Violence Against Women Scale (see glossary, p 147) at 6 months (threats score 27.3 v 33.4; actual violence 33.1 v 35.9) and 12 months (threats score 27.0 v 33.6; actual violence 32.6 v 37.1) compared with women in the control group (P = 0.052), although it is unclear to which comparison the statistical test refers to. At 12 months, the safety planning group had used significantly more relevant safety behaviours than women in the control group (P < 0.001).

Harms: None reported. However, a potential harm for any intervention targeting victims of domestic violence is escalation of violence as a result of reprisal. In the RCT, one woman committed suicide after 3 weeks. The study did not report which treatment she was assigned. However, it is not clear that the suicide was related to treatment.[34]

Comment: The RCT recruited participants from a district attorney's office, a setting to which healthcare providers may refer people who have experienced domestic violence.[34] Less than 3% of women refused to participate (4/154). Nearly all women completed the study at 6 months (149/150). The occurrence of intimate partner violence during the trial was not assessed. The intervention ceased at 8 weeks, and a subsequent assessment of effect size showed a decrease between 3–6 months. The authors noted that this may reflect a ceiling effect or a need for reinforcement with additional intervention services. In the non-randomised study, the intervention group was recruited during prenatal care, whereas the comparison group was recruited postpartum.[35] The influence of different periods of recruitment on recall of abuse was not explored.

Mental health

GLOSSARY

Advocacy involves providing information to a client on her legal, medical, and financial options; facilitating her access to and utilisation of community resources such as shelters, counselling, and protection orders; accessing and mobilising her natural support networks; assisting in goal setting and making choices; validating her feelings of being victimised; and providing emotional support.[6]

Beck Depression Inventory in its short version has 13 items. Scores above 4 indicate increasing levels of depression.

CES-D (Centers for Epidemiological Studies Depression) Scale Twenty item 4 point Lickert scale, with scores that range from 0 to 60. Higher scores indicate more symptoms of depression.

Counselling usually involves professional guidance in solving a client's problems. Counselling services tend to focus on providing information rather than the use of psychological techniques. However, counselling, as used in one of the controlled trials referred to above,[25] may also include referral to services and assistance in accessing these services (overlapping with advocacy).

Hudson's Index of Self-esteem Scores vary from 0–100. Higher scores indicate lower self esteem.

Index of Spouse Abuse Scale is a 30 item, self report scale measuring the frequency with which respondents have experienced 11 types of physical abuse and 19 types of non-physical abuse inflicted by a male partner. In scoring the measure, items are weighted differentially based on severity. Scores range from 0–100 on each subscale, with high scores indicating high frequency of severe abuse and low scores indicating relative absence of abuse.

Modified Conflict Tactics Scale (CTS2) has 78 items measuring the frequency (on an 8 point scale from never to more than 20 times) with which partners engage in psychological and physical attacks on each other.

Peer support groups Sometimes facilitated by a professional, peer support groups are hypothesised to help women exposed to domestic violence by reducing social isolation (risk factor for or effect of domestic violence) and providing encouragement and support, for example by allowing women to see that they are not alone in their experience and that there are available alternatives to changing their situation.

Rosenberg's Self-esteem Scale A 10 item scale with a four point response format resulting in a score range of 10 to 40, with higher scores representing higher self steem.

Safety planning helps participants to identify behaviours that might signal increased danger and prepare, ahead of time, codes of communication with family or friends, as well as needed documents, keys, and clothing should a quick exit become necessary.

Self-efficacy Scale Scores on the original 23 item scale vary from 14 to 322, with a mean of 230 ± 39. Higher scores indicate higher self efficacy.[27]

Severity of Violence Against Women Scale Scores on the physical violence component range from 27 to 108, where 27 would equal never being exposed to any of the behaviours and 108 would equal being exposed many times to all of the behaviours in the inventory.

Shelters provide housing, food, and clothing, usually for 30–90 days, to victims and their children under 12 who leave their abuser. Many shelters also offer individual or group therapy or counselling, advocacy, child care, job training, and assistance in finding transitional housing.

Spielberger's 20 item State-Trait Anxiety Inventory Scores range from 20–80, where 20 equals not feeling like that at all (state anxiety) or ever (trait anxiety) and 80 would equal feeling like that very much (state anxiety) or always (trait anxiety).

REFERENCES

1. National Center for Injury Prevention and Control. *Injury fact book 2001–2002.* Atlanta, GA: Centers for Disease Control and Prevention, 2001.

2. Krug EG, Dahlberg LL, Mercy JA, et al. *World report on violence and health.* Geneva: World Health Organization, 2002.

3. Tjaden P, Thoennes N. *Full report of the prevalence, incidence, and consequences of violence against women.* Washington, DC: National Institute of Justice, 2000.

4. Gazmarian JA, Lazorick S, Spitz AM, et al. Prevalence of violence against pregnant women. *JAMA* 1996;275:1915–1920.

5. Savona-Ventura C, Savona-Ventura M, Dregsted-Nielsen S, et al. Domestic abuse in a central Meditarranean pregnant population. *Eur J Obstet Gynecol Reprod Biol* 2001;98:3–8.

6. Purwar MB, Jeyaseelan L, Varhadpande U, et al. Survey of physical abuse during pregnancy GMCH, Nagpur, India. *J Obstet Gynaecol Res* 1999;25:165–171.

7. Lueng WC, Lueng TW, Lam YY, et al. The prevalence of domestic violence against pregnant women in a Chinese community. *Int J Gynaecol Obstet* 1999;66:23–30.

8. Hedin LW, Grimstad H, Moller A, et al. Prevalne of physical and sexual abuse before and during pregnany among Swedish couples. *Acta Obstet Gynecol Scand* 1999;78:310–315.

9. Bauer H, Rodriguez MA, Perez-Stable EJ. Prevalence and determinants of intimate partner abuse among public hospital primary care patients. *J Gen Intern Med* 2000;15:811–817.

10. Richardson J, Coid J, Petruckevitch A, et al. Identifying domestic violence: cross-sectional study in primary care. *BMJ* 2002;324:271–277.

11. McCauley J, Kern DE, Kolodner K, et al. The "battering syndrome": prevalence and clinical characteristics of domestic violence in primary care internal medicine practices. *Ann Intern Med* 1995;123:737–746.

12. Gin NE, Ruker L, Frayne S, et al. Prevalence of domestic violence among patients in three ambulatory care internal medicine clinics. *J Gen Intern Med* 1991;6:317–322.

13. Schumacher JA, Felbau-Kohn S, Smith-Slep AM, et al. Risk factors for male to female physical abuse. *Aggress Violent Behav* 2001;6:281–352.

14. Schumacher JA, Smith-Slep AM, Heyman RE. Risk factors for male-to-female psychological abuse. *Aggress Violent Behav* 2001;6:255–268.

15. Gelles RJ. *Intimate violence in families,* 3rd ed. Thousand Oaks, California: Sage, 1997.

16. Rand MR, Saltzman LE. The nature and extent of recurring intimate partner violence against women in the United States. *J Comp Fam Stud* 2003;34:137–149.

17. Caetano R, Schafer J, Fals-Stewart W. Stability and change in intimate partner violence and drinking among white, black, and Hispanic couples over a 5-year interval. *Alcohol Clin Exp Res* 2003;27:292–300.

18. Campbell J, Jones AS, Dienemann J, et al. Intimate partner violence and physical health consequences. *Arch Intern Med* 2002;162:1157–1163.

19. Coker AL, Smith PH, Bethea L, et al. Physical health consequences of physical and psychological intimate partner violence. *Arch Fam Med* 2000;9:451–457.

20. Chalk R, King PA (ed). *Violence in families. assessing prevention and treatment programs.* Washington, DC: National Academy Press, 1998. Search date 1997; primary sources National Criminal Justice Reference Section, National Child Abuse and Neglect Data System, Medline, Legal Resource Index, Criminal Justice Periodical Index, ERIC, Social SciSearch, PsychINFO, Dissertation Abstracts Online, A-V Online, PAIS Online, IAC Business, ARTS, US Political Science Documents, British Education Index, Ageline, Religion Index, Public Opinion Online, National Center on Child Abuse and Neglect Clearinghouse, Family Violence and Sexual Assault Institute, National Clearinghouse for the Defense of Battered Women, National Resource enter on Domestic Violence, Family Violence Prevention Fund.

21. Ramsay J, Richardson J, Carter Y, et al. Should health professionals screen women for domestic violence? Systematic review. *BMJ* 2002;325:314–327. Search date 2001; primary sources Medline, Embase, Cinahl.

22. Centre for Clinical Effectiveness. *Is therapy/counseling/group work more effective than no treatment for women who are victims of domestic violence?* Melbourne: Southern Health/Monash Institute of Public Health, 2001. Search date 2001; primary sources Cochrane Library, Best Evidence, Medline, Cinahl, Current Contents, Premedline, PsychINFO, SocioFile, Journals OVID, National Guideline Clearinghouse, Australasian Medical Index.

23. Bergman B, Brismar B. A 5-year follow-up of 117 battered women. *Am J Public Health* 1991;81:1486–1489.

24. McFarlane J, Soeken K, Wiist W. An evaluation of interventions to decrease intimate partner violence to pregnant women. *Public Health Nurs* 2000;17:443–451.

25. Kim S, Kim J. The effects of group intervention for battered women in Korea. *Arch Psychiatr Nurs* 2001;15:257–264.

26. Mancoske RJ, Standifer D, Cauley C. The effectiveness of brief counseling services for battered women. *Res Soc Work Pract* 1994;4:53–63.

27. Laverde DI. Effects of cognitive-behavioural therapy in controlling wife abuse [in Spanish]. *Revista de Analisis del Comportamieno* 1987;3:193–200.

28. Brannen SJ, Rubin A. Comparing the effectiveness of gender-specific and couples groups in court-mandated spouse abuse treatment program. *Res Soc Work Pract* 1996;6:405–424.

29. O'Leary KD, Heyman RE, Neidig PH. Treatment of wife abuse: a comparison of gender-specific and conjoint approaches. *Behav Ther* 1999;30:475–505.

30. Wathen C, MacMillan H. Interventions for violence against women: scientific review. *JAMA* 2003;289:589–600. Search date 2002; primary sources Medline, PsychINFO, Cinahl, HealthStar, Sociological Abstracts, and hand searches of reference lists from key articles.

31. Sullivan CM, Bybee DI. Reducing violence using community based advocacy for women with abusive partners. *J Consult Clin Psychol* 1999;67:43–53.

32. Bell ME, Goodman LA. Supporting battered women involved with the court system: an evaluation of a law school-based advocacy intervention. *Violence Women* 2001;7:1377–1404.

33. Berk RD, Newton PJ, Berk SF. What a difference a day makes: an empirical study of the impact of

shelters for battered women. *J Marriage Fam* 1986;48:481–490.

34. McFarlane J, Malecha A, Gist J, et al. An intervention to increase safety behaviours of abused women: results of a randomised clinical trial. *Nurs Res* 2002;51:347–354.

35. Parker B, McFarlane J, Soeken K, et al. Testing an intervention to prevent further abuse to pregnant women. *Res Nurs Health* 1999;22:59–66.

Joanne Klevens
Epidemiologist
Centers for Disease Control, National
Center for Injury Prevention and Control,
Division of Violence Prevention
Atlanta
USA

Laura Sadowski
Co-Director/Associate Professor
Collaborative Research Unit, Cook
County Hospital/Department of Internal
Medicine, Rush Medical College
Chicago
USA

Competing interests: None declared.

TABLE 1	Risks for reported conditions in women experiencing psychological abuse (see text, p 139).[19]
Complaint	**RR (95% CI)**
Poor physical health	1.69 (1.20 to 2.29)
Poor mental health	1.74 (1.07 to 2.73)
Disability preventing work	1.49 (1.06 to 2.14)
Arthritis	1.67 (0.20 to 2.22)
Chronic pain	1.91 (1.49 to 2.36)
Migraine	1.54 (1.16 to 1.93)
Other frequent headaches	1.41 (1.05 to 1.82)
Sexually transmitted infections	1.82 (1.19 to 2.68)
Chronic pelvic pain	1.62 (1.03 to 2.48)
Stomach ulcers	1.72 (1.02 to 2.84)
Spastic colon	3.62 (1.63 to 7.50)
Frequent indigestion, diarrhoea, or constipation	1.30 (1.03 to 1.63)

Generalised anxiety disorder

Search date June 2003

Christopher Gale and Mark Oakley-Browne

INTERVENTIONS

Key Messages

- **Buspirone** RCTs have found that buspirone improves symptoms over 4–9 weeks compared with placebo. RCTs found no significant difference in symptoms over 6–8 weeks between buspirone and antidepressants, diazepam, or hydroxyzine, but the studies may have lacked power to detect clinically important differences among treatments.

- **Certain antidepressants (imipramine, opipramol, paroxetine, and venlafaxine)** RCTs have found that antidepressants (imipramine, opipramol, paroxetine, and venlafaxine) improve symptoms over 4–28 weeks compared with placebo. RCTs found no significant difference among these antidepressants or between antidepressants and benzodiazepines or buspirone. RCTs and observational studies have found that antidepressants are associated with sedation, dizziness, nausea, falls, and sexual dysfunction.

- **Cognitive behavioural therapy** Two systematic reviews and two subsequent RCTs have found that cognitive behavioural therapy (using a combination of interventions, such as exposure, relaxation, and cognitive restructuring) improves anxiety and depression over 4–12 weeks compared with waiting list control, anxiety management alone, relaxation alone, or non-directive psychotherapy. Three subsequent RCTs, two in people aged ≥60 years, found no significant difference in symptoms at 13 weeks, 6 months, or 24 months between cognitive therapy and applied relaxation.

- **Hydroxyzine** Three RCTs comparing hydroxyzine versus placebo found different results. Two RCTs found that, compared with placebo, hydroxyzine improved symptoms of anxiety at 4 or 12 weeks, but a third RCT found no significant difference in the proportion of people with improved symptoms of anxiety at 5 weeks. One of the RCTs found that hydroxyzine increased somnolence and headaches compared with placebo. One RCT found no significant difference between hydroxyzine and bromazepam in the proportion of people who responded after 6 weeks. Another RCT found no significant difference between hydroxyzine and buspirone in the proportion of people who responded after 4 weeks.

- **Benzodiazepines** One systematic review and one subsequent RCT found that benzodiazepines reduced symptoms over 2–9 weeks compared with placebo. RCTs found no significant difference in symptoms over 3–8 weeks between alprazolam and bromazepam or mexazolam, or between benzodiazepines and buspirone, hydroxyzine, abecarnil, or antidepressants. RCTs and observational studies found that benzodiazepines increased the risk of dependence, sedation, industrial accidents, and road traffic accidents and that, if used in late pregnancy or while breast feeding, benzodiazepines may cause adverse effects in neonates. One systematic review of poor quality RCTs provided insufficient evidence to assess long term treatment with benzodiazepines.

- **Kava** One systematic review in people with a variety anxiety disorders, including generalised anxiety disorder, found that kava reduced symptoms of anxiety over 1–24 weeks compared with placebo. It is unclear whether results of the review are generalisable to people with generalised anxiety disorder. Observational evidence suggests that kava may be associated with hepatotoxicity.

- **Trifluoperazine** One large RCT found that trifluoperazine reduced anxiety after 4 weeks compared with placebo, but caused more drowsiness, extrapyramidal reactions, and other movement disorders.

- **Abecarnil** One RCT found limited evidence that low dose abecarnil improved symptoms compared with placebo. Another RCT found no significant difference in symptoms at 6 weeks between abecarnil and placebo or diazepam. Both RCTs found that abecarnil increased drowsiness compared with placebo.

- **Applied relaxation** We found no RCTs comparing applied relaxation versus placebo or no treatment. Three RCTs found no significant difference in symptoms at 13 weeks, 6 months, or 24 months between applied relaxation and cognitive behavioural therapy.

- **β Blockers** We found no RCTs on the effects of β blockers in people with generalised anxiety disorder.

DEFINITION   Generalised anxiety disorder (GAD) is defined as excessive worry and tension about every day events and problems, on most days, for at least 6 months, to the point where the person experiences distress or has marked difficulty in performing day-to-day tasks.[1] It may be characterised by the following symptoms and signs: increased motor tension (fatigability, trembling, restlessness, and muscle tension); autonomic hyperactivity (shortness of breath, rapid heart rate, dry mouth, cold hands, and dizziness); and increased vigilance and scanning (feeling keyed up, increased startling, and impaired concentration), but not panic attacks.[1] One non-systematic review of epidemiological and clinical studies found marked reduction of quality of life and psychosocial functioning in people with anxiety disorders (including GAD).[2] It also found that people with GAD had low overall life satisfaction and some impairment in ability to fulfil roles, social tasks, or both.[2]

INCIDENCE/   One overview of observational studies found that the prevalence of
PREVALENCE GAD among adults in the community was 1.5–3.0%.[3] It found that 3–5% of adults had had GAD in the past year and 4–7% had had GAD during their lives. The US National Comorbidity Survey found that over 90% of people diagnosed with GAD had a co-morbid diagnosis,

including dysthymia (22%), depression (39–69%), somatisation, other anxiety disorders, bipolar disorder, or substance abuse.[4] The Harvard Brown Anxiety Research Program also found that only 30/180 people (17%) had GAD alone.[5] Subgroup analysis suggested that 46/122 people with GAD (38%) had co-morbid personality disorder.[6] A systematic review of the comorbidity of eating disorders and anxiety disorders (search date 2001, 2 observational studies, 55 people) found a lifetime prevalence of GAD among people with anorexia nervosa of 24% in one study and 31% in the other.[7] The lifetime prevalence of GAD in the control group of one of the studies (44 people) was 2%. The reliability of the measures used to diagnose GAD in epidemiological studies is unsatisfactory.[8,9] One US study, with explicit diagnostic criteria (DSM-III-R), estimated that 5% of people will develop GAD at some time during their lives.[9] A recent cohort study of people with depressive and anxiety disorders found that 49% of people initially diagnosed with GAD retained this diagnosis over 2 years.[10] The incidence of GAD in men is only half the incidence in women[11] and is lower in older people.[12] A non-systematic review (20 observational studies in younger and older adults) suggested that autonomic arousal to stressful tasks was decreased in older people, and that older people became accustomed to stressful tasks more quickly than younger people.[13]

AETIOLOGY/ RISK FACTORS GAD is believed to be associated with an increase in the number of minor stressors, independent of demographic factors,[14,15] but this finding is also common in people with other diagnoses.[10] One non-systematic review (5 case control studies) of psychological sequelae to civilian trauma found that rates of GAD reported in four of the five studies were significantly increased compared with a control population (rate ratio 3.3, 95% CI 2.0 to 5.5).[16] One systematic review (search date 1997) of cross-sectional studies found that bullying (or peer victimisation) was associated with a significant increase in the incidence of GAD (effect size 0.21, CI not reported).[17] Genetic factors are also implicated. One systematic review (search date not reported, 2 family studies, 45 index cases, 225 first degree relatives) found a significant association between GAD in the index cases and in their first degree relatives (OR 6.1, 95% CI 2.5 to 14.9).[18] The review also identified three twin studies (13 305 people), which estimated that 32% (95% CI 24% to 39%) of the variance to liability to GAD was explained by genetic factors.

PROGNOSIS One systematic review found that 25% of adults with GAD will be in full remission after 2 years, and 38% will have a remission after 5 years.[3] The Harvard-Brown anxiety research program reported 5 year follow up of 167 people with GAD.[19] In this period, the weighted probability for full remission was 38% and for at least partial remission was 47%: the probability of relapse from full remission was 27% and relapse from partial remission was 39%.

AIMS OF INTERVENTION To reduce symptoms of anxiety; to minimise disruption of day-to-day functioning; and to improve quality of life, with minimum adverse effects.

OUTCOMES Severity of symptoms and effects on quality of life, as measured by symptom scores on continuous rating scales, usually the Hamilton Anxiety Scale, State-Trait Anxiety Inventory, or Clinical Global

Impression Scale. Other continuous scales include the Penn State Worry Questionnaire and the GAD Severity Scale. Most RCTs define a 20% reduction in symptoms scores on the relevant scale as a clinical response. Where numbers needed to treat are given, these represent the number of people requiring treatment within a given time period (usually 6–12 weeks) for one additional person to achieve a certain improvement in symptom score. The method for obtaining numbers needed to treat was not standardised across studies. Some RCTs defined a reduction by, for example, 20 points in the Hamilton Anxiety Scale as a clinical response, others defined a clinical response as a reduction, for example, by 50% of the premorbid score. The authors have not attempted to standardise methods, but instead have used the response rates reported in each study to calculate numbers needed to treat. Similarly, the authors have calculated numbers needed to harm from original trial data.

METHODS   *Clinical Evidence* search and appraisal June 2003. Recent changes in diagnostic classification make it hard to compare older studies with more recent ones. In the earlier classification system (DSM-III-R) the diagnosis was made only in the absence of other psychiatric disorders. In current systems (DSM-IV and ICD-10), GAD can be diagnosed in the presence of any comorbid condition.

QUESTION   What are the effects of treatments?

OPTION   COGNITIVE BEHAVIOURAL THERAPY

Two systematic reviews and two subsequent RCTs have found that cognitive behavioural therapy (using a combination of interventions such as exposure, relaxation, and cognitive restructuring) improves anxiety and depression over 4–12 weeks compared with waiting list control, anxiety management alone, relaxation alone, or non-directive psychotherapy. Three subsequent RCTs, two in people aged ≥ 60 years, found no significant difference in symptoms at 13 weeks, 6 months, or 24 months between cognitive therapy and applied relaxation.

Benefits: We found two systematic reviews[20,21] and five subsequent RCTs[22–26] comparing cognitive behavioural therapy (see glossary, p 164) versus waiting list control (no treatment) or versus other psychotherapies in people with generalised anxiety disorder (GAD). The first systematic review (search date 1996, 13 RCTs, 722 people aged 18–60 years, 60% women) compared cognitive behavioural therapy (which involved, alone or in combination, cognitive restructuring, relaxation, exposure, and systematic desensitisation) versus control (remaining on a waiting list, anxiety management alone, relaxation alone, and non-directive psychotherapy).[20] It found that cognitive behavioural therapy significantly improved symptoms over 4–12 weeks compared with control (effect size for anxiety 0.70, 95% CI 0.57 to 0.83 and for depression 0.77, 95% CI 0.64 to 0.90; dichotomous data not reported). The second systematic review (search date not reported, 5 RCTs, 313 people aged 18–60 years) included three RCTs identified by the first review.[21] It found that cognitive behavioural therapy (including relaxation, cognitive therapy, behavioural therapy, and anxiety management training, alone or in combination) or analytical psychotherapy were associated with an improvement in symptoms compared with waiting list control (median effect size 0.9; CI not reported).[21] The first subsequent RCT (75 people aged > 55 years) compared three interventions: cognitive therapy, attending a discussion group on worrying topics, and waiting list control for 12 weeks.[25] It found that, compared with waiting list control, either cognitive therapy or a discussion group significantly increased the proportion of people who no longer met criteria for GAD immediately after treatment (people without GAD: 54% with cognitive therapy v 50% with discussion group v 13% with control; P < 0.01 for either treatment v control; absolute numbers not reported). It found no significant difference between cognitive therapy and a discussion group in the proportion of people who no longer met criteria for GAD immediately after treatment (P = 0.78) or at 6 months (72% with cognitive therapy v 53% with discussion group; P = 0.23). The second subsequent RCT (80 people aged > 60 years) compared cognitive therapy versus minimal contact for 15 weeks.[24] Minimal contact involved one telephone call a week (see comment below). Symptoms were assessed by Hamilton Anxiety Scale (HAM-A), State-Trait Anxiety Inventory, Penn State Worry Questionnaire, and GAD Severity Scale. It found that cognitive therapy significantly increased the proportion of people who responded immediately after treatment compared with minimal contact (response defined as a 20% reduction in symptoms on 3 of the 4 assessment scales: 13/29 [45%] with cognitive therapy v 3/35 [8%] with minimal contact; RR 5.2, 95% CI 1.6 to 16.5; NNT 3, 95% CI 2 to 8). The third subsequent RCT (36 people aged 18–60 years) found no significant difference between 12 weekly sessions of cognitive therapy and applied relaxation (see glossary, p 164) in the proportion of people who responded after 13 weeks (response defined as improvement to score 3 or 4 on Cognitive Global Impression Scale, 10/18 [56%] with cognitive therapy v 8/15 [53%] with applied relaxation; RR 1.04, 95% CI 0.55 to 1.95).[22] The fourth subsequent RCT (76 people aged mean 37 years, 69 people completed) compared 15 weekly sessions of cognitive therapy, applied relaxation, and a combination of these methods.[23] It found that similar proportions of people in each group no longer met criteria for GAD immediately after treatment and at 24 months (people without GAD at follow up: 8.7% in each group immediately after treatment; 14.3% with cognitive therapy v 19.1% with applied relaxation v 19.1% with combination of treatments at 24 months; P value not reported).[23] The fifth subsequent RCT (45 people aged 17–70 years) found no significant difference between cognitive therapy and applied relaxation for 12 weeks in the proportion of people who responded at 6 months (response defined as a score of ≤ 46 on the State-Trait Anxiety Inventory: 55% with cognitive therapy v 53.3% with applied relaxation; results not intention to treat, reported as non-significant, absolute numbers not reported).[26]

Harms: The reviews and subsequent RCTs gave no information on harms.[20–27]

Comment: In the second subsequent RCT, the control group received minimal contact rather than usual care without cognitive therapy; this may have overestimated the effect of cognitive therapy.[24] A third systematic review (search date 1998, 6 RCTs comparing cognitive therapy versus a variety of other psychological treatments, 404 people) did not compare treatments directly.[28] It reanalysed the raw data from individual RCTs to calculate the proportion of people who experienced a clinically important improvement in symptoms after treatment and maintained that improvement for 6 months. It found limited evidence that more people who had individual cognitive therapy maintained recovery after 6 months than people who had other psychological treatments, with the exception of applied relaxation (proportion of people who maintained improvement: 41% with individual cognitive therapy, 19% with non-directive treatment, 18% with group cognitive therapy, 12% with group behaviour therapy, 18% with individual behaviour therapy, 0% with analytical psychotherapy, and 52% with applied relaxation; P values not reported).[28] Many of the RCTs were small and were not analysed on an intention to treat basis.

OPTION   APPLIED RELAXATION

We found no RCTs comparing applied relaxation versus placebo or no treatment. Three RCTs found no significant difference in symptoms at 13 weeks, 6 months, or 24 months between applied relaxation and cognitive therapy.

Benefits: **Versus placebo or no treatment:** We found no systematic review or RCTs. **Versus other psychological treatments:** See benefits of cognitive therapy, p 153.

Harms: **Versus other psychological treatments:** See harms of cognitive therapy, p 153.

Comment: We found one systematic review (search date 1998, 6 RCTs comparing cognitive therapy (see glossary, p 164) versus a variety of other psychological treatments, 404 people), which did not compare treatments directly (see comment on cognitive therapy, p 155).[28]

OPTION   BENZODIAZEPINES

One systematic review and one subsequent RCT found that benzodiazepines reduced symptoms over 2–9 weeks compared with placebo. RCTs found no significant difference in symptoms over 3–8 weeks between alprazolam and bromazepam or mexazolam, or between benzodiazepines and buspirone, hydroxyzine, abecarnil, or antidepressants. RCTs and observational studies found that benzodiazepines increased the risk of dependence, sedation, industrial accidents, and road traffic accidents and that, if used in late pregnancy or while breast feeding, benzodiazepines may cause adverse effects in neonates. One systematic review of poor quality RCTs provided insufficient evidence to assess long term treatment with benzodiazepines.

Benefits: **Versus placebo:** We found one systematic review (search date 1996, 17 RCTs, 2044 people)[20] and one subsequent RCT.[29] The review found that benzodiazepines significantly improved symptoms over 2–9 weeks compared with placebo (pooled mean effect size 0.70; CI not reported).[20] The subsequent RCT (310 people) compared three interventions: diazepam (15–35 mg/day), abecarnil (7.5–17.5 mg/day), and placebo.[29] It found that diazepam significantly increased the proportion of people with moderate improvement on the Clinical Global Impression (CGI) scores at 6 weeks compared with placebo (73% with diazepam v 56% with placebo; $P < 0.01$).[29] **Versus each other:** The systematic review did not compare different benzodiazepines directly.[20] We found two RCTs.[30,31] The first RCT (121 people) compared sustained release alprazolam versus bromazepam.[30] It found no significant difference in Hamilton Anxiety Scale scores or CGI scores over 5 weeks between alprazolam and bromazepam (reported as non-significant, results presented graphically).[30] The second RCT (64 people) comparing mexazolam versus alprazolam found no significant difference in the proportion of people who had "highly improved" or "moderately improved" CGI scores at 3 weeks (98% with "highly improved" v 87% "moderately improved"; $P > 0.05$; absolute numbers presented graphically).[31] **Long term treatment:** We found one systematic review (search date 1998, 8 RCTs, any benzodiazepine medication, > 2 months' duration).[32] It found that the weak methods of the RCTs prevented firm conclusions being made.[32] **Versus buspirone:** See benefits of buspirone, p 157. **Versus hydroxyzine:** See benefits of hydroxyzine, p 158. **Versus abecarnil:** See benefits of abecarnil, p 159. **Versus antidepressants:** See benefits of antidepressants, p 160.

Harms: **Versus placebo:** The review gave no information on harms.[20] The subsequent RCT found that, compared with placebo, both diazepam and abecarnil significantly increased drowsiness (52% with diazepam v 47% with abecarnil v 14% with placebo; $P < 0.05$ for either drug v placebo) and dizziness (11% with diazepam v 16% with abecarnil v 3% with placebo; $P < 0.05$ for either drug v placebo).[29] **Dependence and sedation:** One non-systematic review of the harms of benzodiazepines found that rebound anxiety on withdrawal has been reported in 15–30% of people.[33] It also found that there is a high risk of substance abuse and dependence with benzodiazepines. Benzodiazepines have been found to cause impairment in attention, concentration, and short term memory. One RCT identified by the review found an increased rate of drowsiness (71% with diazepam v 13% with placebo; $P = 0.001$) and dizziness (29% with diazepam v 11% with placebo; $P = 0.001$).[20] Sedation can interfere with concomitant psychotherapy. **Memory:** Thirty one people with agoraphobia/panic disorder in an RCT comparing alprazolam versus placebo for 8 weeks were reviewed after 3.5 years.[34] Five people were still taking benzodiazepines and had significant impairment in memory tasks. There was no clear difference in memory performance between those who had been in the placebo group and those who had been given alprazolam but were no longer taking the drug.[34] **Road traffic accidents:** We found one systematic review (search date 1997) examining the relation between benzodiazepines and road traffic accidents.[35] In the case control studies, the odds ratio for death or emergency medical treatment in those who had taken benzodiazepines compared with those who had not taken them was 1.45–2.40. The odds ratio increased with higher doses and more recent intake. In the police and emergency ward studies, benzodiazepine use was a factor in 1–65% of accidents (usually 5–10%). In two studies in which people had blood alcohol concentrations under the legal limit, benzodiazepines were found in 43% and 65% of people. For drivers over 65 years of age, the risk of being involved in reported road traffic accidents was higher if they had taken longer acting and larger quantities of benzodiazepines. These results are from case control studies and are, therefore, subject to confounding. **Pregnancy and breast feeding:** One systematic review (search date 1997) of 23 case series and reports found no association between cleft lip and palate and benzodiazepines in the first trimester of pregnancy.[36] However, case reports in one non-systematic review suggested that benzodiazepines taken in late pregnancy may be associated with neonatal hypotonia and withdrawal syndrome.[37] Benzodiazepines are secreted in breast milk, and there have been reports of sedation and hypothermia in infants.[38] **Other:** One non-systematic industry funded review (8 RCTs) comparing benzodiazepines versus placebo or buspirone found that recent use of benzodiazepines limited the effectiveness of buspirone in people with generalised anxiety disorder.[38]

Comment: All of the RCTs assessing benzodiazepines were short term (at most 12 weeks).[20,29,30]

OPTION BUSPIRONE

RCTs have found that buspirone improves symptoms over 4–9 weeks compared with placebo. RCTs found no significant difference in symptoms over 6–8 weeks between buspirone and antidepressants, diazepam, or hydroxyzine, but the studies may have lacked power to detect clinically important differences among treatments.

Benefits: **Versus placebo:** We found one systematic review (search date 1996, 9 RCTs)[20] and two subsequent RCTs.[39,40] The systematic review found that buspirone significantly improved symptoms over 4–9 weeks compared with placebo (pooled mean effect size 0.39; CI not reported, withdrawal rate 17%).[20] The first subsequent RCT (162 people) comparing buspirone versus placebo found similar results (55% with buspirone v 35% with placebo; P < 0.05).[39] The second subsequent RCT (365 people) compared four interventions: buspirone (30 mg/day), venlafaxine (75 mg/day), venlafaxine (150 mg/day), and placebo over 8 weeks (see also benefits of antidepressants, p 160).[39] It found that, compared with placebo, buspirone significantly increased the proportion of people who responded after 8 weeks of treatment (response defined as score of 1 or 2 on the Clinical Global Impression Scale; 52/95 [55%] with buspirone v 38/98 [39%] with placebo; P = 0.03).[39] **Versus benzodiazepines:** One large RCT (240 people) identified by the review[20] compared three interventions: buspirone, diazepam, and placebo.[41] It found that a similar proportion of people responded over 6 weeks with buspirone compared with diazepam (response

defined as $\geq 40\%$ reduction in Hamilton Anxiety Scale score; 54% with buspirone *v* 61% with diazepam; P values not reported).[41]
Versus antidepressants: See benefits of antidepressants, p 160.
Versus hydroxyzine: See benefits of hydroxyzine, p 158.

Harms:
The systematic review gave no information on harms.[20] One subsequent RCT found that, compared with placebo, buspirone significantly increased the proportion of people with nausea (27/80 [34%] with buspirone *v* 11/82 [13%] with placebo; RR 2.5, 95% CI 1.3 to 4.7; NNH 5, 95% CI 4 to 14), dizziness (51/80 [64%] with buspirone *v* 10/82 [12%] with placebo; RR 5.2, 95% CI 2.9 to 9.6; NNH 2, 95% CI 2 to 3), and somnolence (15/80 [19%] with buspirone *v* 6/82 [7%] with placebo; RR 2.6, 95% CI 1.0 to 6.3; NNH 9, 95% CI 5 to 104).[39] Diazepam was associated with more fatigue and weakness compared with buspirone but less headache and dizziness.[41] **Pregnancy and breast feeding:** We found no evidence on the effects of buspirone during pregnancy or breast feeding..

Comment:
We found one non-systematic review (8 RCTs, 520 people) that was sponsored by pharmaceutical companies and had been included in regulatory submissions for buspirone.[42] It found that buspirone significantly increased the proportion of people "much or very much improved" as rated by their physician compared with placebo (54% with buspirone *v* 28% with placebo; P ≤ 0.001). Another non-systematic industry funded review (8 RCTs) comparing benzodiazepines versus placebo or buspirone found that recent use of benzodiazepines limited the effectiveness of buspirone in people with generalised anxiety disorder.[38]

OPTION   HYDROXYZINE

Three RCTs comparing hydroxyzine versus placebo found different results. Two RCTs found that, compared with placebo, hydroxyzine improved symptoms of anxiety at 4 or 12 weeks, but a third RCT found no significant difference in the proportion of people with improved symptoms of anxiety at 5 weeks. One of the RCTs found that hydroxyzine increased somnolence and headaches compared with placebo. One RCT found no significant difference between hydroxyzine and bromazepam in the proportion of people who responded after 6 weeks. Another RCT found no significant difference between hydroxyzine and buspirone in the proportion of people who responded after 4 weeks.

Benefits:
Versus placebo: We found one non-systematic review (2 RCTs, 354 people)[43] and one additional RCT.[44] The first RCT (110 people) identified by the review found that hydroxyzine (50 mg/day) significantly improved Clinical Global Impression Scale scores after 4 weeks compared with placebo (mean improvement 1.53 with hydroxyzine *v* 0.95 with placebo; P < 0.02).[43] The second RCT (244 people entered, 213 people analysed) identified by the review compared three interventions: hydroxyzine, buspirone, and placebo for 28 days, followed by placebo in all groups for 7 days. It found no significant difference between hydroxyzine 50 mg/day and placebo in the proportion of people with a Hamilton Anxiety Scale (HAM-A) score reduction of 50% or greater at 35 days (30/71 [42%] with

hydroxyzine v 20/70 [29%] with placebo; RR 1.50, 95% CI 0.93 to 2.23; not intention to treat).[43] The additional RCT (369 people) also compared three interventions: hydroxyzine, bromazepam, and placebo for 12 weeks, followed by placebo in all groups for 1 week.[44] It found that, compared with placebo, hydroxyzine significantly increased the proportion of people who responded at 42 days (response defined as ≥50% reduction in HAM-A scores from baseline; P = 0.022; absolute numbers presented graphically). **Versus benzodiazepines:** The additional RCT found no significant difference in the proportion of people who responded at 42 days between hydroxyzine and bromazepam (response defined as a HAM-A score reduction of ≥50%; reported as non-significant, no further data provided).[44] **Versus buspirone:** The second RCT identified by the non-systematic review also found no significant difference between hydroxyzine and buspirone in the proportion of people who responded at 28 days (response defined as HAM-A score reduction of ≥50%: 30/71 [42%] with hydroxyzine v 26/72 [36%] with buspirone; RR 1.20, 95% CI 0.78 to 1.80).[43]

Harms: **Versus placebo:** The second RCT (244 people) identified by the review found that, compared with placebo, more people taking hydroxyzine had somnolence (AR 10% with hydroxyzine v 0% with placebo) and headaches (AR 6% with hydroxyzine v 1% with placebo).[43] Overall adverse effects were reported in 40% of people taking hydroxyzine and 28% taking placebo.

Comment: None.

OPTION   ABECARNIL

One RCT found limited evidence that low dose abecarnil improved symptoms compared with placebo. Another RCT found no significant difference in symptoms at 6 weeks between abecarnil and placebo or diazepam. Both RCTs found that abecarnil increased drowsiness compared with placebo.

Benefits: We found no systematic review, but found two multicentre RCTs of abecarnil (an anxiolytic).[29,45] The first RCT (129 people) compared 3 weeks of treatment with abecarnil (3–9, 7.5–15, and 15–30 mg/day) versus placebo.[45] Within each group the dose was escalated from the minimum to the maximum over the length of the trial. It found that lower doses of abecarnil (3–9 mg/day) significantly improved symptoms compared with placebo (outcome 50% reduction in Hamilton Anxiety Scale score 19/31 [61%] with abecarnil v 8/26 [31%] with placebo; RR 1.99, 95% CI 1.05 to 3.78), but found no significant difference in symptoms between higher doses of abecarnil and placebo. Results were not calculated by intention to treat (12/34 [35%] people withdrew with abecarnil 15–30 mg/day v 4/35 [11%] with abecarnil 7.5–15 mg/day v 1/32 [3%] with abecarnil 3–9 mg/day v 2/28 [7%] with placebo).[45] The second RCT (310 people) compared three interventions: abecarnil (7.5–17.5 mg/day), diazepam (15–35 mg/day), and placebo.[29] It found no significant difference between abecarnil and placebo or diazepam in the proportion of people with moderate improvement on the Clinical Global Impression scores at 6 weeks (AR for moderate improvement 62% with abecarnil v 56% with placebo v 73% with diazepam; reported as non-significant; P values not reported).[29]

Harms: The first RCT found that abecarnil (3–9 mg/day) was associated with fatigue (4/32 [13%] with abecarnil v 0/28 [0%] with placebo), equilibrium loss (2/32 [6%] with abecarnil v 0/28 [0%] with placebo), and drowsiness (10/32 [31%] with abecarnil v 4/28 [14%] with placebo). Higher doses were associated with more adverse effects (62% of people taking abecarnil 15–30 mg experienced at least 1 adverse effect v 51% of people taking abecarnil 7.5–15 mg v 22% with abecarnil 3–9 mg v 21% with placebo).[45]

Comment: None.

OPTION **ANTIDEPRESSANTS**

RCTs have found that antidepressants (imipramine, opipramol, paroxetine, and venlafaxine) improve symptoms over 4–28 weeks compared with placebo. RCTs found no significant difference among these antidepressants or between antidepressants and benzodiazepines or buspirone. RCTs and observational studies have found that antidepressants are associated with sedation, dizziness, nausea, falls, and sexual dysfunction.

Benefits: **Versus placebo:** We found one systematic review (search date 2002, 8 RCTs, 2058 people),[46] one subsequent[47] and one additional RCT.[48] The review found that antidepressants (imipramine, paroxetine, and venlafaxine) significantly increased the proportion of people who responded at 8–28 weeks compared with placebo (4 RCTs, proportion of people who failed to respond 277/606 [46%] with antidepressants v 280/449 [62%] with placebo; RR of not responding 0.70, 95% CI 0.62 to 0.79; NNT 6, 95% CI 5 to 9).[46] It also found that each antidepressant significantly increased response rates compared with placebo: imipramine (1 RCT; RR 0.67, 95% CI 0.50 to 0.91; NNT 4, 95% CI 3 to 14), venlafaxine (2 RCTs; RR 0.68, 95% CI 0.46 to 0.99; NNT 5, 95% CI 4 to 9), and paroxetine (1 RCT; RR 0.72, 95% CI 0.56 to 0.92; NNT 7, 95% CI 4 to 25).[46] The subsequent RCT compared paroxetine (20 or 40 mg/day) versus placebo.[47] It found that, compared with placebo, paroxetine at either dose significantly increased response rates (response defined as Clinical Global Impression [CGI] scores ≤2: paroxetine 20 mg/day: 116/188 [62%] v 82/180 [45%]; RR 1.36, 95% CI 1.11 to 1.64; NNT 6, 95% CI 4 to 13; paroxetine 40 mg/day: 134/197 [68%] v 82/180 [45%]; RR 1.49, 95% CI 1.24 to 1.79; NNT 4, 95% CI 3 to 6).[47] The additional RCT (318 people) compared three treatments: opipramol (a tricyclic antidepressant with minimal serotonin reuptake blocking properties), alprazolam, or placebo over 28 days.[48] It found that opipramol significantly increased response rate after 28 days compared with placebo (response defined as CGI scale score of < 2; 63/100 [63%] with opipramol v 50/107 [47%] with placebo; RR 1.35, 95% CI 1.05 to 1.69; NNT 7; 95% CI 1 to 26). **Versus each other:** The systematic review[46] identified one RCT (56 people) that found no significant difference between paroxetine and imipramine in the proportion of people who responded over 8 weeks of treatment (proportion who failed to respond 3/36 [8%] with paroxetine v 2/30 [7%] with imipramine; RR of failing to respond 1.73, 95% CI 0.31 to 9.57). **Versus benzodiazepines:** The systematic review[46] identified two RCTs[49,50] and we found one additional RCT.[48] The first RCT (230 people) identified by the review compared variable doses of four interventions: imipramine, trazodone, diazepam, and placebo.[49] It found similar improvements among groups in participant assessed global improvement after 8 weeks of treatment (results not intention to treat; 73% of people improved with imipramine v 67% with trazodone v 66% with diazepam).[49] The RCT did not directly compare the significance of differences between groups. The second RCT (81 people) identified by the review compared paroxetine, imipramine, and 2'-chlordesmethyldiazepam for 8 weeks.[50] It found that paroxetine and imipramine significantly improved anxiety after 8 weeks compared with 2'-chlordesmethyldiazepam (mean Hamilton Anxiety Scale score: 11.1 with paroxetine v 10.8 with imipramine v 12.9 with 2'-chlordesmethyldiazepam; P = 0.05 for either comparison v 2'-chlordesmethyldiazepam). The additional RCT found no significant difference between opipramol and alprazolam in response rate over 28 days (63/100 [63%] with opipramol v 67/105 [64%] with alprazolam; RR 1.01, 95% CI 0.79 to 1.25).[48] **Versus buspirone:** One RCT (365 people) identified by the review[46] compared four interventions: venlafaxine at two different doses (75 or 150 mg/day), buspirone (30 mg/day), and placebo over 8 weeks. It found similar response rates between venlafaxine and buspirone after 8 weeks of treatment (response defined as CGI score of 1 or 2; 54/87 [62%] with venlafaxine 75 mg v 44/89 [49%] with venlafaxine 150 mg v 52/95 [55%] with buspirone; P values not reported).[40]

Harms: **Withdrawals:** The review found no significant difference between antidepressants and placebo in the proportion of people who withdrew for any cause (403/1273 [31%] with antidepressants v 240/678 [35%] with placebo; RR 0.95, 95% CI 0.73 to 1.24).[46] A survival analysis of the two RCTs of venlafaxine (767 people) identified by the review[46] found no significant difference between venlafaxine and placebo in the proportion of people who withdrew because of adverse effects over 6 months (36/253 [14%] with venlafaxine v 91/514 [18%] with placebo; RR 1.24, 95% CI 0.87 to 1.77).[51] **Common adverse events:** The review found that people taking venlafaxine were more likely to report nausea, dry mouth, insomnia, constipation, flatulence, anorexia, somnolence, and sexual dysfunction than people taking placebo.[46] One RCT found sedation, confusion, dry mouth, and constipation with both imipramine and trazodone.[49] RCTs reported nausea, somnolence, dry mouth, sweating, constipation, anorexia, and sexual dysfunction with venlafaxine. Most of the adverse effects (apart from dizziness and sexual dysfunction) decreased over 6 months in those who continued to take the medication. There have been case reports of nausea in people taking paroxetine.[50] **Adverse effects when discontinuing treatment:** Abrupt discontinuation of selective serotonin reuptake inhibitors has been associated with adverse effects including dizziness, headache, nausea, vomiting, diarrhoea, movement disorders, insomnia, irritability, visual disturbance, lethargy, anorexia, and lowered mood. One RCT (120 people receiving maintenance selective serotonin reuptake inhibitors for depression) found that significantly more people had adverse effects when discontinuing paroxetine or sertraline compared with people discontinuing fluoxetine (60% with paroxetine v 66% with sertraline v 16% taking fluoxetine; P < 0.01 for paroxetine or sertraline v fluoxetine).[52] **Overdose:** In a series of 239 coroner directed necropsies from 1970–1989, tricyclic antidepressants were considered to be a causal factor in 12% of deaths and hypnosedatives (primarily benzodiazepines and excluding barbiturates) in 8% of deaths.[53] **Accidental poisoning:** Tricyclic antidepressants are a major cause of accidental poisoning.[54] A study estimated that there was one death for every 44 children admitted to hospital after ingestion of tricyclic antidepressants.[55] **Hyponatraemia:** One case series reported 736 incidents of hyponatraemia in people taking selective serotonin reuptake inhibitors; 83% of episodes were in hospital inpatients aged over 65 years.[56] It is not possible to establish causation from this type of data. **Falls:** One retrospective cohort study (2428 elderly residents of nursing homes) found an increased risk of falls in new users of antidepressants (665 people taking tricyclic antidepressants; adjusted RR 2.0, 95% CI 1.8 to 2.2; 612 people taking selective serotonin reuptake inhibitors; adjusted RR 1.8, 95% CI 1.6 to 2.0; and 304 people taking trazodone; adjusted RR 1.2, 95% CI 1.0 to 1.4).[57] The increased rate of falls persisted through the first 180 days of treatment and beyond. One case control study (8239 people aged ≥66 years, treated in hospital for hip fracture) found an increased risk of hip fracture in those taking antidepressants (adjusted OR, selective serotonin reuptake inhibitors 2.4, 95% CI 2.0 to 2.7; secondary amine tricyclic antidepressants such as nortriptyline 2.2, 95% CI 1.8 to 2.8; and tertiary amine tricyclic antidepressants such as amitriptyline 1.5, 95% CI 1.3 to 1.7).[58] This study could not control for confounding factors; people taking antidepressants may be at increased risk of hip fracture for other reasons. **In pregnancy:** We found no reports of harmful effects in pregnancy. One case control study found no evidence that imipramine or fluoxetine increased the rate of malformations in pregnancy.[59] **Sexual dysfunction:** A survey (1022 people mostly suffering from depression; 610 women) of people using antidepressants with acceptable sexual function before antidepressant treatment has reported the incidence of sexual dysfunction (decreased desire, delayed ejaculation, and anorgasmia) to be 71% with paroxetine, 67% with venlafaxine, and 63% with fluvoxamine.[60]

Comment: None.

OPTION   ANTIPSYCHOTIC DRUGS

One large RCT found that trifluoperazine reduced anxiety after 4 weeks compared with placebo, but caused more drowsiness, extrapyramidal reactions, and other movement disorders.

Mental health

Benefits: We found no systematic review. We found one RCT (415 people) comparing 4 weeks of trifluoperazine treatment (2–6 mg/day) versus placebo.[61] It found that trifluoperazine significantly reduced the total score on the Hamilton Anxiety Scale compared with placebo (difference 14 points; P < 0.001).

Harms: The RCT reported more cases of drowsiness (43% with trifluoperazine v 25% with placebo) and extrapyramidal reactions and movement disorders (17% with trifluoperazine v 8% with placebo) with trifluoperazine compared with placebo.[61] A cohort study found that in the longer term, rates of tardive dyskinesia are increased if trifluoperazine treatment is frequently interrupted.[62]

Comment: None.

OPTION   β BLOCKERS

We found no RCTs on the effects of β blockers in people with generalised anxiety disorder.

Benefits: We found no systematic review or RCTs.

Harms: We found no RCTs.

Comment: None.

OPTION   KAVA

One systematic review in people with a variety anxiety disorders, including generalised anxiety disorder, found that kava reduced symptoms of anxiety over 1–24 weeks compared with placebo. It is unclear whether results of the review are generalisable to people with generalised anxiety disorder. Observational evidence suggests that kava may be associated with hepatotoxicity.

Benefits: **Versus placebo:** We found one systematic review (search date 2002, 11 RCTs, 645 people with a variety of anxiety disorders, including generalised anxiety disorder, preoperative anxiety, and climacteric).[63] It found that kava significantly improved Hamilton Anxiety Scale scores over 1–24 weeks compared with placebo (6 RCTs, 345 people: WMD 4.97, 95% CI 1.14 to 8.81).

Harms: The review gave little information on adverse effects.[63] Eight RCTs identified by the review found that kava was associated with adverse effects, including stomach complaints, restlessness, drowsiness, tremor, headache, and tiredness.[63] We found one systematic review (search date 2000, 30 studies including 9 clinical trials) assessing adverse effects associated with kava.[64] Adverse effects in the clinical trials were gastrointestinal symptoms, tiredness, restlessness, tremor, and headache. Post-marketing surveillance (4049 adults taking 150 mg/day kava extract) found an adverse reaction rate of 1.5% (61/4094). Case reports included five cases of dermatological reactions, four cases of acute dyskinesias, nine cases of liver damage, and one case of myoglobulinuria (the incidence of these adverse effects was not reported).[64] One case was found where kava may have interacted with alprazolam, leading to decreased in level of consciousness.[64]

Comment: It is unclear whether results of the review are generalisable to people with generalised anxiety disorder as we were unable to ascertain how many people in the RCTs included in the review had generalised anxiety disorder.[63] The review found that, although research about kava has been published in languages other than English, there was a trend for positive results to be published in English and negative results in other languages and that this could lead to a bias when extracting data.[63] There have been concerns that kava may cause liver damage.[65]

GLOSSARY

Applied relaxation A technique involving training in relaxation techniques and self monitoring of symptoms without challenging beliefs.

Cognitive behavioural therapy Brief (20 sessions over 12–16 weeks) structured treatment incorporating elements of cognitive therapy and behavioural therapy. Covers a variety of techniques. *Behavioural therapy* is based on learning theory and concentrates on changing behaviour. *Cognitive therapy* is aimed at identifying anxiety associated thoughts and beliefs, changing over monitoring of physical symptoms, and minimising the catastophising that characterises generalised anxiety disorder. This is combined with relaxation, exercise, and testing the validity of beliefs in real life situations. *Cognitive restructuring* involves systematic challenging of thought processes and underlying assumptions related to the symptoms. *Exposure* entails being confronted (through visualisation, image, or the stimulus) with an anxiogenic stimulus in a repetitive and prolonged manner. *Relaxation* involves practising techniques that lead to muscular or bodily relaxation. *Systematic desensitisation* is a type of exposure.

REFERENCES

1. American Psychiatric Association. *Diagnostic and statistical manual of mental disorders*, 4th ed. Washington, DC: American Psychiatric Association, 1994.
2. Mendlowicz MV, Stein MB. Quality of life in individuals with anxiety disorders. *Am J Psychiatry* 2000;157:669–682.
3. Kessler RD Wittchen HU. Patterns and correlates of generalized anxiety disorder in community samples. *J Clin Psychiatry* 2002;63(suppl 8):4–10.
4. Stein D. Comorbidity in generalised anxiety disorder: impact and implications. *J Clin Psychiatry* 2001;62(suppl 11):29–34 [review].
5. Goldenberg IM, White K, Yonkers K, et al. The infrequency of "pure culture" diagnoses among the anxiety disorders. *J Clin Psych* 1996:57:528–533.
6. Dyck IR, Phillips KA, Warshaw MG, et al. Patterns of personality pathology in patients with generalized anxiety disorder, panic disorder with and without agoraphobia, and social phobia. *J Personal Disord* 2001;15:60–71.
7. Godart NT, Flament MF, Perdereau F, et al. Comorbidity between eating disorders and anxiety disorders: a review. *Int J Eat Disord* 2002;32:253–270. Search date 2001; primary source Medline.
8. Judd LL, Kessler RC, Paulus MP, et al. Comorbidity as a fundamental feature of generalised anxiety disorders: results from the National Comorbidity Study (NCS). *Acta Psychiatry Scand* 1998;98(suppl 393):6–11.
9. Andrews G, Peters L, Guzman AM, et al. A comparison of two structured diagnostic interviews: CIDI and SCAN. *Aust N Z J Psychiatry* 1995;29:124–132.
10. Kessler RC, McGonagle KA, Zhao S, et al. Lifetime and 12-month prevalence of DSM-III-R psychiatric disorders in the United States: results from the national comorbidity survey. *Arch Gen Psychiatry* 1994;51:8–19.
11. Seivewright N, Tyrer P, Ferguson B, et al. Longitudinal study of the influence of life events and personality status on diagnostic change in three neurotic disorders. *Depression Anx* 2000;11:105–113.
12. Pigott T. Gender differences in the epidemiology and treatment of anxiety disorders. *J Clin Psychiatry* 1999;60(suppl 18):4–15.
13. Jorm AF. Does old age reduce the risk of anxiety and depression? A review of epidemiological studies across the adult life span. *Psychol Med* 2000;30:11–22.
14. Lau AW, Edelstein BA, Larkin KT. Psychophysiological arousal in older adults: a critical review. *Clin Psychol Rev* 2001;21:609–630 [review].
15. Brantley PJ, Mehan DJ Jr, Ames SC, et al. Minor stressors and generalised anxiety disorders among low income patients attending primary care clinics. *J Nerv Ment Dis* 1999;187:435–440.
16. Brown ES, Fulton MK, Wilkeson A, et al. The psychiatric sequelae of civilian trauma. *Comp Psychiatry* 2000;41:19–23.
17. Hawker DSJ, Boulton MJ. Twenty years' research on peer victimisation and psychosocial maladjustment: a meta-analytic review of cross-sectional studies. *J Child Psychol Psychiatr* 2000;41:441–445. Search date 1997; primary sources Psychlit, Social Science Citation Index, OCLC Firstsearch, hand searches of relevant journals, bibliographies, reviews, reference lists of relevant articles, and book chapters, and personal contact with authors.

18. Hettema JM, Neale MC, Kendler KS. A review and meta-analysis of the genetic epidemiology of anxiety disorders. *Am J Psychiatry* 2001;158:1568–1578. Search date not reported; primary source Medline.

19. Yonkers KA, Dyck IR, Warshaw M, et al. Factors predicting the clinical course of generalised anxiety disorder. *Br J Psychiatry* 2000;176:544–549.

20. Gould RA, Otto MW, Pollack MH, et al. Cognitive behavioural and pharmacological treatment of generalised anxiety disorder: a preliminary meta-analysis. *Behav Res Ther* 1997;28:285–305. Search date 1996; primary sources Psychlit, Medline, examination of reference lists, and unpublished articles presented at national conferences.

21. Westen D, Morrison K. A multidimensional meta-analysis of treatments for depression, panic and generalized anxiety disorder: an empirical examination of the status of empirically supported therapies. *J Consult Clin Psychol* 2001;69:875–889. Search date not reported but only included studies published 1990–1999; primary source hand searches of 10 journals and psychological abstracts.

22. Ost L, Breitholts E. Applied relaxation vs. cognitive therapy in the treatment of generalized anxiety disorder. *Behav Res Ther* 2000;38:777–790.

23. Borkovec TD, Newman MG, Pincus AL. A component analysis of cognitive-behavioural therapy for generalized anxiety disorder and the role of interpersonal process. *J Consult Clin Psychology* 2002;20:288–298.

24. Stanley MA, Beck JG, Novy DM, et al. Cognitive-behavioural treatment of late-life generalized anxiety disorder. *J Consult Clin Psychol* 2003;71:309–319.

25. Wetherall JL, Gatx M, Craske MG. Treatment of generalized anxiety disorder in older adults. *J Consult Clin Psychol* 2003;71:31–40.

26. Arntz A. Cognitive therapy versus applied relaxation as treatment for generalized anxiety disorder. *Behav Res Ther* 2003;41:633–646.

27. Barrowclough C, King P, Russell E, et al. A randomized trial of effectiveness of cognitive-behavioural therapy and supportive counselling for anxiety disorders in older adults. *J Consult Clin Psychol* 2001;69;756–762.

28. Fisher PL, Durham RC. Recovery rates in generalised anxiety disorder following psychological therapy: an analysis of clinically significant change in the STAI-T across outcome studies since 1990. *Psychol Med* 1999;29:1425–1434. Search date 1998; primary sources Medline, Psychlit, and Cochrane Controlled Trials Register.

29. Rickels K, DeMartinis N, Aufdembrinke B. A double-blind, placebo controlled trial of abecarnil and diazepam in the treatment of patients with generalized anxiety disorder. *J Clin Psychopharmacol* 2000;20:12–18.

30. Figueira ML. Alprazolam SR in the treatment of generalised anxiety: a multicentre controlled study with bromazepam. *Hum Psychother* 1999;14:171–177.

31. Vaz-Serra A, Figuerra L, Bessa-Peixoto A, et al. Mexazolam and alprazolam in the treatment of generalized anxiety disorder. *Clin Drug Invest* 2001;21:257–263.

32. Mahe V, Balogh A. Long-term pharmacological treatment of generalized anxiety disorder. *Int Clin Psychopharmacol* 2000;15:99–105. Search date 1998; primary sources Medline, Biosis, and Embase.

33. Tyrer P. Current problems with the benzodiazepines. In: Wheatly D, ed. *The anxiolytic jungle: where next?* Chichester: Wiley, 1990:23–47.

34. Kilic C, Curran HV, Noshirvani H, et al. Long-term effects of alprazolam on memory: a 3.5 year follow-up of agoraphobia/panic patients. *Psychol Med* 1999;29:225–231.

35. Thomas RE. Benzodiazepine use and motor vehicle accidents. Systematic review of reported association. *Can Fam Physician* 1998;44:799–808. Search date 1997; primary source Medline.

36. Dolovich LR, Addis A, Regis Vaillancourt JD, et al. Benzodiazepine use in pregnancy and major malformations of oral cleft: meta-analysis of cohort and case-control studies. *BMJ* 1998;317:839–843. Search date 1997; primary sources Medline, Embase, Reprotox, and references of included studies and review articles.

37. Bernstein JG. *Handbook of drug therapy in psychiatry*, 3rd ed. St Louis, Missouri: Mosby Year Book, 1995:401.

38. DeMartinis N, Rynn M, Rickels K, et al. Prior benzodiazepine use and buspirone response in the treatment of generalized anxiety disorder. *J Clin Psychiatry* 2000;61:91–94.

39. Sramek JJ, Transman M, Suri A, et al. Efficacy of buspirone in generalized anxiety disorder with coexisting mild depressive symptoms. *J Clin Psychiatry* 1996;57:287–291.

40. Davidson JR, DuPont RL, Hedges D, et al. Efficacy, safety and tolerability of venlafaxine extended release and buspirone in outpatients with generalised anxiety disorder. *J Clin Psychiatry* 1999;60:528–535.

41. Rickels K, Weisman K, Norstad N, et al. Buspirone and diazepam in anxiety: a controlled study. *J Clin Psychiatry* 1982;12:81–86.

42. Gammans RE, Stringfellow JC, Hvisdos AJ, et al. Use of buspirone in patients with generalized anxiety disorder and coexisting depressive symptoms: a meta-analysis of eight randomized, controlled trials. *Pharmacopsychiatry* 1992;25:193–201.

43. Lader M, Anxiolytic effect of hydroxyzine: a double-blind trial versus placebo and buspirone. *Hum Psychopharmacol Clin Exp* 1999;14;S94–S102.

44. Llorca PM, Spadone C, Sol O, et al. Efficacy and safety of hydroxyzine in the treatment of generalized anxiety disorder: a 3-month double-blind study. *J Clin Psychiatry* 2002;63:1020–1027.

45. Ballenger JC, McDonald S, Noyes R, et al. The first double-blind, placebo-controlled trial of a partial benzodiazepine agonist, abecarnil (ZK 112–119) in generalised anxiety disorder. *Adv Biochem Psychopharmacol* 1992;47:431–447.

46. Kapczinski F, Schmitt R, Lima MS Antidepressants for generalized anxiety disorder. In: The Cochrane Library, Issue 2, 2003. Oxford: Update Software. Search date 2002; primary sources CCDAN and CSG Controlled Trials Register, Medline, Lilacs, reference searching, personal communication, conference abstracts, pharmaceutical industry, and book chapters on the treatment of generalised anxiety disorder.

47. Rickels K, Zaninelli R, McCafferty J, et al. Paroxetine treatment of generalized anxiety disorder: a double-blind, placebo-controlled study. *Am J Psychiatry* 2003;160:749–756.

48. Moller HJ, Volz HP, Reimann IW, et al. Opipramol for the treatment of generalised anxiety disorder: a placebo-controlled trial including an alprazolam-treated group. *J Clin Psychopharmacol* 2001;21:51–65.

49. Rickels K, Downing R, Schweizer E, et al. Antidepressants for the treatment of generalised anxiety disorder: a placebo-controlled comparison of imipramine, trazodone and diazepam. *Arch Gen Psychiatry* 1993;50:884–895.

50. Rocca P, Fonzo V, Scotta M, et al. Paroxetine efficacy in the treatment of generalized anxiety disorder. *Acta Psychiatr Scand* 1997;95:444–450.

51. Montgomery SA, Mahe V, Haudiquet V, et al. Effectiveness of venlafaxine, extended release formulation, in the short-term and long-term treatment of generalized anxiety disorder: results of a survival analysis. *J Clin Psychopharmacol* 2002;22:561–567.

52. Rosenbaum JF, Fava M, Hoog SL, et al. Selective serotonin reuptake inhibitor discontinuation syndrome: a randomized clinical trial. *Biol Psychiatry* 1998;44:77–87.

53. Dukes PD, Robinson GM, Thomson KJ, et al. Wellington coroner autopsy cases 1970–89: acute deaths due to drugs, alcohol and poisons. *N Z Med J* 1992;105:25–27. [Erratum in *N Z Med J* 1992;105:135.]

54. Kerr GW, McGuffie AC, Wilkie S. Tricyclic antidepressant overdose: a review. *Emerg Med J* 2001;18:236–241.

55. Pearn J, Nixon J, Ansford A, et al. Accidental poisoning in childhood: five year urban population study with 15 year analysis of fatality. *BMJ* 1984;288:44–46.

56. Liu BA, Mittmann N, Knowles SR, et al. Hyponatremia and the syndrome of inappropriate secretion of antidiuretic hormone associated with the use of selective serotonin reuptake inhibitors: a review of spontaneous reports. *Can Med Assoc J* 1995;155:519–527. [Erratum in *Can Med Assoc J* 1996;155:1043.]

57. Thapa PB, Gideon P, Cost TW, et al. Antidepressants and the risk of falls among nursing home residents. *N Engl J Med* 1998;339:875–882.

58. Liu B, Anderson G, Mittmann N, et al. Use of selective serotonin-reuptake inhibitors of tricyclic antidepressants and risk of hip fractures in elderly people. *Lancet* 1998;351:1303–1307.

59. Kulin NA, Pastuszak A, Koren G. Are the new SSRIs safe for pregnant women? *Can Fam Physician* 1998;44;2081–2083.

60. Montejo AL, Llorca G, Izquierdo JA, et al. Incidence of sexual dysfunction associated with antidepressant agents: a prospective multicentre study of 1022 outpatients. *J Clin Psychiatry* 2000;62(suppl 3):10–21.

61. Mendels J, Krajewski TF, Huffer V, et al. Effective short-term treatment of generalized anxiety with trifluoperazine. *J Clin Psychiatry* 1986;47:170–174.

62. Van Harten PN, Hoek HW, Matroos GE, et al. Intermittent neuroleptic treatment and risk of tardive dyskinesia: Curacao Extrapyramidal Syndromes study III. *Am J Psychiatry* 1998;155:565–567.

63. Pittler MH, Ernst E. Kava extract for treating anxiety. In: The Cochrane Library, Issue 2, 2003. Oxford: Update Software. Search date 2002; primary sources Medline, Embase, Biosis, Amed, Ciscom, Cochrane Library, hand searches of references, personal files, and contact with manufacturers of kava preparations and experts.

64. Stevensin C, Huntley A, Ernst E. A systematic review of the safety of Kava extract in the treatment of anxiety. *Drug Saf* 2002;25;251–256. Search date 2000; primary sources Medline, Embase, Amed, Cochrane Library, reference lists, departmental files, contact with colleagues in herbal medicine, World Health Organization, USA Food and Drug Administration, UK Committee on Safety of Medicines, German Bundesinstitut fur Arzneimittel und Medizinprodukte, and 10 manufacturers of kava preparations.

65. National Center for Complimentary and Alternative Medicine. Consumer Advisory. Kava linked to liver damage. Internet 2003 [cited February 10]; http://www.nccam.nih.gov/health/alerts/kava/index.htm (last accessed 20 October 2003).

Christopher Gale

Consultant Psychiatrist, Clinical Senior Lecturer
Faculty of Medicine and Health Sciences
University of Auckland, Auckland, New Zealand

Mark Oakley-Browne

Professor of Rural Psychiatry
University of Monash, Victoria, Australia

Competing interests: CG has been paid by Eli Lilly, the manufacturer of Prozac (fluoxetine), and by Janssen to attend symposia. MOB has been paid by GlaxoSmithKline, the manufacturer of Aropax (paroxetine) for contributing to educational sessions for general practitioners. MOB has also been reimbursed by Pfizer for attending a conference.

Obsessive compulsive disorder

Search date September 2003

G Mustafa Soomro

INTERVENTIONS

Key Messages

Initial treatment

- **Behavioural therapy** We found no RCTs comparing behavioural therapy versus no treatment. One systematic review and subsequent RCTs have found that behavioural therapy improves symptoms compared with relaxation. The review and one subsequent RCT found no significant difference in symptoms over 4–16 weeks between behavioural therapy and cognitive therapy. One subsequent RCT found limited evidence that group behavioural therapy improved symptoms after 12 weeks compared with group cognitive behavioural therapy.

- **Cognitive or cognitive behavioural therapy** We found no RCTs comparing cognitive therapy versus no treatment. One RCT found that cognitive behavioural group therapy improved symptoms and quality of life compared with no treatment after 12 weeks. One systematic review and one subsequent RCT found no significant difference in symptoms over 4–16 weeks between behavioural therapy and cognitive therapy. Another subsequent RCT found limited evidence that group behavioural therapy improved symptoms over 12 weeks compared with group cognitive behavioural therapy.

- **Serotonin reuptake inhibitors (citalopram, clomipramine, fluoxetine, fluvoxamine, paroxetine, sertraline)** RCTs have found that selective and non-selective serotonin reuptake inhibitors (citalopram, clomipramine, fluoxetine, fluvoxamine, paroxetine) improve symptoms compared with placebo. Two systematic reviews found inconsistent results about the effects of sertraline compared with placebo. RCTs have found that selective and non-selective serotonin reuptake inhibitors (citalopram, clomipramine, fluoxetine, fluvoxamine, paroxetine, sertraline) improve symptoms compared with tricyclic antidepressants or monoamine oxidase inhibitors. RCTs have found no consistent evidence of a difference in efficacy among serotonin reuptake inhibitors, but have found that the non-selective serotonin reuptake inhibitor clomipramine is associated with more adverse effects than selective serotonin reuptake inhibitors.

- **Behavioural or cognitive therapy plus serotonin reuptake inhibitors (compared with behavioural or cognitive therapy alone)** RCTs provided insufficient evidence to assess the effects of adding serotonin reuptake inhibitors to behavioural or cognitive therapy.

- **Electroconvulsive therapy** We found no RCTs of electroconvulsive therapy in people with obsessive compulsive disorder.

- **Venlafaxine** One RCT provided insufficient evidence to compare venlafaxine versus clomipramine.

Maintenance treatment

- **Optimum duration of treatment with serotonin reuptake inhibitors** RCTs provided insufficient evidence to define the optimum duration of treatment with serotonin reuptake inhibitors.

In people who do not respond to selective and non-selective serotonin reuptake inhibitors

- **Addition of antipsychotics in people who have not responded to serotonin reuptake inhibitors** Three small RCTs in people unresponsive to serotonin reuptake inhibitors found that the addition of antipsychotics improved symptoms compared with placebo.

DEFINITION Obsessive compulsive disorder involves obsessions, compulsions, or both, that are not caused by drugs or a physical disorder, and which cause significant personal distress or social dysfunction.[1,2] The disorder may have a chronic or an episodic course (see glossary, p 179). **Obsessions** are recurrent and persistent ideas, images, or impulses that cause pronounced anxiety and that the person perceives to be self produced. **Compulsions** are repetitive behaviours or mental acts performed in response to obsessions or according to certain rules, which are aimed at reducing distress or preventing certain imagined dreaded events. People with obsessive compulsive disorder may have insight into their condition, in that obsessions and compulsions are usually recognised and resisted. There are minor differences in the criteria for obsessive compulsive disorder between the third, revised third, and fourth editions of the *Diagnostic and Statistical Manual* (DSM-III, DSM-III-R, and DSM-IV)[1] and *The ICD-10 Classification of Mental and Behavioural Disorders*.[2]

INCIDENCE/ PREVALENCE One national, community based survey of obsessive compulsive disorder in the UK (1993, 10 000 people) found that 1% of men and 1.5% of women reported symptoms in the past month.[3] An epidemiological catchment area (ECA) survey carried out in the USA in 1984 (about 10 000 people) found age and sex standardised annual prevalence of obsessive compulsive disorder in people aged 26–64 years of 1.3%, and lifetime prevalence of 2.3%.[4] Subsequent cross national surveys using methodology comparable to ECA found age and sex standardised annual and lifetime prevalence in people aged 26–64 years as follows: Canada (survey size about 2200 people), annual prevalence 1.4% (SE 0.25), and lifetime prevalence 2.3% (SE 0.32); Puerto Rico (survey size about 1200 people), annual prevalence 1.8% (SE 0.39), and lifetime prevalence 2.5% (SE 0.46); Germany (survey size 4811 people), annual prevalence 1.6% (SE 0.57), and lifetime prevalence 2.1% (SE 0.66); Taiwan (survey size about 7400 people), annual prevalence 0.4% (SE 0.07), and lifetime prevalence 0.7% (SE 0.10); Korea (survey size about 4000 people), annual prevalence 1.1% (SE 0.10), and lifetime prevalence 1.9% (SE 0.20); and New Zealand (survey size about 1200 people), annual prevalence 1.1% (SE 0.31), and lifetime prevalence 2.2% (SE 0.42).[4]

AETIOLOGY/ RISK FACTORS The cause of obsessive compulsive disorder is uncertain. Behavioural, cognitive, genetic, and neurobiological factors have been implicated.[5–11] Risk factors include a family history of obsessive compulsive disorder, being single (which could be a consequence of the disorder), and belonging to a higher socioeconomic class.[12] Other risk factors include cocaine abuse, female sex, not being in paid employment, past history of alcohol dependence, affective disorder, and phobic disorder.[4]

PROGNOSIS One study (144 people followed for a mean of 47 years) found that an episodic course of obsessive compulsive disorder was more common during the initial years (about 1–9 years), but a chronic course was more common afterwards.[13] Over time, the study found that 39–48% of people had symptomatic improvement. A 1 year prospective cohort study found that 46% of people had an episodic course and 54% had a chronic course.[14]

AIMS OF INTERVENTION To improve symptoms, and to reduce the impact of illness on social functioning and quality of life, with minimal adverse effects of treatment.

OUTCOMES Severity of symptoms; social functioning; and adverse effects of treatment. Commonly used instruments for measuring symptoms include the Hamilton Anxiety Rating scale; the Hamilton Depression Rating scale; and the Yale-Brown Obsessive Compulsive Scale, which is observer rated and well validated. It rates severity of both obsessions and compulsions across five dimensions (time spent, interference with functioning, distress, resistance, and control), each on a five point scale from 0–4 (0 means that the dimension is absent and 4 means that the dimension is present to extremely severe degree). The total score range of obsessions and compulsions combined is 0–40 (the higher the score the more severe the condition).[15–17] Most trials use a 25% reduction in Yale-Brown scale scores from baseline as indicative of clinically important improvement, but some studies use a 35% reduction.[17]

METHODS *Clinical Evidence* search and appraisal September 2003.

Mental health

| OPTION | SEROTONIN REUPTAKE INHIBITORS (CITALOPRAM, CLOMIPRAMINE, FLUOXETINE, FLUVOXAMINE, PAROXETINE, SERTRALINE) |

RCTs have found that selective and non-selective serotonin reuptake inhibitors (citalopram, clomipramine, fluoxetine, fluvoxamine, paroxetine) improve symptoms compared with placebo. Two systematic reviews found inconsistent results about the effects of sertraline compared with placebo. RCTs have found that selective and non-selective serotonin reuptake inhibitors (citalopram, clomipramine, fluoxetine, fluvoxamine, paroxetine, sertraline) improve symptoms compared with tricyclic antidepressants or monoamine oxidase inhibitors. One RCT found no significant difference in symptoms between clomipramine and venlafaxine, but it is likely to have been underpowered to detect a clinically important difference. RCTs have found no consistent evidence of a difference in efficacy among serotonin reuptake inhibitors, but have found that the non-selective serotonin reuptake inhibitor clomipramine is associated with more adverse effects than selective serotonin reuptake inhibitors.

Benefits: **Versus placebo:** We found two systematic reviews (search dates 1994[18] and not reported[19]) and three subsequent RCTs.[20–22] The two systematic reviews and three subsequent RCTs found that selective or non-selective serotonin reuptake inhibitors (citalopram, clomipramine, fluoxetine, fluvoxamine, paroxetine) significantly improved symptoms compared with placebo (see comment below).[18–22] One of the reviews found that sertraline significantly improved symptoms compared with placebo,[18] and the other review found no significant difference in symptoms (see table 1, p 182).[19]

Versus each other: We found two systematic reviews[18,19] and five subsequent RCTs.[23–27] All found no significant difference in symptoms between different selective and non-selective serotonin reuptake inhibitors.[18,19,23–27] The first review (search date 1994, 85 people, 3 RCTs) found no significant difference in symptoms among clomipramine, fluoxetine and fluvoxamine (SMD −0.04, 95% CI −0.43 to +0.35).[18] The second review (search date not reported) found no significant difference in symptoms between clomipramine and fluvoxamine (4 RCTs, including 2 RCTs from the first review; change in Yale-Brown scale score; SMD +1.23, 95% CI −1.11 to +3.56).[19] It also found no significant difference in symptoms between clomipramine and fluoxetine (1 RCT, not included in the first review, 55 people; change in Yale-Brown scale score; SMD +1.40, 95% CI −5.74 to +2.94) or clomipramine and paroxetine (1 RCT not included in the first review, 300 people; change in Yale-Brown scale score; SMD 0.00, 95% CI −1.94 to +1.94).[19] The first subsequent RCT (170 people) found that sertraline significantly improved symptoms compared with clomipramine (8% greater mean reduction in Yale-Brown scale score, P = 0.036; see comment below).[23] The second subsequent RCT (133 people) found no significant difference in symptoms between clomipramine and fluvoxamine (change in Yale-Brown scale score, 12.6 with clomipramine v 12.3 with fluvoxamine; reported as non-significant, no further data reported).[24] The third subsequent RCT (227 people, double blind) found no significant difference between clomipramine (150–300 mg) and fluvoxamine (150–300 mg) in severity of symptoms after 10 weeks (mean reduction in Yale-Brown scale score about 12 in both groups; P value not reported; proportion of people achieving at least 35% reduction in Yale-Brown scale score 65% with clomipramine v 62% with fluvoxamine, reported as non-significant).[25] The fourth subsequent RCT (150 people) compared sertraline (50–200 mg) versus fluoxetine (20–80 mg).[26] It found similar symptom severity at 24 weeks between sertraline and fluoxetine (reduction in Yale-Brown scale score 9.6 with sertraline v 9.7 with fluoxetine, CI not reported). The fifth subsequent RCT (30 people, observer blinded) compared three interventions: fluvoxamine, paroxetine, and citalopram.[27] It found no significant difference in symptoms among drugs, but was too small to exclude a clinically important difference. **Versus tricyclic antidepressants and monoamine oxidase inhibitors:** We found one systematic review[18] and two subsequent RCTs.[28,29] These found that serotonin reuptake inhibitors significantly improved symptoms compared with tricyclic antidepressants or monoamine oxidase inhibitors. The systematic review (search date 1994, 7 RCTs, 147 people with obsessive compulsive disorder, including 67 children/adolescents) found that, compared with tricyclic antidepressants (desipramine, imipramine, nortripytyline) or monoamine oxidase inhibitors (clorgiline, phenelzine), clomipramine significantly improved symptoms (SMD 0.65, 95% CI 0.36 to 0.92).[18] The first subsequent RCT (54 people) compared three interventions: fluoxetine, phenelzine (a monoamine oxidase inhibitor), and placebo.[28] It found that fluoxetine significantly improved symptoms over 10 weeks compared with phenelzine or placebo (mean reduction in Yale-Brown scale score 2.8 with fluoxetine v 1.7 with phenelzine v 0.2 with placebo; P < 0.05 for fluoxetine v either comparator). The second subsequent RCT (164 people with concurrent obsessive compulsive disorder and major depressive disorder) found that sertraline significantly increased the proportion of people who had a clinically important reduction in obsessive compulsive symptoms compared with desipramine (> 40% improvement on Yale-Brown scale, 38/79 [48%] with sertraline v 26/85 [31%] with desipramine; P = 0.01) and significantly increased the proportion of people with remission of depressive symptoms (< 7 on Hamilton Depression Rating Scale, 39/79 [49%] with sertraline v 30/85 [35%] with desipramine; P = 0.04).[29] **Versus venlafaxine:** We found one RCT (73 people), which compared clomipramine (150–225 mg daily, 47 people) versus venlafaxine (225–350 mg daily, 26 people).[30] It found no significant difference in response at 12 weeks between clomipramine and venlafaxine (response defined as ≥ 35% reduction in Yale-Brown scale score and Clinical Global Impression Scale score of ≥ 2, 9/25 [36%] v 20/40 [50%]; RR 1.39, 95% CI 0.76 to 2.55). **Versus behavioural therapy:** We found one systematic review (search date 1997, number of studies and people not reported).[31] It found no significant difference in symptoms among serotonin reuptake inhibitors, behavioural therapy (see glossary, p 179), and placebo, but these conclusions must be treated with caution as the review made indirect comparisons of effect sizes (standardised mean differences).[31] **Plus behavioural or cognitive therapy:** See behavioural or cognitive therapy plus serotonin reuptake inhibitors, p 176.

Harms: **Versus placebo:** One systematic review (search date 1995, 16 RCTs) found that serotonin reuptake inhibitors significantly increased overall adverse effects (unspecified) compared with placebo (RRI v placebo: 54% with clomipramine, 11% with fluoxetine, 19% with fluvoxamine, and 27% with sertraline).[32] The other systematic reviews gave no information on adverse effects.[18,19] The first subsequent RCT found that fluoxetine significantly increased tremor ($P < 0.001$), dry mouth ($P < 0.001$), and nausea ($P < 0.01$) compared with placebo (absolute numbers presented graphically).[20] The second subsequent RCT found that citalopram significantly increased nausea, insomnia, fatigue, sweating, dry mouth, and ejaculatory failure compared with placebo ($P < 0.05$).[21] The third subsequent RCT (253 people) found that more people withdrew because of adverse effects with controlled release fluvoxamine than with placebo (20% with fluvoxamine v 7% with placebo; P value not reported).[22] Compared with placebo, fluvoxamine increased insomnia (35% with fluvoxamine v 20% with placebo), somnolence (27% v 11%), asthenia (25% v 8%, nausea (34% v 13%), diarrhoea (18% v 8%), anorexia (13% v 5%), and decreased libido (7% v 3%). **Versus each other:** The systematic reviews gave no information on adverse effects.[18,19] Three subsequent RCTs found that clomipramine increased adverse effects compared with selective serotonin reuptake inhibitors,[23–25] and one subsequent RCT[26] found no significant difference in adverse effects between the selective serotonin reuptake inhibitors sertraline and fluoxetine. The first subsequent RCT (170 people) found that significantly more people withdrew because of adverse effects with clomipramine than with sertraline ($P < 0.05$).[23] Clomipramine was associated with dry mouth, nausea, tremor, anxiety, and constipation, whereas sertraline was associated with nausea and diarrhoea. The second subsequent RCT (133 people) found that clomipramine significantly increased dry mouth (38% v 10%) and constipation (26% v 10%) compared with fluvoxamine ($P < 0.05$).[24] The third subsequent RCT comparing clomipramine versus fluvoxamine (227 people) found that more people stopped clomipramine prematurely (16% withdrew with clomipramine v 8% with fluvoxamine; CI not reported), and found that clomipramine significantly increased the proportion of people who had anticholinergic adverse effects (dry mouth 43% with clomipramine v 10% with fluvoxamine; constipation 25% v 9%; tremor 22% v 9%; and dizziness 18% v 7%; $P = 0.05$ for frequency of all anticholinergic adverse effects with clomipramine v fluvoxamine).[25] The fourth subsequent RCT found no significant difference in adverse effects between sertraline and fluoxetine.[26] The fifth subsequent RCT gave no information on adverse effects.[27] One systematic review (search date 1997) of controlled and uncontrolled studies found that the withdrawal rate because of adverse effects was 11% with clomipramine, 10% with fluoxetine, 13% with fluvoxamine, 9% with sertraline, and 11% with paroxetine.[31] One non-systematic review of three prospective cohort studies and five surveys found that fluoxetine during pregnancy did not increase the risk of spontaneous abortion or major malformation (numerical values not provided).[33] The review included one prospective cohort study (174 people) and three surveys that found similar outcomes with other selective serotonin reuptake inhibitors (sertraline, paroxetine, and fluvoxamine). One prospective cohort study of 55 preschool children exposed to fluoxetine *in utero* found no significant difference from unexposed children in global IQ, language, or behaviour. It included no information on long term harms for the other selective serotonin reuptake inhibitors. The non-systematic review of effects in pregnancy did not describe how articles were selected.[33] **Versus tricyclic antidepressants and monoamine oxidase inhibitors:** The systematic review gave no information on adverse effects.[18] The second subsequent RCT (164 people) found that significantly more people discontinued treatment because of adverse effects with desipramine than with sertraline (26% v 10%; P = 0.009).[29] One systematic review comparing the harms of selective serotonin reuptake inhibitors versus tricyclic antidepressants found that selective serotonin reuptake inhibitors were associated with fewer anticholinergic adverse effects but more nausea, diarrhoea, anxiety, agitation, insomnia, and headache.[34] **Versus venlafaxine:** The RCT (73 people) found that significantly more people had overall adverse effects with clomipramine than with venlafaxine (43/47 [92%] with clomipramine v 16/26 [62%] with venlafaxine; P = 0.002).[30] It found that, compared with venlafaxine, clomipramine significantly increased the proportion of people who had dry mouth (16/47 [34%] with clomipramine v 3/26 [12%] with venlafaxine; P = 0.036) and constipation (17/47 [36%] v 2/26 [8%]; P = 0.008).

Comment: One of the reviews found that sertraline was more effective than placebo,[18] whereas the other did not.[19] This may have been due to different methods of meta analysis. The reviews found heterogeneity in the selection of participants and duration of treatment in the RCTs identified; the first review[18] found that this heterogeneity reached significance in RCTs comparing clomipramine versus placebo. Two RCTs comparing clomipramine versus placebo in the first review included 73 children, but the review did not analyse these RCTs separately.[18] Some RCTs identified by the reviews included people with depression associated with obsessive compulsive disorder. The first systematic review performed a subgroup analysis in people with obsessive compulsive disorder without depression and found that, compared with placebo, clomipramine improved symptoms of obsessive compulsive disorder in people without depression (5 RCTs, 594 people, standardised mean differences 1.37, 95% CI 1.19 to 1.55).[18] This suggests that the effect of serotonin reuptake inhibitors on obsessive compulsive symptoms is independent of their effect on symptoms of depression. In the first subsequent RCT comparing sertraline versus clomipramine, people taking clomipramine received very low doses (median 90 mg/day). This makes the results of the RCT difficult to interpret. **Factors predicting outcome:** Four RCTs found that people who did not respond to serotonin reuptake inhibitors had younger age of onset, longer duration of the condition, higher frequency of symptoms, coexisting personality disorders, and a greater likelihood of previous hospital admission. Predictors of good response were older age of onset, history of remissions, no previous drug treatment, more severe obsessive compulsive disorder, and either high or low score on the Hamilton Depression Rating Scale.[35-38] Two cohort studies of people with obsessive compulsive disorder found that poor response to serotonin reuptake inhibitors was predicted by concomitant schizotypal personality disorder, by tic disorder (see glossary, p 179), and also by severe obsessive compulsive disorder with cleaning rituals (OR 4.9, 95% CI 1.1 to 21.2).[39,40]

OPTION   BEHAVIOURAL THERAPY

We found no RCTs comparing behavioural therapy versus no treatment. One systematic review and subsequent RCTs have found that behavioural therapy improves symptoms compared with relaxation. The review and one subsequent RCT found no significant difference in symptoms over 4–16 weeks between behavioural therapy and cognitive therapy. Another subsequent RCT found limited evidence that group behavioural therapy may improve symptoms over 12 weeks compared with group cognitive behavioural therapy.

Benefits: **Versus no treatment:** We found no systematic review or RCTs. **Versus relaxation:** We found one systematic review (search date 1995, 2 RCTs, 121 people), which found that behavioural therapy (see glossary, p 179) significantly improved symptoms over 4–16 weeks of treatment compared with relaxation (standardised mean differences 1.18, CI not reported; P < 0.01).[32] One subsequent RCT (218 people with DSM-IV obsessive compulsive disorder, 49% of whom were also taking a serotonin reuptake inhibitor) compared three treatments: behavioural therapy guided by a computer, behavioural therapy guided by a clinician, and relaxation.[41] It found that both types of behavioural therapy significantly improved Yale-Brown scale score after 10 weeks of treatment compared with relaxation (mean reduction 5.6 with computer guided behavioural therapy v 8.0 with clinician guided behavioural therapy v 1.7 with relaxation; P = 0.001 for relaxation v either type of behavioural therapy; P = 0.035 for clinician guided v computer guided behavioural therapy; analysis not by intention to treat).[41] **Versus cognitive or cognitive behavioural therapy:** We found one systematic review[32] and two subsequent RCTs.[42,43] The systematic review (search date 1995, 4 RCTs, 92 people) found no significant difference in symptoms over 4–16 weeks between behavioural therapy and cognitive therapy (see glossary, p 179) (SMD –0.19; reported as P > 0.05, no further data reported).[32] The first subsequent RCT (76 people) found no significant difference between group behavioural therapy (exposure with response prevention) and group cognitive behavioural therapy in recovery (defined as ≥6 point Yale-Brown scale score reduction and score ≤12) immediately after 12 weeks of treatment (AR 12/32 [38%] with behavioural therapy v 5/31 [16%] with cognitive behavioural therapy; P = 0.09), but found that behavioural therapy significantly improved recovery at 3 months follow up compared with cognitive behavioural therapy (AR 14/31 [45%] with behavioural therapy v 4/31 [13%] with cognitive behavioural therapy; P = 0.01; analysis not by intention to treat). The second subsequent RCT (63 people) found no significant difference between behavioural therapy and cognitive therapy in the proportion of people achieving at least 25% improvement in Yale-Brown scale score after 16 weeks of treatment (OR 0.7, 95% CI 0.2 to 2.0).[43] **Versus serotonin reuptake inhibitors:** See benefits of serotonin reuptake inhibitors, p 170. **Plus serotonin reuptake inhibitors:** See behavioural therapy or cognitive therapy plus serotonin reuptake inhibitors, p 176.

Harms: We found no evidence from RCTs or cohort studies of adverse effects from behavioural therapy. Case reports have described unbearable and unacceptable anxiety in some people receiving behavioural therapy.

Comment: **Factors predicting outcome:** We found two RCTs of behavioural therapy (total 96 people, duration 2.5 months and 32 weeks) and two retrospective cohort studies (total 346 people, duration 1 year and 11 weeks), which assessed factors predicting outcome.[44–47] These found that poorer outcome was predicted by initial severity, depression, longer duration, poorer motivation, and dissatisfaction with the therapeutic relationship. Good outcome was predicted by early adherence to exposure homework (see glossary, p 179), employment, living with one's family, no previous treatment, having fear of contamination, overt ritualistic behaviour, and absence of depression.[44–46] Good outcome for women was predicted by having a co-therapist (someone, usually related to the woman concerned, who is enlisted to help with treatment outside regular treatment sessions; OR 19.5, 95% CI 2.7 to 139).[47] Two systematic reviews of drug, behavioural, cognitive, and combination treatments for obsessive compulsive disorder are being prepared. **Maintenance of improvement:** A prospective follow up (20 people with obsessive compulsive disorder, specific diagnostic criteria not provided) after a 6 month RCT of behavioural therapy found that 79% maintained improvement in obsessive compulsive symptoms at 2 years follow up.[48] A prospective non-inception cohort study of behavioural therapy in 21 people with obsessive compulsive disorder (specific diagnostic criteria not provided) found that, after 2 weeks of treatment, 68–79% maintained complete or much improvement in symptoms at 3 months follow up.[49] In both RCTs, some people received additional behavioural therapy during follow up.

OPTION **COGNITIVE OR COGNITIVE BEHAVIOURAL THERAPY**

We found no RCTs comparing cognitive therapy versus no treatment. One RCT found that cognitive behavioural group therapy improved symptoms and quality of life compared with no treatment after 12 weeks. One systematic review and one subsequent RCT found no significant difference in symptoms over 4–16 weeks between behavioural therapy and cognitive therapy. Another subsequent RCT found limited evidence that group behavioural therapy improved symptoms over 12 weeks compared with group cognitive behavioural therapy.

Benefits: **Versus no treatment:** We found one RCT (47 people with DSM-IV obsessive compulsive disorder, 45% of whom were also taking a serotonin reuptake inhibitor), which compared cognitive behavioural group therapy versus no therapy.[50] It found that cognitive behavioural group therapy significantly increased the proportion of people achieving at least 35% improvement in Yale-Brown scale score after 12 weeks treatment, and significantly improved quality of life compared with no treatment (16/23 [69.6%] with cognitive behavioural group therapy v 1/24 [4.2%] with no treatment; OR 16.7, 95% CI 2.2 to 115.9; mean reduction in Yale-Brown scale score 11.6 with cognitive behavioural group therapy v 1.5 with no treatment, P value not reported; difference in quality of life: P < 0.04 in favour of cognitive behavioural therapy).[50] **Versus behavioural therapy:** See behavioural therapy, p 174. **Plus serotonin reuptake inhibitors:** See behavioural therapy or cognitive therapy plus serotonin reuptake inhibitors, p 176.

Harms: **Versus no treatment:** The RCT reported that one person withdrew from the treatment group owing to to severe anxiety during response prevention and exposure homework (see glossary, p 179) exercises.[50]

Comment: None.

OPTION	BEHAVIOURAL OR COGNITIVE THERAPY PLUS SEROTONIN REUPTAKE INHIBITORS

RCTs provided insufficient evidence to assess the effects of adding serotonin reuptake inhibitors to behavioural or cognitive therapy.

Benefits: We found one systematic review[31] and two subsequent RCTs.[51,52] The systematic review (search date 1997, 77 studies, number of people not reported) did not make direct comparisons between treatments.[31] It included all types of study with the exception of case control studies. In indirect comparisons, it found similar reductions in symptoms with behavioural therapy alone versus placebo, behavioural therapy plus serotonin reuptake inhibitors (clomipramine, fluoxetine, fluvoxamine, paroxetine, or sertraline) versus placebo, and serotonin reuptake inhibitors alone versus placebo. One subsequent RCT (99 people in an outpatient setting) compared four interventions: behavioural therapy, cognitive therapy (see glossary, p 179), behavioural therapy plus fluvoxamine (a selective serotonin reuptake inhibitor), and cognitive therapy plus fluvoxamine. It found no significant difference among interventions in symptoms after 16 weeks of treatment (mean reduction in Yale-Brown scale score 17.1 with behavioural therapy v 13.5 with cognitive therapy v 12.6 with behavioural therapy plus fluvoxamine v 15.6 with cognitive therapy plus fluvoxamine, reported as non-significant, no further data reported).[51] Another subsequent RCT (49 people in a hospital setting) found that behavioural therapy plus fluvoxamine significantly increased the proportion of people with improved symptoms after 9 weeks of treatment compared with behavioural therapy plus pill placebo (number of people with > 35% reduction of Yale-Brown scale score 21/24 [88%] v 15/25 [60%]; RR 1.46, 95% CI 1.02 to 2.08).[52]

Harms: We found no evidence from RCTs or cohort studies of adverse effects from behavioural therapy. Case reports have described unbearable and unacceptable anxiety in some people receiving behavioural therapy. See harms of serotonin reuptake inhibitors, p 172. See harms of cognitive therapy, p 176.

Comment: None.

OPTION **ELECTROCONVULSIVE THERAPY**

We found no RCTs of electroconvulsive therapy in people with obsessive compulsive disorder.

Benefits: We found no systematic review or RCTs.

Harms: We found no RCTs.

Comment: People with obsessive compulsive disorder who also have depression may be treated with electroconvulsive therapy. The evidence for the effects of electroconvulsive therapy in depression is summarised elsewhere in *Clinical Evidence* (see depressive disorders in adults, p 114).

QUESTION   **What are the best forms of maintenance treatment in adults?**

OPTION   **OPTIMUM DURATION OF MAINTENANCE TREATMENT WITH SEROTONIN REUPTAKE INHIBITORS**

RCTs provided insufficient evidence to define the optimum duration of treatment with serotonin reuptake inhibitors.

Benefits: Most RCTs lasted only 10–12 weeks.[53] We found two RCTs that assessed maintenance of serotonin reuptake inhibitors for 1 year in people who had responded to treatment.[54,55] The first RCT (70 people who had responded to a 20 week course of fluoxetine) found no significant difference between maintenance of fluoxetine and replacement by placebo for 1 year in relapse rate over 1 year (21% with fluoxetine v 32% with placebo; P = 0.137).[54] The second RCT compared sertraline versus placebo in 223 people with obsessive compulsive disorder, who had all previously responded to 1 year's treatment with sertraline (response defined as at least 25% reduction in Yale-Brown scale score from baseline).[55] People continuing on sertraline were prescribed their previous dose (mean 183 mg). The RCT found that, compared with placebo, sertraline significantly reduced the proportion of people who withdrew because of relapse or insufficient clinical response over 24 weeks (9% with sertraline v 24% with placebo; P = 0.006). It found that sertraline reduced the proportion of people who had worsening of symptoms compared with placebo (12% with sertraline v 35% with placebo; P = 0.001), but found no significant difference in relapse rate over 24 weeks (2.7% with sertraline v 4.4% with placebo; P = 0.34).[55]

Harms: The first RCT found no significant difference between fluoxetine and placebo in overall adverse effects (reported as non-significant, adverse effects not specified, absolute numbers and CI not reported) or in the proportion of people who withdrew from the trial for any cause over 52 weeks (16/36 [44%] with fluoxetine v 23/35 [66%] with placebo; P = 0.072).[54] The second RCT found that upper respiratory infection, headache, and malaise were reported in

≥ 10% of people taking sertraline, and that people taking placebo had dizziness and depression (no further data reported).[55] It found that fewer people taking sertraline withdrew because of adverse effects than people taking placebo (5/109 [5%] with sertraline v 12/114 [11%] with placebo; P value not reported).

Comment: One prospective, 1 year study found further improvement after a 40 week open label extension of the study, with continuing adverse effects.[56] One observational study found that 16/18 (89%) of people relapsed within 7 weeks of replacing clomipramine with placebo treatment.[57]

QUESTION **What are the effects of treatments in adults who have not responded to initial treatment with serotonin reuptake inhibitors?**

OPTION **ADDITION OF ANTIPSYCHOTICS TO SEROTONIN REUPTAKE INHIBITORS**

Three small RCTs in people unresponsive to serotonin reuptake inhibitors found that the addition of antipsychotics improved symptoms compared with placebo.

Benefits: We found no systematic review, but found three small RCTs that assessed combined antipsychotics and serotonin reuptake inhibitors in people who did not respond to serotonin reuptake inhibitors alone.[58–60] The first RCT (34 people with obsessive compulsive disorder who had not responded to 8 weeks of treatment with fluvoxamine) compared fluvoxamine (a selective serotonin reuptake inhibitor) plus haloperidol (an antipsychotic; maximum dose of haloperidol 10 mg/day) versus fluvoxamine plus placebo.[58] It found that fluvoxamine plus haloperidol significantly increased the proportion of people who met two out of three different response criteria compared with fluvoxamine plus placebo (11/17 [65%] v 0/17 [0%]; NNT 2, 95% CI 2 to 3; P < 0.0002). The second RCT (36 people with obsessive compulsive disorder who did not respond to 12 weeks of treatment with a serotonin reuptake inhibitor) found that, compared with addition of placebo, addition of 6 weeks of risperidone (an antipsychotic) to the prior serotonin reuptake inhibitor significantly improved symptoms of obsessive compulsive disorder (reduction in the Yale-Brown scale score 36% v 9%; P = 0.001), depression (reduction in the Hamilton Depression Rating Scale 35% v 20%; P = 0.002), and anxiety (reduction in the Hamilton Anxiety Rating Scale 31% v 12%; P = 0.007).[59] People taking risperidone were more likely to have met two of the response criteria (8/18 [44%] with serotonin reuptake inhibitor plus risperidone v 0/15 [0%] with serotonin reuptake inhibitor plus placebo; NNT 2, 95% CI 2 to 3; P < 0.005). The third RCT (27 people who did not respond to 3 months of treatment with fluoxetine, fluvoxamine, or clomipramine in an open label trial) compared a serotonin reuptake inhibitor plus quetiapine (an atypical antipsychotic 50–200 mg daily) versus a serotonin reuptake inhibitor plus placebo for 8 weeks.[60] People received the same serotonin reuptake inhibitors in the RCT as they had in the open label phase of the study. The RCT found that a serotonin reuptake inhibitor plus quetiapine significantly increased the proportion of people who responded compared with a serotonin reuptake inhibitor plus placebo (response defined as 30% or greater reduction in the Yale-Brown scale score; 10/14 [71%] with a serotonin reuptake inhibitor plus quetiapine v 0/14 [0%] with a serotonin reuptake inhibitor plus placebo; P < 0.0001).

Harms: Extrapyramidal adverse effects are common with haloperidol, which can also cause prolactinaemia. The RCT of serotonin reuptake inhibitors plus risperidone found that sedation, restlessness, increased appetite, dry mouth, or tinnitus were experienced by at least 10% of people taking serotonin reuptake inhibitors plus risperidone, and that blurred vision, excessive perspiration, headache, increased appetite, lightheadedness, restlessness, and sedation were experienced by at least 10% of people taking placebo.[59] Risperidone is commonly associated with hypotension and prolactinaemia. The RCT of serotonin reuptake inhibitors plus quetiapine found that people taking a serotonin reuptake inhibitor plus quetiapine had nausea (6/14), sedation (3/14), and dizziness (1/14), and people taking a serotonin reuptake inhibitor plus placebo had sedation (2/13), headache (1/13), and nervousness (1/13).[60]

Comment: None.

GLOSSARY

Behavioural therapy Consists of exposure to the anxiety provoking stimuli and prevention of ritualistic behaviour (engaging in compulsions).

Chronic obsessive compulsive disorder Continuous course without periods of remission since first onset.

Cognitive therapy Aims to correct distorted thoughts (such as exaggerated sense of harm and personal responsibility) by Socratic questioning, logical reasoning, and hypothesis testing.

Episodic obsessive compulsive disorder Episodic course with periods of remission since first onset.

Exposure homework Tasks involving contact with anxiety provoking situations to be carried out outside regular psychotherapy sessions.

Schizotypal personality disorder Characterised by discomfort in close relationships, cognitive and perceptual distortions, and eccentric behaviour.

Tic disorder Characterised by motor tics, vocal tics, or both.

REFERENCES

1. American Psychiatric Association. *Diagnostic and statistical manual of mental disorders,* 4th ed. Washington, DC: APA, 1994:669–673.
2. World Health Organization. *The ICD-10 classification of mental and behavioural disorders.* Geneva: World Health Organization, 1992.
3. Bebbington PE. Epidemiology of obsessive–compulsive disorder. *Br J Psychiatry* 1998;35(suppl.):2–6.
4. Horwath E, Weissman MM. The epidemiology and cross-national presentation of obsessive-compulsive disorder. *Psychiatr Clin North Am* 2000;23:493–507.
5. Baer L, Minichiello WE. Behavior therapy for obsessive–compulsive disorder. In: Jenike MA, Baer L, Minichiello WE, eds. *Obsessive–compulsive disorders.* St Louis: Mosby, 1998: 337–367.
6. Steketee GS, Frost RO, Rheaume J, et al. Cognitive theory and treatment of obsessive–compulsive disorder. In: Jenike MA, Baer L, Minichiello WE, eds. *Obsessive–compulsive disorders.* St Louis: Mosby, 1998: 368–399.
7. Alsobrook JP, Pauls DL. The genetics of obsessive–compulsive disorder. In: Jenike MA, Baer L, Minichiello WE, eds. *Obsessive–compulsive disorders.* St Louis: Mosby, 1998:276–288.
8. Rauch SL, Whalen PJ, Dougherty D, et al. Neurobiologic models of obsessive compulsive disorder. In: Jenike MA, Baer L, Minichiello WE, eds. *Obsessive–compulsive disorders.* St Louis: Mosby, 1998: 222–253.
9. Delgado PL, Moreno FA. Different roles for serotonin in anti-obsessional drug action and the pathophysiology of obsessive–compulsive disorder. *Br J Psychiatry* 1998;35(suppl.):21–25.

10. Saxena S, Brody AL, Schwartz JM, et al. Neuroimaging and frontal–subcortical circuitry in obsessive–compulsive disorder. Br J Psychiatry 1998;35(suppl.):26–37.

11. Rauch SL, Baxter LR Jr. Neuroimaging in obsessive–compulsive disorder and related disorders. In: Jenike MA, Baer L, Minichiello WE, eds. Obsessive–compulsive disorders. St Louis: Mosby, 1998:289–317.

12. Yaryura-Tobias JA, Neziroglu FA. Obsessive-compulsive disorder spectrum. Washington, DC: American Psychiatric Press, Inc., 1997.

13. Skoog G, Skoog I. A 40-year follow up of patients with obsessive–compulsive disorder. Arch Gen Psychiatry 1999;56:121–127.

14. Ravizza L, Maina G, Bogetto F. Episodic and chronic obsessive–compulsive disorder. Depress Anxiety 1997;6:154–158.

15. Goodman WK, Price LH, Rasmussen SA, et al. The Yale-Brown obsessive compulsive scale. I. Development, use, and reliability. Arch Gen Psychiatry 1989;46:1006–1011.

16. Goodman WK, Price LH, Rasmussen SA, et al. The Yale-Brown obsessive compulsive scale. II. Validity. Arch Gen Psychiatry 1989;46:1012–1016.

17. Goodman WK, Price LH. Rating scales for obsessive–compulsive disorder. In: Jenike MA, Baer L, Minichiello WE, eds. Obsessive–compulsive disorders. St Louis: Mosby, 1998:97–117.

18. Piccinelli M, Pini S, Bellantuono C, et al. Efficacy of drug treatment in obsessive–compulsive disorder. A meta-analytic review. Br J Psychiatry 1995;166:424–443. Search dates 1994; primary sources Medline and Excerpta Medica-Psychiatry.

19. Ackerman DL, Greenland S. Multivariate meta-analysis of controlled drug studies for obsessive–compulsive disorder. J Clin Psychopharmacol 2002;22:309–317. Search date not reported; primary sources Medline, Psycinfo, and hand searches of bibliographies of published reviews and previous meta-analyses.

20. Tollefson GD, Rampey AH, Potvin JH, et al. A multicenter investigation of fixed-dose fluoxetine in the treatment of obsessive–compulsive disorder. Arch Gen Psychiatry 1994;51:559–567.

21. Montgomery SA, Kasper S, Stein DJ, et al. Citalopram 20 mg, 40 mg and 60 mg are all effective and well tolerated compared with placebo in obsessive-compulsive disorder. Int Clin Psychopharmacol 2001;16:75–86.

22. Hollander E, Koran LM, Goodman WK, et al. A double-blind, placebo-controlled study of the efficacy and safety of controlled-release fluvoxamine in patients with obsessive-compulsive disorder. J Clin Psychiatry 2003;64:640–647.

23. Bisserbe JC, Lane RM, Flament MF. A double blind comparison of sertraline and clomipramine in outpatients with obsessive–compulsive disorder. Eur Psychiatry 1997;12:82–93.

24. Mundo E, Maina G, Uslenghi C. Multicentre, double-blind, comparison of fluvoxamine and clomipramine in the treatment of obsessive–compulsive disorder. Int Clin Psychopharmacol 2000;15:69–76.

25. Mundo E, Rouillon F, Figuera L, et al. Fluvoxamine in obsessive-compulsive disorder: Similar efficacy but superior tolerability in comparison with clomipramine. Hum Psychopharmacol 2001;16:461–468.

26. Bergeron R, Ravindran AV, Chaput Y, et al. Sertraline and fluoxetine treatment of obsessive-compulsive disorder: Results of a double-blind, 6-month treatment study. J Clin Psychopharmacol 2002;22:148–154.

27. Mundo E, Bianchi L, Bellodi L. Efficacy of fluvoxamine, paroxetine, and citalopram in the treatment of obsessive compulsive disorder: a single-blind study. J Clin Psychopharmacol 1997;17:267–271.

28. Jenike MA, Baer L, Minichiello WE, et al. Placebo-controlled trial of fluoxetine and phenelzine for obsessive–compulsive disorder. Am J Psychiatry 1997;154:1261–1264.

29. Hoehn-Saric R, Ninan P, Black DW, et al. Multicenter double-blind comparison of sertraline and desipramine for concurrent obsessive–compulsive and major depressive disorders. Arch Gen Psychiatry 2000;57:76–82.

30. Albert U, Aguglia E, Maina G, et al. Venlafaxine versus clomipramine in the treatment of obsessive-compulsive disorder: a preliminary single-blind, 12-week, controlled study. J Clin Psychiatry 2002;63:1004–1009.

31. Kobak KA, Greist JH, Jefferson JW, et al. Behavioral versus pharmacological treatments of obsessive compulsive disorder: a meta-analysis. Psychopharmacology (Berl) 1998;136:205–216. Search date 1997; primary sources Medline, PsycINFO, Dissertations, and Abstracts International databases.

32. Abramowitz JS. Effectiveness of psychological and pharmacological treatments for obsessive–compulsive disorder: a quantitative review. J Consult Clin Psychol 1997;65:44–52. Search date 1995; primary sources Medline and PsycLIT.

33. Goldstein DJ, Sundell K. A review of safety of selective serotonin reuptake inhibitors during pregnancy. Hum Psychopharmacol Clin Exp 1999;14:319–324.

34. Trindade E, Menon D. Selective serotonin reuptake inhibitors differ from tricyclic antidepressants in adverse events [abstract]. Selective serotonin reuptake inhibitors for major depression. Part 1. Evaluation of clinical literature. Ottawa: Canadian Coordinating Office for Health Technology Assessment, August 1997 Report 3E. Evid Based Ment Health 1998;1:50.

35. Ravizza L, Barzega G, Bellino S, et al. Predictors of drug treatment response in obsessive–compulsive disorder. J Clin Psychiatry 1995;56:368–373.

36. Cavedini P, Erzegovesi S, Ronchi P, et al. Predictive value of obsessive–compulsive personality disorder in antiobsessional pharmacological treatment. Eur Neuropsychopharmacol 1997;7:45–49.

37. Ackerman DL, Greenland S, Bystritsky A. Clinical characteristics of response to fluoxetine treatment of obsessive–compulsive disorder. J Clin Psychopharmacol 1998;18:185–192.

38. Ackerman DL, Greenland S, Bystritsky A, et al. Predictors of treatment response in obsessive–compulsive disorder: multivariate analyses from a multicenter trial of clomipramine. J Clin Psychopharmacol 1994;14:247–254.

39. Mundo E, Erzegovesi S, Bellodi L. Follow up of obsessive-compulsive patients treated with proserotonergic agents [letter]. J Clin Psychopharmacol 1995;15:288–289.

40. Alarcon RD, Libb JW, Spitler D. A predictive study of obsessive-compulsive disorder response to clomipramine. J Clin Psychopharmacol 1993;13:210–213.

41. Greist JH, Marks IM, Baer L, et al. Behavior therapy for obsessive-compulsive disorder guided by a computer or by a clinician compared with relaxation as a control. J Clin Psychiatry 2002;63:138–145.

42. McLean PD, Whittal ML, Thordarson DS, et al. Cognitive versus behavior therapy in the group treatment of obsessive-compulsive disorder. J Consult Clin Psychol 2001;69:205–214.

43. Cottraux J, Note I, Yao SN, et al. A randomized controlled trial of cognitive therapy versus

intensive behavior therapy in obsessive compulsive disorder. *Psychother Psychosom* 2001;70:288–297.

44. Keijsers GP, Hoogduin CA, Schaap CP. Predictors of treatment outcome in the behavioural treatment of obsessive–compulsive disorder. *Br J Psychiatry* 1994;165:781–786.

45. De Araujo LA, Ito LM, Marks IM. Early compliance and other factors predicting outcome of exposure for obsessive–compulsive disorder. *Br J Psychiatry* 1996;169:747–752.

46. Buchanan AW, Meng KS, Marks IM. What predicts improvement and compliance during the behavioral treatment of obsessive compulsive disorder? *Anxiety* 1996;2:22–27.

47. Castle DJ, Deale A, Marks IM, et al. Obsessive–compulsive disorder: prediction of outcome from behavioural psychotherapy. *Acta Psychiatr Scand* 1994;89:393–398.

48. Marks IM, Hodgson R, Rachman S. Treatment of chronic obsessive–compulsive neurosis by in-vivo exposure. A two-year follow up and issues in treatment. *Br J Psychiatry* 1975;127:349–364.

49. Foa EB, Goldstein A. Continuous exposure and complete response prevention in obsessive–compulsive neurosis. *Behav Ther* 1978;9:821–829.

50. Cordioli AV, Heldt E, Bochi DB, et al. Cognitive–behavioral group therapy in obsessive-compulsive disorder: A randomized clinical trial. *Psychother Psychosom* 2003;72:211–216.

51. van Balkom AJ, de Haan E, van Oppen P, et al. Cognitive and behavioral therapies alone versus in combination with fluvoxamine in the treatment of obsessive compulsive disorder. *J Nerv Ment Dis* 1998;186:492–499.

52. Hohagen F, Winkelmann G, Rasche-Ruchle H, et al. Combination of behaviour therapy with

fluvoxamine in comparison with behaviour therapy and placebo. Results of a multicentre study. *Br J Psychiatry* 1998;35(suppl):71–78.

53. Rauch SL, Jenike MA. Pharmacological treatment of obsessive compulsive disorder. In: Nathan PE, Gorman JM, eds. *Treatments that work*. New York: Oxford University Press, 1998:359–376.

54. Romano S, Goodman W, Tamura R, et al. Long-term treatment of obsessive-compulsive disorder after an acute response: a comparison of fluoxetine versus placebo. *J Clin Psychopharmacol* 2001;21:46–52.

55. Koran LM, Hackett E, Rubin A, et al. Efficacy of sertraline in the long-term treatment of obsessive-compulsive disorder. *Am J Psychiatry* 2002;159:88–95.

56. Rasmussen S, Hackett E, DuBoff E, et al. A 2-year study of sertraline in the treatment of obsessive–compulsive disorder. *Int Clin Psychopharmacol* 1997;12:309–316.

57. Pato MT, Zohar-Kadouch R, Zohar J, et al. Return of symptoms after discontinuation of clomipramine in patients with obsessive–compulsive disorder. *Am J Psychiatry* 1988;145:1521–1525.

58. McDougle CJ, Goodman WK, Leckman JF, et al. Haloperidol addition in fluvoxamine-refractory obsessive-compulsive disorder. A double-blind, placebo-controlled study in patients with and without tics. *Arch Gen Psychiatry* 1994;51:302–308.

59. McDougle CJ, Epperson CN, Pelton GH, et al. A double-blind, placebo-controlled study of risperidone addition in serotonin reuptake inhibitor-refractory obsessive-compulsive disorder. *Arch Gen Psychiatry* 2000;57:794–801.

60. Atmaca M, Kuloglu M, Tezcan E, et al. Quetiapine augmentation in patients with treatment resistant obsessive-compulsive disorder: a single-blind, placebo-controlled study. *Int Clin Psychopharmacol* 2002;17:115–119.

G Mustafa Soomro
Honorary Research Fellow
Section of Community Psychiatry
St George's Hospital Medical School
London
UK

Competing interests: None declared.

TABLE 1 Serotonin reuptake inhibitors (clomipramine, citalopram, fluoxetine, fluvoxamine, paroxetine, sertraline) versus placebo (see text, p 170).

Intervention and reference	Study design	Symptom improvement
Citalopram** 21	RCT (401 people)	AR 57% with citalopram 20 mg v 52% with 40 mg v 65% with 60 mg v 37% with placebo; NNT for 20 mg citalopram v placebo 5, 95% CI 3 to 14
Clomipramine*¶ 18 19	SR (9 RCTs; 668 people) SR (7 RCTs; 808 people)	SMD 1.31 (95% CI 1.15 to 1.47) SMD −8.19 (95% CI −10.53 to −5.85)
Fluoxetine†¶ 18 19 20	SR (1 RCT; 287 people) SR (3 RCTs; 329 people) RCT (350 people)	SMD 0.57 (95% CI 0.33 to 0.81) SMD −1.61 (95% CI −2.18 to −1.04) Mean reduction in score 4.6 with fluoxetine 20 mg, 5.5 with 40 mg, 6.5 with 60 mg v 0.9 with placebo (P < 0.001 for all doses v placebo)
Fluvoxamine‡ 18 19 22	SR SR RCT (253 people)	SMD 0.57 (95% CI 0.37 to 0.77) SMD −4.84 (95% CI −7.78 to −1.83) (measured as a change in raw score of Yale Brown) Mean reduction in score 8.5 with fluvoxamine controlled release 100–300 mg v 5.6 with placebo (P = 0.001)
Paroxetine¶ 19	SR (1 RCT; 300 people)	SMD −3.00 (95% CI −4.91 to −1.09)
Sertraline§¶ 18 19	SR (3 RCTs; 270 people) SR (4 RCTs; 598 people)	SMD 0.52 (95% CI 0.27 to 0.77) SMD −2.57 (95% CI −6.13 to +1.20 [NS])

*The total number of different RCTs identified was 11; †the total number of different RCTs identified was 5; ‡the total number of different RCTs identified was 6; §the total number of different RCTs identified was 4; ¶symptoms assessed by Yale-Brown scale score; **25% reduction in Yale-Brown score; NS, non-significant.

QUESTIONS

INTERVENTIONS

Key Messages

- **Selective serotonin reuptake inhibitors** Systematic reviews and one additional RCT have found that selective serotonin reuptake inhibitors improve symptoms in panic disorder compared with placebo. One subsequent RCT found that discontinuation of sertraline in people with a good response increased exacerbation of symptoms. A second subsequent RCT found that paroxetine plus cognitive behavioural therapy improved symptoms compared with placebo plus cognitive behavioural therapy.

- **Tricyclic antidepressants (imipramine)** One systematic review, one subsequent RCT, and one additional RCT have found that imipramine improves symptoms compared with placebo. One subsequent RCT found that imipramine reduced relapse rates over 12 months.

- **Benzodiazepines** One systematic review and one additional RCT have found that alprazolam reduces the number of panic attacks and improves symptoms compared with placebo. However, benzodiazepines are associated with a wide range of adverse effects, both during and after treatment.

- **Buspirone** We found insufficient evidence to assess the effects of buspirone.

- **Monoamine oxidase inhibitors** We found no RCTs on the effects of monoamine oxidase inhibitors.

DEFINITION A panic attack is a period in which there is sudden onset of intense apprehension, fearfulness, or terror often associated with feelings of impending doom. Panic disorder occurs when there are recurrent, unpredictable attacks followed by at least 1 month of persistent concern about having another panic attack, worry about the possible implications or consequences of the panic attacks, or a significant behavioural change related to the attacks.[1] The term panic disorder excludes panic attacks attributable to the direct physiological effects of a general medical condition, a substance, or another mental disorder. Panic disorder is sometimes categorised as being with or without agoraphobia.[1] Alternative categorisations focus on phobic anxiety disorders and specify agoraphobia with or without panic disorder.[2]

INCIDENCE/ PREVALENCE Panic disorder often starts at around 20 years of age (between late adolescence and the mid-30s).[3] Lifetime prevalence is 1–3%, and panic disorder is more common in women than in men.[4] An Australian community study found 1 month prevalence rates for panic disorder (with or without agoraphobia) of 0.4% using International Classification of Diseases (ICD)-10 diagnostic criteria, and of 0.5% using Diagnostic and Statistical Manual (DSM)-IV diagnostic criteria.[5]

AETIOLOGY/ RISK FACTORS Stressful life events tend to precede the onset of panic disorder,[6,7] although a negative interpretation of these events in addition to their occurrence has been suggested as an important causal factor.[8] Panic disorder is associated with major depression,[9] social phobia, generalised anxiety disorder, obsessive compulsive disorder,[10] and a substantial risk of drug and alcohol abuse.[11] It is also associated with avoidant, histrionic, and dependent personality disorders.[10]

PROGNOSIS The severity of symptoms in people with panic disorder fluctuates considerably, and patients commonly experience periods of no attacks, or only mild attacks with few symptoms. There is often a long delay between the initial onset of symptoms and presentation for treatment. Recurrent attacks may continue for several years, especially if associated with agoraphobia. Reduced social or occupational functioning varies among people with panic disorder and is worse in people with associated agoraphobia. Panic disorder is also associated with an increased rate of attempted, but unsuccessful, suicide.[12] One study analysing data from RCTs and systematic reviews found that co-existence of anxiety and depressive features adversely affected treatment response at 12 years compared with treatment of panic disorder alone.[13]

AIMS OF INTERVENTION To reduce the severity and frequency of panic attacks, phobic avoidance, and anticipatory anxiety; to improve social and occupational functioning, with minimal adverse effects of treatment.

OUTCOMES Measures of panic attacks, agoraphobia, and associated disability (self reported and clinician rated, before and after treatment, and longer term) using general or specific scales for panic disorder (e.g. the panic and agoraphobia scale, the mobility inventory for agoraphobia).

METHODS   *Clinical Evidence* search and appraisal September 2003. Studies with follow up periods of less than 6 months were excluded.

| QUESTION | What are the effects of drug treatments for panic disorder? |

| OPTION | TRICYCLIC ANTIDEPRESSANTS |

One systematic review, one subsequent RCT, and one additional RCT have found that imipramine improves symptoms in people with panic disorder compared with placebo. One subsequent RCT found that imipramine reduced relapse rates after 12 months in people with panic disorder compared with placebo.

Benefits: We found one systematic review (search date not reported, 27 RCTs, 2348 people),[14] one additional RCT,[15] and two subsequent RCTs.[16,17] The systematic review compared imipramine, selective serotonin reuptake inhibitors (SSRIs; paroxetine, fluvoxamine, zimelidine, and clomipramine; see comment below), and alprazolam verssu placebo and versus each other (see benefits of SSRIs, p 186 and benzodiazepines, p 188).[14] It found that imipramine significantly increased the proportion of people judged to have improved compared with placebo ($P < 0.0001$; see comment below). The additional RCT (181 people with panic disorder with or without agoraphobia) compared three treatments: oral imipramine (maximum dose 225 mg; see comment below), oral alprazolam (maximum dose 10 mg; see comment below), and placebo (see benefits of benzodiazepines, p 188).[15] It found that imipramine reduced the number of panic attacks after 8 months compared with placebo (results presented graphically, significance not calculated). The first subsequent RCT (56 adults with panic disorder and agoraphobia in stable remission after 24 weeks' treatment with oral imipramine) comparing oral imipramine 2.25 mg/kg daily versus placebo found that significantly fewer people taking imipramine relapsed after 12 months (see comment below; 1/29 [3%] with imipramine v 10/27 [37%] with placebo; RR 0.09, 95% CI 0.01 to 0.68; NNT 5, 95% CI 3 to 14).[16] The second subsequent RCT (312 people) compared five groups: oral imipramine (maximum dose 300 mg/day; see comment below), cognitive behavioural therapy (see glossary, p 189), placebo, cognitive behavioural therapy plus oral imipramine (maximum dose 300 mg/day; see comment below), and cognitive behavioural therapy plus placebo.[17] It found that imipramine significantly increased the proportion of people judged to have responded (using the panic disorder severity scale) compared with placebo after 6 months (response rate: 38% with imipramine v 13% with placebo; absolute numbers not provided; $P = 0.02$).

Harms: Adverse effects associated with imipramine treatment included blurred vision, tachycardia, palpitations, blood pressure changes, insomnia, nervousness, malaise, dizziness, headache, nausea, vomiting, and reduced appetite (see harms of prescription antidepressant drugs under depressive disorders, p 114).[15,18]

Comment: The review included clomipramine as an SSRI. This drug is also often described as a tricyclic antidepressant.[14] The review used improvement as an outcome measure without a clear definition of this term. In the additional RCT and the second subsequent RCT, flexible dosing was used according to tolerance and therapeutic need.[15,17] In the subsequent RCT comparing imipramine versus placebo, relapse rate was not clearly defined.[16] **Short term effects:** We found one systematic review (search date 1999, 43 studies including 34 RCTs, 2367 people, drop-out rate 24%, analysis based on completers) that compared the short term efficacy of SSRIs (fluoxetine, fluvoxamine, paroxetine, citalopram, and sertraline) versus tricyclic antidepressants (imipramine, desipramine, nortryptiline, and clomipramine) and analysed effect size within treatment group rather than within studies.[19] It found no significant difference between treatments in the proportion of people who were free of panic attacks at 6–10 weeks, but found that tricyclic antidepressants significantly increased drop-out rates (free of panic attacks: 60% with tricyclic antidepressants v 55% with SSRIs, P value not reported; drop-outs: 31% with tricyclic antidepressants v 18% with SSRIs, P < 0.001).

OPTION   SELECTIVE SEROTONIN REUPTAKE INHIBITORS

Systematic reviews and one additional RCT have found that selective serotonin reuptake inhibitors improve symptoms compared with placebo in panic disorder. One subsequent RCT found that discontinuation of sertraline in people with a good response increased exacerbation of symptoms. A second subsequent RCT found that paroxetine plus cognitive behavioural therapy improved symptoms compared with placebo plus cognitive behavioural therapy.

Benefits: **Versus placebo:** We found two systematic reviews (see benefits of tricyclic antidepressants, p 185 and benzodiazepines, p 188),[14,20] one additional RCT,[21] and two subsequent RCTs.[22,23] The first systematic review (search date not reported, 27 RCTs, 2348 people) found that selective serotonin reuptake inhibitors (SSRIs; paroxetine, fluvoxamine, zimelidine, and clomipramine; see comment below) significantly increased the proportion of people who improved compared with placebo (P < 0.0001; see comment below).[14] The second systematic review (search date not reported, 12 RCTs, 1741 people) only reported combined results as an effect size against placebo (effect size 0.55), and did not report statistical significance.[20] The additional RCT (279 people) compared five groups: oral citalopram 10 or 15 mg daily, oral citalopram 20 or 30 mg daily, oral citalopram 40 or 60 mg daily, oral clomipramine 60 or 90 mg daily, and placebo.[21] It found that citalopram (at all doses) significantly increased the proportion of people who responded (defined as no panic attacks and either no episodic increases in anxiety or only slight increases in anxiety precipitated by definite events or activities) compared with placebo after 12 months (citalopram 10 or 15 mg/day v placebo, P = 0.05; citalopram 20 or 30 mg/day v placebo, P = 0.001; citalopram 40 or 60 mg/day v placebo, P = 0.003; results presented graphically). The first subsequent RCT (182 people who had responded to open label sertraline for 52 weeks) compared double blind placebo (discontinuation of sertraline) versus sertraline for 28 weeks.[22] It found that significantly more people on placebo had exacerbation of symptoms (33% with placebo v 13% with sertraline; P = 0.005; CI not reported). The second subsequent RCT (43 people with panic disorder with or without agoraphobia who had been unsuccessfully treated with 15 sessions of manual guided cognitive behavioural therapy [CBT; see glossary, p 189] alone) compared paroxetine 40 mg plus CBT versus placebo plus CBT (see comment below).[23] Success was defined as no panic attacks for a 2 week period or achieving cut-off scores or lower on panic disorder scales. It found that combined treatment significantly increased success compared with placebo plus CBT (12/19 [63%] with combined treatment v 5/19 [26%] with placebo plus CBT; RR 2.4, 95% CI 1.1 to 5.6; NNT 3, 95% CI 2 to 21).

Harms: The additional RCT reported that harms associated with citalopram included headache, tremor, dry mouth, and somnolence (see harms of prescription antidepressant drugs under depressive disorders, p 114).[21] The first subsequent RCT found the highest incidence of adverse events with sertraline in the first 12 weeks of the study, and tolerability seemed to improve with time.[22] The most common adverse events over the 52 week trial period were headache, malaise, insomnia, upper respiratory infection, diarrhoea, nausea, and dizziness. The second subsequent RCT did not report on adverse events.[23]

Comment: The first review included clomipramine as an SSRI, although this drug is often described as a tricyclic antidepressant.[14] It also included the SSRI zimelidine, which is rarely used these days. In addition, the review used improvement as an outcome measure, without defining this term clearly. In the additional RCT, only 28/54 (52%) completed the trial; analysis was by intention to treat and people who withdrew from the trial were counted as treatment failures.[21] The RCT used flexible dosing according to tolerance and therapeutic need. SSRIs can cause initial increased anxiety, which can exacerbate a tendency to focus on internal sensations and to avoid situations that trigger these sensations (catastrophise somatic sensations). Education about this event is likely to improve adherence with medication. The second systematic review found that smaller RCTs were associated with larger effect sizes, suggesting the possibility of publication bias.[20] The second subsequent RCT only used 8 weeks of medication as opposed to a more common 12 weeks, it only used clinician rated outcomes, and most people in both the placebo and paroxetine groups guessed correctly which treatment they had been allocated (62% with placebo v 79% with paroxetine).[23] **Tricyclic antidepressants versus selective serotonin reuptake inhibitors:** See comment under tricyclic antidepressants, p 186.

OPTION	MONOAMINE OXIDASE INHIBITORS

We found no RCTs on the effects of monoamine oxidase inhibitors in panic disorder.

Benefits: We found no systematic review and no RCTs.

Mental health

Harms: We found no evidence of harms associated specifically with the use of monoamine oxidase inhibitors in the long term treatment of panic disorder.

Comment: Our search strategy excluded studies with follow up of less than 6 months.

OPTION   BUSPIRONE

We found insufficient evidence to assess the effects of buspirone in people with panic disorder.

Benefits: We found no systematic review but found two RCTs.[24,25] The first RCT (48 people) compared oral buspirone (maximum 60 mg/day) plus (CBT; see glossary, p 189) versus placebo plus CBT for 16 weeks.[24] It found that oral buspirone plus CBT significantly improved self rated panic and agoraphobia scores after 1 year (using a 90 point symptom scale where each symptom was graded from $0 =$ not present to $4 =$ severe; $P = 0.03$; absolute numbers not reported).[24] The second RCT (41 people with panic disorder and agoraphobia) compared 16 weeks of oral buspirone 30 mg daily plus CBT versus 16 weeks of placebo plus CBT.[25] It found no significant difference in the proportion of people who had a reduction of at least 50% in their agoraphobic symptoms after 68 weeks (44% with buspirone plus CBT v 68% with placebo plus CBT; absolute numbers of people not provided).

Harms: The RCTs did not report harms (see harms of buspirone under generalised anxiety disorder, p 150).

Comment: The first RCT used a flexible dosing regimen with maximum dose adjustment according to tolerance and therapeutic need.[24]

OPTION   BENZODIAZEPINES

One systematic review and one additional RCT have found that alprazolam reduces the number of panic attacks and improves symptoms compared with placebo. However, benzodiazepines are associated with a wide range of adverse effects, both during and after treatment.

Benefits: We found one systematic review (search date not reported, 27 RCTs, 2348 people; see benefits of tricyclic antidepressants, p 185 and selective serotonin reuptake inhibitors, p 186)[14] and one additional RCT.[15] The review found that alprazolam significantly increased the proportion of people judged to have improved compared with placebo ($P < 0.0001$; see comment below).[14] The additional RCT (181 people with panic disorder with or without agoraphobia) compared three treatments: oral alprazolam (maximum 10 mg/day; see comment below), oral imipramine (maximum 225 mg/day; see comment below), and placebo (see benefits of tricyclic antidepressants, p 185 and selective serotonin reuptake inhibitors, p 186).[15] It found that alprazolam was associated with fewer panic attacks after 8 months compared with placebo (results presented graphically; significance not calculated).

Mental health

Harms: The systematic review did not report harms.[14] Adverse effects associated with alprazolam include sedation, insomnia, memory lapses, nervousness, irritability, dry mouth, tremor, impaired coordination, constipation, urinary retention, altered libido, and altered appetite (see harms of benzodiazepines under generalised anxiety disorder, p 150).[15] We found one non-systematic review of the effects of benzodiazepines in anxiety disorder in people with a history of substance abuse or dependence.[26] The review reported that the mortality of long term benzodiazepine users was no higher than that of matched controls. It reported that the most pronounced adverse effects followed sudden withdrawal and included tinnitus, paraesthesia, vision disturbance, depersonalisation, seizures, withdrawal psychosis, and persistent discontinuation syndrome.

Comment: The review used improvement as an outcome measure without clearly defining this term.[14] The additional RCT used flexible dosing according to tolerance and therapeutic need.[15] Many RCTs of psychological and pharmacological treatments (even those not involving benzodiazepines) allowed people to receive small amounts of anxiolytic drugs during the study because benzodiazepine abuse is quite prevalent in people who suffer from panic disorder.

GLOSSARY

Cognitive behavioural therapy (CBT) Brief structured treatment using relaxation and exposure procedures, and aimed at changing dysfunctional beliefs and negative automatic thoughts (typically 20 sessions over 12–16 weeks).

REFERENCES

1. American Psychiatric Association. *Diagnostic and statistical manual of mental disorders*, 4th ed. Washington, DC: American Psychiatric Association, 1994.

2. World Health Organization. *The ICD-10 classification of mental and behavioural disorders.* Geneva: World Health Organization, 1992.

3. Robins LN, Regier DA, eds. *Psychiatric disorders in America: the epidemiologic catchment area study.* New York, NY: Free Press, 1991.

4. Weissman MM, Bland MB, Canino GJ, et al. The cross-national epidemiology of panic disorder. *Arch Gen Psychiatry* 1997;54:305–309.

5. Andrews G, Henderson S, Hall W. Prevalence, comorbidity, disability and service utilisation. Overview of the Australian National Mental Health Survey. *Br J Psychiatry* 2001;178:145–153.

6. Last CG, Barlow DH, O'Brien GT. Precipitants of agoraphobia: role of stressful life events. *Psychol Rep* 1984;54:567–570.

7. De Loof C, Zandbergen H, Lousberg T, et al. The role of life events in the onset of panic disorder. *Behav Res Ther* 1989;27:461–463.

8. Rapee RM, Mattick RP, Murrell E. Impact of life events on subjects with panic disorder and on comparison subjects. *Am J Psychiatry* 1990;147:640–644.

9. Hirschfeld RMA. Panic disorder: diagnosis, epidemiology and clinical course. *J Clin Psychiatry* 1996;57:3–8.

10. Andrews G, Creamer M, Crino R, et al. *The treatment of anxiety disorders.* Cambridge: Cambridge University Press, 1994.

11. Page AC, Andrews G. Do specific anxiety disorders show specific drug problems? *Aust N Z J Psychiatry* 1996;30:410–414.

12. Gorman JM, Coplan JD. Comorbidity of depression and panic disorder. *J Clin Psychiatry* 1996;57:34–41.

13. Tyrer P, Seivewright H, Simmonds S, et al. Prospective studies of cothymia (mixed anxiety-depression): how do they inform clinical practice? *Eur Arch Psychiatry Clin Neurosci* 2001;251:II53–II56.

14. Boyer W. Serotonin uptake inhibitors are superior to imipramine and alprazolam in alleviating panic attacks: a meta-analysis. *Int Clin Psychopharmacol* 1995;10:45–49. Search date not reported; primary sources Medline, Embase, Psychlit, and sponsoring agencies of two trials contacted for supplementary statistical information.

15. Curtis GC, Massana J, Udina C, et al. Maintenance drug therapy of panic disorder. *J Psychiatr Res* 1993;27:127–142.

16. Mavissakalian MR, Perel JM. Long-term maintenance and discontinuation of imipramine therapy in panic disorder with agoraphobia. *Arch Gen Psychiatry* 1999;56:821–827.

17. Barlow DH, Gorman J, Shear MK, et al. Cognitive-behavioral therapy, imipramine, or their combination for panic disorder: a randomized controlled trial. *JAMA* 2000;283:2529–2536.

18. Cassano GB, Toni C, Petracca A, et al. Adverse effects associated with the short-term treatment of panic disorder with imipramine, alprazolam or placebo. *Eur Neuropsychopharmacol* 1994;4:47–53.

19. Bakker A, van Balkom AJLM, Spinhoven P. SSRIs vs TCAs in the treatment of panic disorder: a meta-analysis. *Acta Psychiatr Scand* 2002;106:163–167. Search date 1999; primary sources Medline, Embase, PsychInfo, and hand searches of reference lists of articles obtained.

20. Otto M, Tuby K, Gould R, et al. An effect-size analysis of the relative efficacy and tolerability of serotonin selective reuptake inhibitors for panic disorder. *Am J Psychiatry* 2001;158:1989–1992. Search date not reported; primary sources Medline, Psychlit, and hand searches of references.

21. Lepola UM, Wade AG, Leinonen EV, et al. A controlled, prospective, 1-year trial of citalopram in the treatment of panic disorder. *J Clin Psychiatry* 1998;59:528–534.

22. Rapaport M, Wolkow R, Rubin A, et al. Sertraline treatment of panic disorder: results of a long term study. *Acta Psych Scand* 2001;104:289–298.

23. Kampman M, Keijsers GP, Hoogduin CA, et al. A randomized, double-blind, placebo-controlled study of the effects of adjunctive paroxetine in panic disorder patients unsuccessfully treated with cognitive-behavioral therapy alone. *J Clin Psychiatry* 2002;63:772–777.

24. Bouvard M, Mollard E, Guerin J, et al. Study and course of the psychological profile in 77 patients expressing panic disorder with agoraphobia after cognitive behaviour therapy with or without buspirone. *Psychother Psychosom* 1997;66:27–32.

25. Cottraux J, Note ID, Cungi C, et al. A controlled study of cognitive behaviour therapy with buspirone or placebo in panic disorder with agoraphobia. *Br J Psychiatry* 1995;167:635–641.

26. Posternak M, Mueller T. Assessing the risks and benefits of benzodiazepines for anxiety disorders in patients with a history of substance abuse or dependence. *Am J Addict* 2001;10:48–68.

Shailesh Kumar
Division of Psychiatry
Auckland Medical School
Auckland
New Zealand

Mark Oakley-Browne
Professor of Rural Psychiatry
Monash University
Gippsland, Victoria
Australia

Competing interests: SK was reimbursed by Eli-Lilly, the manufacturers of Prozac (fluoxetine), for attending several conferences. MOB has been paid by GlaxoSmithKline for contributing to educational sessions for general practitioners. The programme topic was "the recognition and management of generalised anxiety disorder". MOB has received reimbursement from Pfizer for attending a symposium.

INTERVENTIONS

Key Messages

- **Antidepressants (fluoxetine)** Limited evidence from one small RCT suggests that fluoxetine may improve postnatal depression at 4 and 1)2 weeks compared with placebo. The RCT had problems with recruitment and a high drop out rate, and it excluded breastfeeding women. We found no RCTs that satisfactorily compared fluoxetine versus psychological treatment.

- **Cognitive behavioural therapy (individual)** One RCT provided limited evidence that individual cognitive behavioural therapy and ideal standard care both improved depressive symptoms, but that there was no difference between the two interventions. Limited evidence from one RCT suggests that individual cognitive behavioural therapy may improve postnatal depression in the short term (immediately after treatment) compared with routine primary care. The RCT found no clear longer term benefits (9 months to 5 years post partum) from individual cognitive behavioural therapy in comparison with routine primary care, non-directive counselling, or psychodynamic therapy.

- **Interpersonal psychotherapy** One RCT found that interpersonal psychotherapy improved postnatal depression compared with waiting list controls at 12 weeks.

- **Non-directive counselling** Limited evidence from two RCTs suggests that in the short term (immediately after treatment) non-directive counselling may improve postnatal depression compared with routine primary care. The one RCT with follow up beyond 12 weeks found no clear longer term benefits (from 9 months to 5 years post partum) from non-directive counselling compared with routine primary care, individual cognitive behavioural therapy, or psychodynamic therapy.

Postnatal depression

- **Psychodynamic therapy** Limited evidence from one RCT suggests that psychodynamic therapy may improve postnatal depression in the short term (immediately after treatment) compared with routine primary care. The RCT found no clear longer term benefits (9 months to 5 years post partum) from psychodynamic therapy compared with routine primary care, non-directive counselling, or cognitive behavioural therapy.

- **Antidepressants other than fluoxetine** We found no RCTs on the effects of antidepressants in women with postnatal depression, and no RCTs that satisfactorily compared antidepressants other than fluoxetine versus psychological treatments.

- **Cognitive behavioural therapy (group)** One small RCT in women with a high level of depressive symptoms on screening found that group cognitive behavioural therapy improved symptoms at 6 months compared with routine primary care.

- **Hormones** Limited evidence from one small RCT in women with severe postnatal depression suggests that oestrogen treatment may improve postnatal depression at 3 and 6 months compared with placebo.

- **Light therapy** We found no RCTs evaluating light therapy.

- **Mother–infant interaction coaching** One small RCT found that mother–infant interaction coaching had no significant effect on maternal depression scores compared with usual treatment, but it improved maternal responsiveness to the infant within 10 weeks of starting treatment.

- **Psychoeducation with partner** One small RCT found that psychoeducation with partner reduced patients' depression scores and partners' psychiatric morbidity compared with psychoeducation without partner.

- **Telephone based peer support (mother to mother)** One small RCT found that telephone based peer support reduced depression scores after 8 weeks compared with usual treatment.

DEFINITION Postnatal depression (PND) is broadly defined as non-psychotic depression occurring during the first 6 months post partum. Puerperal mental disorders have only recently been categorised separately in psychiatric classifications, but both the International Classification of Diseases (ICD-10)[1] and the Diagnostic and Statistical Manual of mental disorders, fourth edition (DSM-IV) require certain qualifications to be met that limit their use: ICD-10 categorises mental disorders that occur post partum as puerperal but only if they cannot otherwise be classified, and DSM-IV allows "postpartum onset" to be specified for mood disorders starting within 4 weeks' post partum.[2] In clinical practice and research the broader definition above is often used, because whether or not PND is truly distinct from depression in general, depression in the postpartum period raises treatment issues for the nursing mother and has implications for the developing infant (see prognosis below). The symptoms are similar to symptoms of depression at other times of life, but in addition to low mood, sleep disturbance, change in appetite, diurnal variation in mood, poor concentration, and irritability, women with postnatal depression also experience guilt about their inability to look after their new baby. In many countries, health visitors screen for PND using the Edinburgh Postnatal Depression Scale (see glossary, p 203),[3,4] which elicits depressive symptoms.

INCIDENCE/ PREVALENCE	The prevalence of depression in women post partum is similar to that found in women generally. However, the incidence of depression in the first month after childbirth is three times the average monthly incidence in non-childbearing women.[5] Studies across different cultures have shown a consistent incidence of postnatal depression (10–15%),[6] with higher rates in teenage mothers. A meta-analysis of studies mainly based in the developed world found the incidence of postnatal depression to be 12–13%.[7]
AETIOLOGY/ RISK FACTORS	Three systematic reviews have identified the following risk factors for postnatal depression: past history of any psychopathology (including history of previous postnatal depression), low social support, poor marital relationship, and recent life events.[7–9]
PROGNOSIS	Most episodes of PND resolve spontaneously within 3–6 months,[10] but about one in four affected mothers are still depressed on the child's first birthday.[11] In the developed world, suicide is now the main cause of maternal deaths in the first year post partum,[12] but the suicide rate is lower at this time than in age matched non-postpartum women.[13] PND is also associated with reduced likelihood of secure attachment,[14] deficits in maternal–infant interactions,[15] and impaired cognitive and emotional development of the child, particularly in boys living in areas of socioeconomic deprivation.[15–17] These associations remain significant even after controlling for subsequent episodes of depression in the mother.
AIMS OF INTERVENTION	To improve symptoms, quality of life, mother–infant interaction, with minimal adverse effects on mother and child.
OUTCOMES	Symptom scores (e.g. the Edinburgh Postnatal Depression Scale[3,4]) and other scales used in studies of depression at other times in life (see depressive disorders, p 114) quality of life, mother–infant interaction (rated using questionnaires or observer rated videos), effect on marital/family relationship (rated using questionnaires), rates of suicide.
METHODS	*Clinical Evidence* search and appraisal May 2003. We searched Medline (1996 to date), Embase (1980 to date), the Cochrane Library 2003, Issue 2, and two independent critical appraisers appraised the results. We included only RCTs with a minimum of 6 weeks' follow up. We included non-blinded studies as it can be difficult to blind patients and assessors to psychological interventions.

QUESTION   What are the effects of treatments?

OPTION   ANTIDEPRESSANTS

Limited evidence from one small RCT suggests that fluoxetine may improve postnatal depression at 4 and 12 weeks compared with placebo. The RCT had problems with recruitment and a high drop out rate, and it excluded breastfeeding women. We found no RCTs that satisfactorily compared fluoxetine versus psychological treatment. We found no RCTs on the effects of other antidepressants in women with postnatal depression, and no RCTs that satisfactorily compared other antidepressants versus psychological treatments.

Benefits: We found three systematic reviews (search dates 1998,[18] 1999,[19] and 2000[20]). All three reviews found the same single RCT[21] (87 women recruited from community based screening, 51 with a major and 36 with a minor depressive episode defined by research diagnostic criteria[22]). This trial conducted a four way comparison: fluoxetine 20 mg plus one session (the assessment session) of cognitive behavioural counselling (see glossary, p 203), fluoxetine 20 mg plus six sessions of cognitive behavioural counselling, and placebo plus one session of cognitive behavioural counselling, placebo plus six sessions of cognitive behavioural counselling. Outcomes were assessed at 4 and 12 weeks using the Clinical Interview Schedule (revised),[23] the Edinburgh Postnatal Depression Scale (see glossary, p 203),[3,4] and the Hamilton Depression Scale,[24] using an intention to treat analysis. The trial had several weaknesses (see comment below). Fluoxetine significantly reduced depression scores measured as part of the revised Clinical Interview Schedule at 4 and 12 weeks compared with placebo (percentage difference of geometric mean scores between fluoxetine and placebo at 4 weeks: 37.1%, 95% CI 5.7% to 58.0%; at 12 weeks: 40.7%, 95% CI 10.9% to 60.6%). The trial did not report on infant outcomes.

Harms: **Effects on the infant:** The RCT excluded breastfeeding mothers and did not report on adverse effects on the infant.[21] We found some evidence of short term adverse effects in infants whose mothers were using antidepressants while breastfeeding.[25] A review of 95 case reports and small case series on the use of psychotropic medications during breastfeeding found one case of respiratory depression in a nursing infant whose mother was treated with doxepin, which resolved 24 hours after discontinuation of breastfeeding.[25] The review also identified 10 cases of adverse effects in 190 nursing infants whose mothers were treated with fluoxetine. Six infants had unconfirmed and unspecified adverse effects that resolved spontaneously. Three infants were reported to have colic. One infant had an episode of transient seizure-like activity at 3 weeks of age and episodes of unresponsiveness at 4 months of age, with one episode of peripheral cyanosis at 5.5 months of age. The results of neurological monitoring were within normal limits up to 1 year of age. The review found no adverse effects in the infants of breastfeeding mothers taking other tricyclic antidepressants. A review of three controlled follow up studies of antidepressants used during breastfeeding (79 infants) found no infant developmental abnormalities with tricyclics or sertraline.[26] We found no good evidence on long term risks to the developing child from maternal use of antidepressants. **Effects on the mother:** The RCT reported no suicides in the 12 week follow up period.[21] See harms of antidepressants in the chapter on depressive disorders, p 114.

Comment: The RCT had several weaknesses.[21] Most of the women who were approached (101/188 [54%]) refused to participate, most commonly because of reluctance to take antidepressants. A further 26/87 (30%) of the participants dropped out after randomisation.

However, the authors performed an appropriate intention to treat analysis. The design of the trial does not allow comparison between fluoxetine and cognitive behavioural counselling as all the women received one session of cognitive behavioural counselling.

OPTION   HORMONES

Limited evidence from one small RCT in women with severe postnatal depression suggests that oestrogen treatment may improve postnatal depression at 3 and 6 months compared with placebo.

Benefits: We found two systematic reviews (search dates 2000[20] and 2001[27]), both of which found the same single RCT[28] (61 women with major depression beginning within 3 months post partum who, at enrolment, were < 18 months post partum, recruited from outpatient clinics, general practitioners, and self referrals). Women were excluded if they were breastfeeding, had a medical history that would contraindicate oestrogen therapy, or had changed psycho-tropic medication in the previous 6 weeks. The RCT compared oestrogen treatment (oestradiol skin patches for 6 months plus additional dydrogesterone tablets for 12 days each month) versus placebo (patches and tablets). After 3 and 6 months, the women taking oestrogen had significantly lower Edinburgh Postnatal Depression Scale scores (see glossary, p 203) than those taking placebo (WMD at 3 months −3.20, 95% CI −5.97 to −0.43; at 6 months −4.38, 95% CI −1.89 to −6.87). The trial did not report on infant outcomes.

Harms: **Effects on the infant:** The RCT did not report on adverse effects on the infant.[28] **Effects on the mother:** Endometrial curettage at the end of treatment showed endometrial changes (details not reported) in three women in the treatment group, which had resolved by follow up at 9 months.[28] One woman in the oestrogen group, who had been admitted to a psychiatric ward soon after the start of the study because of her worsening mental state, committed suicide. However, her clinical consultant had stopped the oestrogen treatment soon after admission.

Comment: None.

OPTION   LIGHT THERAPY

We found no RCTs evaluating light therapy.

Benefits: We found one systematic review (search date 2000, no RCTs)[20] and no subsequent RCTs.

Harms: We found no good information on adverse effects of light therapy.

Comment: Case studies of two women with postnatal depression found a drop in depression scores with 4 weeks of daily light therapy.[29]

OPTION   NON-DIRECTIVE COUNSELLING

Limited evidence from two RCTs suggests that in the short term (immediately after treatment) non-directive counselling may improve postnatal depression compared with routine primary care. The one RCT

with follow up beyond 12 weeks found no clear longer term benefits (from 9 months to 5 years post partum) from non-directive counselling in comparison with routine primary care, individual cognitive behavioural therapy, or psychodynamic therapy.

Benefits: We found three systematic reviews (search dates 1997,[30] 2000,[20] and 2001[31]), all of which found the same single RCT.[32] We also found one subsequent RCT.[33,34] The RCT identified by all three reviews (55 women with depression defined by research diagnostic criteria,[21] recruited from the community up to 13 weeks' post partum) compared non-directive counselling, delivered by trained health visitors for 8 weeks, versus routine primary care.[32] The subsequent larger RCT (193 women with major depression [DSM-III-R][2] recruited from the community within 8 weeks' post partum) had several methodological flaws (see comment below). It compared non-directive counselling, psychodynamic therapy, individual cognitive behavioural therapy, and routine primary care conducted in the women's homes by trained therapists on a weekly basis from 8 to 18 weeks' post partum.[33,34] Outcomes, assessed at 4.5 months, 9 months, 18 months, and 5 years post partum were: the proportion of women with a diagnosis of depression, using the Structured Clinical Interview for DSM-III-R Diagnoses (SCID) adjusted for mean baseline SCID scores; depression scores, using the Edinburgh Postnatal Depression Scale (EPDS; see glossary, p 203); at 4.5 months: mother–infant interactions, using rated videotapes; maternal management of the infant and problems in mother and infant relationship, both using a checklist; at 18 months: infant emotional and behavioural problems using a modified Behavioural Screening Questionnaire with maternal reports, infant attachment using Ainsworth Strange Situation Procedure and infant cognitive development using the Mental Development Index of the Bayley Scales of Infant Development; at 5 years: child emotional and behavioural difficulties, using maternal reports on the Rutter A[2] Scale and teacher reports using the Preschool Behaviour Checklist; and child cognitive development, using the McCarthy Scales. **Versus routine primary care:** The first, smaller RCT found that after an average of 5 weeks' treatment, non-directive counselling significantly reduced the number of women who were categorised as depressed compared with routine primary care (69% with non-directive counselling v 38% with routine primary care; difference 31.7%, 95% CI 5% to 58%; P = 0.03).[32] The subsequent, larger RCT found that, immediately after treatment (at 4.5 months' post partum), non-directive counselling increased (though not significantly) the proportion of women without depression compared with routine primary care (26/48 [54%] with non-directive counselling v 20/50 [40%] with routine primary care; RR 1.38, 95% CI 0.82 to 1.89).[33,34] It also found that non-directive counselling significantly reduced depression scores compared with routine primary care (mean EPDS score adjusted for mean centred baseline EPDS scores: 9.9 with non-directive counselling v 11.3 with routine primary care; treatment effect for non-directive counselling: –2.1, 95% CI –3.8 to –0.3; P = 0.02). It also found that non-directive counselling significantly reduced the proportion of women with mother–infant relationship difficulties compared with routine primary care (proportion of women reporting problems, adjusted for relationship problems prior to treatment: 53% [23/43] with non-directive counselling v 74% [26/35] with routine primary care; RR 0.63, 95% CI 0.32 to 0.97). After controlling for baseline differences between groups, there were no significant differences between non-directive counselling and routine primary care in terms of behavioural management problems (P = 0.77), nor in terms of maternal sensitivity in mother–infant interactions (P = 0.14), except for women with high social adversity, among whom non-directive counselling significantly improved maternal sensitivity (P = 0.04). In the longer term (at 9 months, 18 months, and 5 years post partum), there were no significant differences in any outcomes except for some evidence that non-directive coun- selling improved infant emotional and behavioural problems com- pared with routine primary care at 18 months post partum (P = 0.001). However, this outcome relied solely on maternal reports (see comment below). **Versus cognitive behavioural therapy (individual):** The RCT[33,34] found no significant difference between non-directive counselling and individual cognitive behav- ioural therapy for any outcomes immediately after treatment or in the longer term. There was some evidence that non-directive counselling improved infant emotional and behavioural problems compared with cognitive behavioural therapy at 18 months post partum. However, this outcome relied solely on maternal reports (see comment below). **Versus psychodynamic therapy:** The RCT[33,34] found no significant difference between non-directive counselling and psychodynamic therapy for any outcomes immedi- ately after treatment or in the longer term. There was some evidence that non-directive counselling improved infant emotional and behavioural problems compared with psychodynamic therapy at 18 months post partum. However, this outcome relied solely on maternal reports (see comment below). **Versus antidepressants:** We found no RCTs comparing non-directive counselling versus antidepressants.

Harms: None reported.

Comment: The subsequent, larger RCT[33,34] had several methodological flaws. It was underpowered to detect differences between treatment groups and there was no adjustment for multiple comparisons. More women in the routine primary care group had experienced social adversity compared with the treatment groups (35% in the routine primary care group v 30% in the non-directive counselling group v 24% in the cognitive behavioural therapy group v 10% in psychodynamic therapy group) and this was not controlled for in some analyses. Ten per cent of the women who were randomised did not complete the trial. More women dropped out of the non-directive counselling and psychodynamic therapy groups (6 from the non-directive counselling group v 8 from the psychody- namic therapy group v 1 from the cognitive therapy group v 4 from the routine primary care group). Reasons for non-completion were not investigated and the authors did not perform an intention to treat analysis. Women who did not complete therapy were younger

(P = 0.004) and more likely to be single or separated (P = 0.05). The infant outcomes which showed a beneficial effect of treatment (i.e. fewer mother–infant relationship problems at 4.5 months and fewer emotional and behavioural problems at 18 months) relied solely on maternal reports.

| OPTION | COGNITIVE BEHAVIOURAL THERAPY (INDIVIDUAL) |

One RCT provided limited evidence that individual cognitive behavioural therapy and ideal standard care both improved depressive symptoms, but that there was no difference between the two interventions. Limited evidence from one RCT suggests that individual cognitive behavioural therapy may improve postnatal depression in the short term (immediately after treatment) compared with routine primary care. The RCT found no clear longer term benefits (9 months to 5 years post partum) from individual cognitive behavioural therapy in comparison with routine primary care, non-directive counselling, or psychodynamic therapy.

Benefits: We found no systematic review. We found two RCTs.[33–35] The first RCT (37 women, 32% major depression, 68% minor, recruited from the community) compared modified cognitive behavioural therapy (CBT) delivered by specifically trained early childhood nurses once a week for 6 weeks versus ideal standard care (weekly 20–60 minute appointments for mothercraft advice and non-specific support delivered by early childhood nurses who had not received specific training).[35] For a description of the second RCT and a comment on its methodology see non-directive counselling, p 196.[33,34] **Versus ideal standard care:** The first RCT found that individual CBT and ideal standard care were both effective in improving depressive symptoms immediately and at 6 months post-treatment but there was no significant difference between the two interventions (Edinburgh Postnatal Depression [EPDS; see glossary, p 203] mean score: 15.9 pretreatment CBT group v 13.7 with ideal standard care, P = 0.03; 8.1 post intervention CBT v 6.5 with ideal standard care, P value not reported, reported as not significant; 6.2 at 6 months with CBT v 7.7 with ideal standard care, P value not reported, reported as not significant).[35] (See comment below.) **Versus routine primary care:** The second RCT found that immediately after treatment (at 4.5 months post partum), individual CBT increased (though not significantly) the proportion of women without depression compared with routine primary care (57% [24/42] with CBT v 40% [20/50] with routine primary care; RR 1.50, 95% CI 0.92 to 1.98).[33,34] It also found that individual CBT significantly reduced depression scores compared with routine primary care (mean EPDS score: 9.2 with CBT v 11.3 with routine primary care; treatment effect for CBT –2.7, 95% CI –4.5 to –0.9; P = 0.003). It also found that individual CBT significantly reduced the proportion of women with mother–infant relationship difficulties compared with routine primary care (proportion of women reporting problems, adjusted for relationship problems prior to treatment: 39% [16/41] with CBT v 74% [26/35] with routine primary care; RR 0.46, 95% CI 0.2 to 0.81).[33,34] After controlling for baseline differences between groups, there were no significant differences between CBT and routine primary care in terms of behavioural management problems (P = 0.60), nor in terms of mother infant interactions (results presented graphically; P value not reported). In the medium to longer term (at 9 months, 18 months, and 5 years post partum), there were no significant differences in any outcome, except for infant emotional and behavioural problems, for which CBT achieved significant improvement at 18 months post partum compared with routine primary care (P = 0.06). However, this outcome relied solely on maternal reports (see comment under non-directive counselling, p 197). **Versus non-directive counselling:** See benefits of non-directive counselling, p 196. **Versus psychodynamic therapy:** The second RCT found no significant difference between CBT and psychodynamic counselling for any outcomes.[33,34] **Versus antidepressants:** We found no satisfactory RCTs comparing CBT versus antidepressants.

Harms: None reported.

Comment: The first RCT was probably underpowered to compare modified CBT versus ideal standard care effectively. There was a trend towards CBT being more effective. Adjusting for baseline EPDS (which was higher in the CBT group) in a multivariate analysis had no impact on results at any time point.[35] For a comment on the methodology of the second RCT, see comment under non-directive counselling, p 197.[33,34]

OPTION   COGNITIVE BEHAVIOURAL THERAPY (GROUP)

One small RCT in women with a high level of depressive symptoms on screening found that group cognitive behavioural therapy improved symptoms at 6 months compared with routine primary care.

Benefits: We found no systematic review but found one RCT (45 women < 1 year post partum, recruited from the community with the Edinburgh Postnatal Depression Scale [EPDS; see glossary, p 203] > 12 but no confirmation of diagnosis of postnatal depression by diagnostic interview, block randomised).[36] The RCT compared group cognitive behavioural therapy including education and relaxation, given by two health visitors for 2 hours each week for 8 weeks, versus routine primary care. At 6 months, group cognitive therapy significantly improved depression scores (proportion of women scoring < 13 on the EPDS: 65% [15/23] with group cognitive therapy v 36% [8/22] with routine primary care; P = 0.05). The RCT did not report on outcomes in infants.

Harms: None reported.

Comment: The RCT's criteria for inclusion (EPDS > 12) and response to treatment (EPDS < 13) meant that a small change in EPDS would count as a response to treatment.

OPTION   PSYCHOEDUCATION WITH PARTNER

One small RCT found that psychoeducation with partner reduced patients' depression scores and partners' psychiatric morbidity compared with psychoeducation without partner.

Postnatal depression

Benefits: We found one systematic review[20] (search date 2000, 1 RCT,[37] 29 women < 12 months post partum, referred to hospital with major depression of postpartum onset). All women in the RCT attended seven clinic visits for assessment of mood, adjustment of medication and psychoeducation. The women in the intervention group brought their partners to four of the visits. The RCT found significantly lower depression scores in the group attending with their partners at 10 weeks' follow up (mean Edinburgh Postnatal Depression Scale [EPDS; see glossary, p 203] 8.6 with partner v 14.7 without partner; P = 0.01). It also found significantly lower psychological morbidity in partners who attended clinics (mean General Health Questionnaire score 18.4 in partners who attended v 43 in the control group; P = 0.01). The RCT did not report on outcomes in infants.

Harms: None reported

Comment: Women taking psychotropic medication were included and no adjustment was made for any potential confounding effect of medication.

OPTION **INTERPERSONAL PSYCHOTHERAPY**

One RCT found that interpersonal psychotherapy improved postnatal depression compared with waiting list controls at 12 weeks.

Benefits: We found one systematic review (search date 2000, 1 RCT).[20] The RCT[38] (120 women recruited from the community with major depression [DSM-IV criteria and > 11 on the Hamilton Depression Rating Scale; HDRS],[24] for an average duration of 7 months) found that interpersonal psychotherapy, performed by experienced psychotherapists for 1 hour once a week for 12 weeks, significantly increased the proportion of women recovering from depression compared with remaining on a waiting list (proportion of women recovering, defined as HDRS < 7: 31% [19/60] with interpersonal psychotherapy v 15% [9/60] with control; RR 2.11, 95% CI 1.04 to 4.28). There were also significant improvements in social adjustments (mean score on the Social Adjustment Scale — Self Report (SAS-SR[39]): 1.93 with interpersonal psychotherapy v 2.35 with waiting list control; P < 0.001). Subscales of the SAS-SR showed significant improvements in relationship with spouse (P < 0.001), relationship with children older than 2 years (P < 0.05), relationship with immediate family (P = 0.002), and relationship with friends (P = 0.003; absolute numbers not reported). The Postpartum Adjustment Questionnaire[40] also showed a significant effect of interpersonal psychotherapy (mean reduction 0.30 with interpersonal psychotherapy v 0.12 with waiting list control; P = 0.001). There were no significant differences between groups for the Dyadic Adjustment Scale, a specific measure of adjustment in relationship with partner.[41] The RCT did not report on outcomes in infants.

Harms: No harms reported.

Comment: The RCT had problems with recruitment (132 women declined to participate) but achieved an 80% follow up (withdrawal rate 20% in the treatment group v 15% among controls; P = 0.47). There were no significant clinical or demographic differences between women who dropped out and women who stayed in the study.

Limited evidence from one RCT suggests that psychodynamic therapy may improve postnatal depression in the short term (immediately after treatment) compared with routine primary care. The RCT found no clear longer term benefits (9 months to 5 years post partum) from psychodynamic therapy compared with routine primary care, non-directive counselling, or cognitive behavioural therapy.

Benefits: We found no systematic review but found one RCT (193 women with major depression [DSM-III-R][2] recruited from the community within 8 weeks post partum).[33,34] For a description of the RCT and a comment on its methodological flaws, see non-directive counselling, p 196. **Versus routine primary care:** The RCT found that immediately after therapy (at 4.5 months post partum), psychodynamic therapy significantly increased the proportion of women without depression compared with routine primary care (71% [32/45] with psychodynamic therapy v 40% [20/50] with routine primary care; RR 1.89, 95% CI 1.33 to 2.33).[33,34] It also found that psychodynamic therapy significantly reduced depression scores compared with routine primary care (mean Edinburgh Postnatal Depression Scores [EPDS; see glossary, p 203]: 8.9 with psychodynamic therapy v 11.3 with routine primary care; treatment effect for psychodynamic therapy −2.6, 95% CI −4.4 to −0.9; P = 0.003). It also found that psychodynamic therapy significantly reduced the proportion of women with mother–infant relationship difficulties compared with routine primary care (proportion of women reporting problems, adjusted for relationship problems prior to treatment: 47% [20/43] with psychodynamic therapy v 74% [26/35] with routine primary care; RR 0.57, 95% CI 0.28 to 0.92). After controlling for baseline differences between groups, there were no significant differences between psychodynamic therapy and routine primary care in behavioural management problems or mother–infant interactions. In the longer term (at 9 months, 18 months, and 5 years post partum), there were no significant differences for any outcomes except for infant emotional and behavioural problems, for which psychodynamic therapy achieved significant improvement at 18 months post partum (P = 0.03) compared with routine primary care. However, this outcome relied solely on maternal reports (see comment under non-directive counselling, p 197). **Versus non-directive counselling:** See benefits of non-directive counselling, p 196. **Versus cognitive behavioural therapy:** See benefits of cognitive behavioural therapy (individual), p 198 and cognitive behavioural therpay (group), p 199. **Versus antidepressants:** We found no satisfactory RCTs comparing psychodynamic therapy versus antidepressants.

Harms: None reported.

Comment: For comments on the RCT's methodology see comment under non-directive counselling, p 197.[33,34]

Postnatal depression

| OPTION | MOTHER–INFANT INTERACTION COACHING |

One small RCT found that mother–infant interaction coaching had no significant effect on maternal depression scores compared with usual treatment, but it improved maternal responsiveness to the infant within 10 weeks of starting treatment.

Benefits: We found no systematic review but found one RCT (122 women recruited from the community with Edinburgh Postnatal Depression Scale see glossary, p 203] > 10 at 4–8 weeks post partum).[42] This compared interaction coaching (see glossary, p 203) using a variable number of 15 minute sessions depending on the needs of the mother and infant, versus treatment as usual. After 6 to 10 weeks there was no significant difference in depression scores between treatment and control groups. However, there was a significant difference in maternal responsiveness in Dyadic Mutuality Code scores,[43,44] based on videotaped mother–infant interactions rated by a researcher blind to randomisation status (mean score at 6 weeks: 9.73 with interaction coaching v 8.77 with usual treatment; $P = 0.02$; mean at 10 weeks: 9.55 with interaction coaching v 8.80 with usual treatment; $P = 0.03$). Baseline scores were not significantly different in the two groups. The RCT did not investigate infant outcomes.

Harms: None reported.

Comment: Additional psychiatric treatment for depression was given to women if required.

| OPTION | TELEPHONE BASED PEER SUPPORT (MOTHER TO MOTHER) |

One small RCT found that telephone based peer support reduced depression scores after 8 weeks compared with usual treatment.

Benefits: We found no systematic review but found one RCT (42 women recruited from the community identifed as high risk for postnatal depression with Edinburgh Postnatal Depression Scale [EPDS see glossary, p 203] > 9 at 8 weeks' post partum) comparing individually tailored mother to mother telephone based support, using trained lay volunteers with a personal history of postnatal depression, versus treatment as usual.[45] It found that telephone support significantly reduced depression scores after 8 weeks compared with usual care (proportion of women with EPDS > 12: 15% [3/20] with telephone support v 52% [11/21] with usual care; OR 6.23, 95% CI 1.40 to 27.8; $P = 0.01$). The RCT did not investigate infant outcomes.

Harms: None reported.

Comment: The acceptance rate for enrolment into the trial was 67%. Over a third of peer volunteers (38%) referred a mother to a professional health service and this was not controlled for in the analysis.

GLOSSARY

Cognitive behavioural counselling is derived from cognitive behavioural therapy and designed to be delivered by professionals such as health visitors who are not specialists in mental health. It is sometimes known as CREST because it incorporates child care advice, reassurance, enjoyment, support from others, and targets.

Interaction coaching for at-risk parents and their infants is a six key element intervention strategy designed to strengthen the early parent–infant relationship.

The Edinburgh Postnatal Depression Scale (EPDS) was designed as a screening questionnaire to identify possible depression in a clinical or research setting. The EPDS has a high sensitivity (95%) and specificity (93%) for postnatal depression[3,4] and is used by many health visitors and in many clinical research studies of postnatal depression.

REFERENCES

1. World Health Organisation. *Tenth Revision of the International Classification of Diseases and Related Health Problems. Clinical Descriptions and Diagnostic Guidelines*. Geneva: WHO, 1992.

2. American Psychiatric Association. *Diagnostic and Statistical Manual of Mental Disorders, fourth edition*. New York: American Psychiatric Association, 1994.

3. Murray L, Carothers AD. The validation of the Edinburgh Post-natal Depression Scale on a community sample. *Br J Psychiatry* 1990;157:288–290.

4. Cox JL, Holden JM, Sagovsky R. Detection of postnatal depression. Development of the 10-item Edinburgh Postnatal Depression Scale. *Br J Psychiatry* 1987;150:782–786.

5. Cox JL, Murray D, Chapman G. A controlled study of the onset, duration and prevalence of postnatal depression. *Br J Psychiatry* 1993;163:27–31.

6. Kumar R. Postnatal mental illness: a transcultural perspective. *Soc Psychiatry Psychiatr Epidemiol* 1994;29:250–264.

7. O'Hara MW, Swain AM. Rates and risks of postpartum depression: a meta-analysis. *Int Rev Psychiatry* 1996;8:37–54.

8. Beck CT. A meta-analysis of predictors of postpartum depression. *Nurs Res* 1996;45:297–303.

9. Wilson LM, Reid AJ, Midmer DK, et al. Antenatal psychosocial risk factors associated with adverse postnatal family outcomes. *CMAJ* 1996;154:785–799.

10. Cooper PJ, Murray L. Course and recurrence of postnatal depression. Evidence for the specificity of the diagnostic concept. *Br J Psychiatry* 1995;166:191–195.

11. Kumar R, Robson KM. A prospective study of emotional disorders in childbearing women. *Br J Psychiatry* 1984;144:35–47.

12. *The fifth report of the Confidential Enquiries into Maternal Deaths in the United Kingdom*. London: Royal College of Obstetricians and Gynaecologists, 2001.

13. Appleby L. Suicide during pregnancy and in the first postnatal year. *BMJ* 1991;302:137–140.

14. Martins C, Gaffan EA. Effects of early maternal depression on patterns of infant-mother attachment: a meta-analytic investigation. *J Child Psychol Psychiatry* 2000;41:737–746.

15. Murray L, Cooper PJ. The impact of postpartum depression on child development. *Int Rev Psychiatry* 1996;8:55–63.

16. Carter AS, Garrity-Rokous EF, Chazan-Cohen R, et al. Maternal depression and comorbidity: Predicting early parenting, attachment security, and toddler social-emotional problems and competencies. *J Am Acad Child Adolesc Psychiatry* 2001;40:18–26.

17. Hay DF, Pawlby S, Sharp D, et al. Intellectual problems shown by 11-year-old children whose mothers had postnatal depression. *J Child Psychol Psychiatry* 2001;42:871–889.

18. Mulrow C, Williams J, Trivedi M, et al. Treatment of depression — newer pharmacotherapies. *Psychopharm Bull* 1998;34:409–795. Search date 1998.

19. Hoffbrand S, Howard LM, Crawley H. Antidepressant drug treatment for postnatal depression. In: The Cochrane Library, Issue 2, 2001. Oxford: Update Software. Search date 1999; primary sources the Cochrane Depression, Anxiety and Neurosis Group's Specialised Register of Controlled Trials, Cochrane Library Controlled Trials Register, Cochrane Pregnancy and Childbirth Group's Specialised Register, Medline, Science Citation Index, MIDIRS Midwifery Database, UK National Research Register, HSRProj, Current Controlled Trials website, search of reference lists and book bibliographies, and contact with pharmaceutical companies, experts and organisations.

20. Boath E, Henshaw C. The treatment of postnatal depression: a comprehensive literature overview. *J Reprod Infant Psychol* 2001;19:215–248. Search date 2000; primary sources Medline, PsychLit, Sociofile, CINAHL, COPAC, published books held by BL, hand search, reference checking and search of Marce Society conference proceedings and abstracts.

21. Appleby L, Warner R, Whitton A, et al. A controlled study of fluoxetine and cognitive-behavioural counselling in the treatment of postnatal depression. *BMJ* 1997;314:932–936.

22. Spitzer RL, Endicott J, Robins E. Research diagnostic criteria: rationale and reliability. *Arch Gen Psychiatry* 1978;35:773–782.

23. Lewis G, Pelosi AJ, Arya R, et al. Measuring psychiatric disorder in the community: a standardised assessment for use by lay interviewers. *Psychol Med* 1992;22:465–486.

24. Hamilton M. Hamilton depression scale. In: Guy W, ed. *ECDEU assessment manual for psychopharmacology, revised edition*. Rockville MD: U.S. National Institute of Mental Health Psychopharmacology Research Branch, 1976:179–192.

25. Burt VK, Suri R, Altshuler L, et al. The use of psychotropic medications during breast-feeding. *Am J Psychiat* 2001;158:1001–1009.

26. Austin M, Mitchell P. Use of psychotropic medications in breastfeeding women: acute and prophylactic treatment. *Aust N Z J Psychiatry* 1998;32:778–784.

27. Lawrie TA, Herxheimer A, Dalton K. Oestrogens and progestogens for preventing and treating postnatal depression. In: The Cochrane Library, Issue 2, 2003. Oxford: Update Software. Search date 2001; primary sources Cochrane Pregnancy and Childbirth Group's Specialised Register of Controlled Trials, Cochrane Controlled Trials Register, reference list check.

28. Gregoire AJP, Kumar R, Everitt B, et al. Transdermal oestrogen for treatment of severe postnatal depression. *Lancet* 1996;347:930–933.

29. Corral M, Kuan A, Kostaras D. Bright light therapy's effect on postpartum depression. *Am J Psychiatry* 2000;157:303–304.

30. Elkan R, Kendrick D, Hewitt M, et al. The effectiveness of domiciliary health visiting: a systematic review of international studies and a selective review of the British literature. *Health Technol Assess* 2000;4:1–339. Search date 1997; primary sources Medline, CINAHL, EMBASE, the internet, the Cochrane Library, index to theses, hand search of *Health Visitor*, reference list check, and contact with key individuals and organisations.

31. Ray KL, Hodnett ED. Caregiver support for postpartum depression. In: The Cochrane Library, Issue 2, 2003. Oxford: Update Software. Search date 2001; primary source Cochrane Pregnancy and Childbirth Group trials register.]

32. Holden JM, Sagovsky R, Crawley H. Counselling in a general practice setting: controlled study of health visitor intervention in treatment of postnatal depression. *BMJ* 1989;298:223–226.

33. Cooper PJ, Murray L, Wilson A, et al. Controlled trial of the short and long-term effect of psychological treatment of postpartum depression. I. Impact on maternal mood. *Br J Psychiatry* 2003;182:412–419.

34. Murray L, Cooper PJ, Wilson A, et al. Controlled trial of the short and long-term effect of psychological treatment of postpartum depression: 2: Impact on the mother–child relationship and child outcome. *Br J Psychiatry* 2003;182:420–427.

35. Prendergast J, Austin M-P. Early childhood nurse-delivered cognitive behavioural counselling for postnatal depression. *Australasian Psychiatry* 2001;9:255–259.

36. Honey K, Bennet P, Morgan M. A brief psycho-educational group intervention for postnatal depression. *Br J Clin Psychol* 2002;41:405–409.

37. Misri S, Kostaras X, Fox D, et al. The impact of partner support in the treatment of postnatal depression. *Can J Psychiatry* 2000;45:554–558.

38. O'Hara MW, Stuart S, Gorman, L, et al. Efficacy of interpersonal psychotherapy for postpartum depression. *Arch Gen Psychiatry* 2000;57:1039–1045.

39. Weissman MM, Bothwell S. Assessment of social adjustment by patient self-report. *Arch Gen Psychiatry* 1976;33:1111–1115.

40. O'Hara MW, Hoffman JG, Phillips LHC, et al. Adjustment in childbearing women: the Postpartum Adjustment Questionnaire. *Psychol Assessment* 1992;4:160–169.

41. Spanier GB. Measuring dyadic adjustment: new scales for assessing the quality of marriage and similar dyads. *J Marriage Family* 1976;38:15–28.

42. Horowitz JA, Bell M, Trybulski J, et al. Promoting responsiveness between mothers with depressive symptoms and their infants. *J Nurs Scholarsh* 2001;33:323–329.

43. Censullo M, Bowler R, Lester B, et al. Development of an instrument to measure infant–adult synchrony. *Nurs Res* 1987;36:244–248.

44. Censullo M. *Dyadic mutuality code manual*. Wellesley MA: Wellesley College Center for Research on Women, 1991.

45. Dennis C. The effect of peer support on postpartum depression: a pilot randomized controlled trial. *Can J Psychiatry* 2003;48:115–124.

Louise Howard
Senior Lecturer
Health Services Research Department
Institute of Psychiatry
London
UK

Competing interests: None declared.

QUESTIONS

INTERVENTIONS

Key Messages

Prevention

- The evidence about the effects of interventions in preventing post-traumatic stress disorder is generally inconclusive.

- **Multiple session cognitive behavioural therapy in people with acute stress disorder** Two small RCTs in people with acute stress disorder after a traumatic event (accident or non-sexual assault) found that five sessions of cognitive behavioural therapy reduced the proportion of people with post-traumatic stress disorder after 6 months compared with supportive counselling.

Post-traumatic stress disorder

- **Hydrocortisone** One small RCT in people in intensive care with septic shock provided insufficient evidence to assess hydrocortisone in preventing post-traumatic stress disorder.

- **Multiple session cognitive behavioural therapy in all people exposed to a traumatic event** One RCT in bus drivers who had been attacked in the past 5 months found that cognitive behavioural therapy improved measures of anxiety and intrusive symptoms at 6 months compared with standard care. It found no significant difference in measures of depression or avoidance symptoms. Another RCT provided insufficient evidence to assess cognitive behavioural therapy plus educational techniques in preventing post-traumatic stress disorder in road traffic accident survivors. A third small RCT provided insufficient evidence to compare memory structuring versus supportive listening in road traffic accident survivors.

- **Multiple session education** One RCT provided insufficient evidence to assess educational techniques plus cognitive behavioural therapy in preventing post-traumatic stress disorder in road traffic accident survivors.

- **Multiple session trauma support** Two RCTs provided insufficient evidence to assess collaborative care interventions involving emotional, social, and practical support in people exposed to a traumatic event in the past 1 day to 1 week.

- **Propranolol** One small RCT provided insufficient evidence to assess propranolol in preventing post-traumatic stress disorder in people with early symptoms of post-traumatic stress disorder after a traumatic event.

- **Temazepam** One small RCT provided insufficient evidence to assess temazepam in preventing post-traumatic stress disorder in people with acute stress disorder or early symptoms of post-traumatic stress disorder after road traffic accident, industrial accident, or non-sexual assault.

- **Single session psychological interventions ("debriefing") in all people exposed to a traumatic event** RCTs in people who had been exposed to a traumatic event in the previous month found no significant difference between a single session of psychological debriefing and no debriefing in the incidence of post-traumatic stress disorder at 3 months or 1 year. One RCT found that debriefing within 10 hours reduced post-traumatic stress disorder compared with debriefing after 48 hours.

Treatment

- **Cognitive behavioural therapy** RCTs have found that cognitive behavioural therapy improves post-traumatic stress disorder symptoms, anxiety, and depression immediately after treatment and at up to 1 year compared with no treatment or supportive counselling.

- **Eye movement desensitisation and reprocessing** RCTs have found that eye movement desensitisation and reprocessing improves symptoms compared with no treatment. RCTs have found no significant difference in symptoms between eye movement desensitisation and reprocessing and cognitive behavioural therapy.

- **Paroxetine** One systematic review and subsequent RCTs found that paroxetine reduced symptoms at 3 months compared with placebo.

- **Sertraline** RCTs found that sertraline reduced symptoms at 3–7 months compared with placebo.

- **Fluoxetine** Two RCTs found that fluoxetine may reduce symptoms at 3 months compared with placebo.

■ **Affect management; benzodiazepines; carbamazepine, drama therapy; eclectic psychotherapy; group therapy; hypnotherapy; inpatient programmes; interapy; lamotrigine; mirtazapine; monoamine oxidase inhibitors (brofaromine, phenelzine); nefazodone; propranolol; psychodynamic psychotherapy; risperidone; supportive counselling; tricyclic antidepressants (amitriptyline, imipramine)** We found insufficient evidence about the effects of these interventions in improving symptoms.

DEFINITION	**Post-traumatic stress disorder (PTSD)** can occur after any major traumatic event. Symptoms include upsetting thoughts and nightmares about the traumatic event, avoidance behaviour, numbing of general responsiveness, increased irritability, and hypervigilance.[1] To fulfil the *Diagnostic and statistical manual of mental disorders* (DSM-IV) criteria for PTSD, an individual must have been exposed to a traumatic event, have at least one re-experiencing, three avoidance and two hyperarousal phenomena, have had the symptoms for at least 1 month, and the symptoms must cause clinically important distress or reduced day to day functioning.[1] People with **sub-syndromal PTSD** have all the criteria for PTSD except one of the re-experiencing, avoidance, or hyperarousal phenomena. **Acute stress disorder** occurs within the first month after a major traumatic event and requires the presence of symptoms for at least 2 days. It is similar to PTSD but dissociative symptoms (see glossary, p 221) are required to make the diagnosis.
INCIDENCE/ PREVALENCE	One large cross-sectional study in the USA found that 1/10 women and 1/20 men experience PTSD at some stage in their lives.[2]
AETIOLOGY/ RISK FACTORS	Risk factors include major trauma, such as rape, a history of psychiatric disorders, acute distress and depression after the trauma, lack of social support, and personality factors.[3]
PROGNOSIS	One large cross-sectional study in the USA found that over a third of sufferers continued to satisfy the criteria for a diagnosis of PTSD 6 years after diagnosis.[2] However, cross-sectional studies provide weak evidence about prognosis.
AIMS OF INTERVENTION	To reduce initial distress after a traumatic event; to prevent PTSD and other psychiatric disorders; to reduce levels of distress in the long term; to improve function and quality of life.
OUTCOMES	Presence or absence of PTSD and severity of symptoms assessed by continuous measures. Continuous measures for assessing changes in symptoms include Impact of Event Scale, Post-traumatic Stress Diagnostic Scale (range 0–51), Clinician Administered PTSD Scale, Trauma Symptom Checklist 40 (range 0–160), Post-Traumatic Stress Disorder Checklist, and Clinical Global Impression Scale (a composite measure of symptoms and everyday functioning). Symptoms assessed include anxiety, depression, intrusion, and avoidance. Changes in continuous measures are often expressed as effect sizes. It is difficult to interpret effect sizes in terms of clinical importance rather than statistical significance. Some categorise effect sizes of less than 0.5 as small, 0.5–0.8 as medium, and greater than 0.8 as large.
METHODS	*Clinical Evidence* search and appraisal May 2003. The prevention question includes RCTs on any intervention commenced within 1 month of a traumatic event.

Post-traumatic stress disorder

OPTION SINGLE SESSION DEBRIEFING

RCTs in people who had been exposed to a traumatic event in the past month found no significant difference between a single debriefing session and no debriefing in the incidence of post-traumatic stress disorder at 3 months or 1 year. One RCT found that debriefing within 10 hours reduced post-traumatic stress disorder compared with debriefing after 48 hours.

Benefits: We found one systematic review (search date 2001, 11 RCTs, 1759 people)[4] and one subsequent RCT[5] comparing early (within 1 month) single session interventions ("debriefing") versus no intervention. The RCTs in the review used psychological debriefing (see glossary, p 221) or similar techniques after traumatic events. The review found no significant difference between debriefing and no debriefing in the risk of post-traumatic stress disorder at 3 months and 1 year, although the risk of post-traumatic stress disorder was higher in people receiving debriefing (OR at 3 months 1.1, 95% CI 0.6 to 2.5; OR at 12 months 2.0, 95% CI 0.9 to 4.5).[4] The subsequent RCT (77 people who had been robbed) compared early group debriefing (within 10 hours) versus delayed group debriefing (after > 48 hours).[5] It found that early debriefing significantly reduced symptom severity measured on the Post-traumatic Stress Diagnostic Scale at 2 weeks compared with delayed debriefing (mean score 6.94 with early debriefing v 33.10 with delayed debriefing; P < 0.001).

Harms: Two RCTs included in the systematic review found an increased risk of subsequent psychological problems in people receiving the intervention.[4] However, initial traumatic exposure had been higher in these people.

Comment: The systematic review of single session debriefing found that the overall quality of RCTs was poor.[4] Problems included lack of blinding, failure to state loss to follow up, and lack of intention to treat analysis despite high withdrawal rates.

OPTION MULTIPLE SESSION COGNITIVE BEHAVIOURAL THERAPY

We found no systematic review or RCT comparing cognitive behavioural therapy alone versus no treatment. One RCT provided insufficient evidence to assess cognitive behavioural therapy plus educational techniques in preventing post-traumatic stress disorder in road traffic accident survivors. One RCT in bus drivers who had been attacked in the past 5 months found that cognitive behavioural therapy improved measures of anxiety and intrusive symptoms at 6 months compared with standard care, but found no significant difference in measures of depression or avoidance symptoms. Another small RCT provided insufficient evidence to compare memory structuring versus supportive listening in road traffic accident survivors. Two RCTs in people with acute stress disorder after a traumatic event (road traffic accident or

non-sexual assault) found that five sessions of either cognitive behavioural therapy or prolonged exposure reduced the proportion of people with post-traumatic stress disorder after 6 months compared with supportive counselling.

Benefits: **Versus no treatment:** We found no systematic review or RCT comparing cognitive behavioural therapy (see glossary, p 221) alone versus no treatment. **Cognitive behavioural therapy plus education versus no treatment:** We found one RCT (151 people who had been involved in a road traffic accident in the past month) that compared 3–6 sessions of cognitive behavioural therapy plus educational techniques versus no psychological intervention (see comment below).[6] The RCT found that people in the treatment group had a significantly higher baseline risk of post-traumatic stress disorder compared with the no intervention group, which makes the results difficult to interpret. The RCT found no significant difference between groups in rates of post-traumatic stress disorder at 6 months. **Versus standard care:** One RCT (132 bus drivers who had been attacked in the past few days) comparing 1–6 sessions of cognitive behavioural therapy versus standard care found that cognitive behavioural therapy significantly improved measures of anxiety and intrusive symptoms at 6 months, but found no significant difference in measures of depression or avoidance symptoms.[7] **Versus supportive counselling:** We found two RCTs.[8,9] The first RCT (24 people with acute stress disorder 2 weeks after a road traffic accident or industrial accident) compared five sessions of cognitive behavioural therapy versus five sessions of supportive counselling (see glossary, p 221).[8] It found that cognitive behavioural therapy significantly reduced the proportion of people who met Post-traumatic Stress Disorder Diagnostic Scale criteria immediately after treatment compared with supportive counselling (AR 8% with cognitive behavioural therapy v 83% with supportive counselling; P < 0.001) and at 6 months (AR 17% with cognitive behavioural therapy v 67% with supportive counselling; P < 0.05). The second RCT (45 survivors of road traffic accidents or non-sexual assault with acute stress disorder) compared three treatments: five 90 minute sessions of prolonged exposure (see glossary, p 221) therapy alone, prolonged exposure therapy plus anxiety management (see glossary, p 220); or supportive counselling.[9] It found that, immediately after completion of treatment, both prolonged exposure alone and prolonged exposure plus anxiety management significantly reduced rates of post-traumatic stress disorder compared with supportive counselling (measured by Clinician Adminis-tered PTSD Scale: AR 2/14 [14%] with prolonged exposure v 3/15 [20%] with prolonged exposure plus anxiety management v 9/16 [56%] with supportive counselling; P < 0.05 for either group v supportive counselling). The differences remained significant at 6 months' follow up (AR 2/13 [15%] with prolonged exposure v 3/13 [23%] with anxiety management v 10/15 [67%] with supportive counselling; P < 0.05 for each group v supportive counselling). **Memory structuring versus supportive listening:** We found one RCT (17 survivors of a road traffic accident in the past 24–48 hours) comparing two sessions of memory structuring versus supportive listening (see glossary, p 221).[10] It found that memory structuring significantly reduced mean scores on the Post-traumatic Stress Diagnostic Scale at 3 months compared with supportive listening (mean score 8.1 with memory structuring v 18.5 with supportive listening; P < 0.05).[10]

Harms: The RCTs gave no information on adverse effects.[6–10]

Comment: The overall quality of RCTs was poor.[6–10] Problems included lack of blinding, failure to state loss to follow up, and lack of intention to treat analysis despite high withdrawal rates. The RCT comparing cognitive behavioural therapy plus educational techniques versus no psychological intervention included multiple types of intervention (help, information, support, and reality testing/confrontation) in the treatment group.[6]

OPTION	MULTIPLE SESSION TRAUMA SUPPORT

Two RCTs provided insufficient evidence to assess collaborative care interventions involving emotional, social, and practical support in people exposed to a traumatic event in the past 1 day to 1 week.

Benefits: We found no systematic review but found two RCTs.[11,12] The first RCT (70 people who had been admitted to hospital after a road traffic accident in the past week) compared three treatments: a social work intervention (emotional, practical, and social support for 2–10 hours in the first 3 months); immediate review (a single debriefing intervention); and no intervention.[11] It found that emotional, practical and social support significantly reduced the risk of a poor outcome (based on Traumatic Neurosis Symptoms) compared with immediate review, although both interventions reduced the risk of a poor outcome compared with no intervention (AR for a poor outcome 30% with social work intervention v 60% with immediate review v 87% with no intervention; ARR for social work v no intervention 57%, NNT 2; ARR for immediate review v no intervention 27%, NNT 4; CI not reported; P < 0.001 for either intervention group v no intervention; P < 0.05 for comparison between the intervention groups). The second RCT (34 survivors of road traffic accidents or assault in the past 24 hours) compared a 4 month collaborative care (see glossary, p 221) intervention (emotional, practical, and social support from a trauma support specialist) versus no intervention.[12] After 4 months, the risk of developing post-traumatic stress disorder was lower with collaborative care than with no intervention, but the difference was not significant (AR for post-traumatic stress disorder assessed by Post-Traumatic Stress Disorder Checklist: 17% with collaborative care v 43% with no intervention; CI not reported; P > 0.1). The RCT might have lacked power to exclude a clinically important difference in outcomes.

Harms: The RCTs gave no information on adverse effects.[11,12]

Comment: The overall quality of RCTs was poor.[11,12] Problems included lack of blinding, failure to state loss to follow up, and lack of intention to treat analysis despite high withdrawal rates.

| OPTION | MULTIPLE SESSION EDUCATION |

One RCT provided insufficient evidence to assess educational techniques plus cognitive behavioural therapy in preventing post-traumatic stress disorder in road traffic accident survivors.

Benefits: **Multiple episode education alone:** We found no systematic review or RCTs. **Multiple session education plus cognitive behavioural therapy:** See benefits of multiple session cognitive behavioural therapy, p 209. See glossary, p 220.

Harms: **Multiple session education alone:** We found no systematic review or RCTs. **Multiple session education plus cognitive behavioural therapy:** See harms of multiple session cognitive behavioural therapy, p 210.

Comment: None.

| OPTION | SUPPORTIVE COUNSELLING |

Two RCTs in people with acute stress disorder after a traumatic event (road traffic accident or non-sexual assault) found that supportive counselling was less effective than five sessions of either cognitive behavioural therapy or prolonged exposure in reducing the proportion of people with post-traumatic stress disorder after 6 months.

Benefits: **Versus no treatment:** We found no systematic review or RCTs comparing supportive counselling (see glossary, p 221) versus no treatment. **Versus cognitive behavioural therapy:** See benefits of cognitive behavioural therapy, p 213. See glossary, p 220.

Harms: **Versus no treatment:** We found no RCTs. **Versus cognitive behavioural therapy:** See harms of cognitive behavioural therapy, p 213.

Comment: None.

| OPTION | HYDROCORTISONE |

One small RCT in people in intensive care with septic shock provided insufficient evidence to assess hydrocortisone in preventing post-traumatic stress disorder.

Benefits: We found no systematic review but found one small RCT (20 people in an intensive care unit with septic shock) comparing intravenous hydrocortisone versus saline.[13] It found that hydrocortisone significantly reduced the proportion of people with post-traumatic stress disorder at 31 months compared with saline (assessed by Structured Clinical Interview using DSM-IV criteria for PTSD: 1/9 [11%] with hydrocortisone v 7/11 [64%] with placebo; RR 0.07, 95% CI 0.01 to 0.80).

Harms: The RCT gave no information on adverse effects.[13]

Comment: None.

PROPRANOLOL

One small RCT provided insufficient evidence to assess propranolol in preventing post-traumatic stress disorder in people with early symptoms of post-traumatic stress disorder after a traumatic event.

Benefits: We found no systematic review but found one RCT (41 people with early symptoms of post-traumatic stress disorder 6 hours after a traumatic event) comparing propranolol 40 mg four times daily versus placebo for 10 days.[14] It found no significant difference between propranolol and placebo in the proportion of people with post-traumatic stress disorder at 1 month (measured by Clinician Administered PTSD Scale 2/11 [18%] with propranolol v 6/20 [30%] with placebo; RR 0.52, 95% CI 0.09 to 3.16) or 3 months (1/11 [9%] with propranolol v 2/15 [13%] with placebo; RR 0.65, 95% CI 0.05 to 8.23; results were not intention to treat).

Harms: The RCT gave no information on adverse effects.[14]

Comment: The RCT had a high withdrawal rate, and results are not intention to treat, which makes them difficult to interpret.[14]

OPTION   TEMAZEPAM

One small RCT provided insufficient evidence to assess temazepam in preventing post-traumatic stress disorder in people with acute stress disorder or early symptoms of post-traumatic stress disorder after road traffic accident, industrial accident, or non-sexual assault.

Benefits: We found no systematic review but found one RCT (22 people with post-traumatic stress disorder symptoms and sleep initiation diffi-culties a mean 14 days after road traffic accident, industrial accident, or non-sexual assault, 7 with acute stress disorder) comparing temazepam 30 mg daily for 5 days followed by 15 mg daily for 2 days versus placebo.[15] It found no significant difference in the proportion of people with post-traumatic stress disorder at 6 weeks (assessed by Structured Clinical Interview using DSM-IV criteria for PTSD: 6/11 [54%] with temazepam v 3/11 [27%] with placebo; RR 3.2, 95% CI 0.54 to 18.98). It found that temazepam significantly improved sleep after one night compared with placebo (P < 0.04), but found similar total sleep patterns after 1 week (P value not reported). The RCT is likely to have been underpowered to detect clinically important differences in outcomes.

Harms: The RCT gave no information on adverse effects.[15]

Comment: The RCT was published as a letter to the editor.[15]

QUESTION   What are the effects of treatments?

OPTION   COGNITIVE BEHAVIOURAL THERAPY

RCTs have found that cognitive behavioural therapy improves post-traumatic stress disorder symptoms, anxiety, and depression immediately after treatment and at up to 1 year compared with no treatment or supportive counselling. RCTs have found no significant difference in symptoms between cognitive behavioural therapy and eye movement desensitisation and reprocessing.

Benefits: **Versus supportive counselling or no treatment:** We found one systematic review (search date not reported)[16] and five subsequent RCTs of cognitive behavioural therapy (see glossary, p 221).[17-21] The review compared a range of specific psychological treatments versus supportive counselling (see glossary, p 221) or no treatment.[16] It identified 17 RCTs (690 people), including six RCTs (232 people) of cognitive behavioural therapy. All RCTs identified by the review found that psychological treatments were associated with a greater improvement immediately after treatment (using a composite score of post-traumatic stress disorder [PTSD] symptoms, anxiety, and depression) compared with supportive counselling or no treatment (17 RCTs, 690 people: overall effect size immediately after treatment 0.54, 95% CI 0.39 to 0.68). The difference was still evident at 1 year (overall effect size from 12 RCTs with long term follow up 0.53, 95% CI 0.37 to 0.69). The first subsequent RCT (87 people) compared exposure, cognitive therapy, or both, versus relaxation treatment (see glossary, p 221).[17] It found that all cognitive behavioural therapies reduced symptoms of PTSD more than relaxation treatment, immediately after treatment and at 3 months (53 people evaluated; no intention to treat analysis performed). The second subsequent RCT (72 people) found no significant difference in symptoms at 1 year between 16 1-hour sessions of imaginal exposure therapy (see glossary, p 221) and cognitive therapy (results not intention to treat; 54 people analysed; effect size 0.88 with imaginal exposure v 1.06 with cognitive therapy; reported as non-significant). It found that overall 21/54 (39%) of people continued to suffer from PTSD at 1 year.[18] The third subsequent RCT (168 female victims of sexual assault or childhood sexual abuse with PTSD and chronic nightmares) compared three sessions of imagery rehearsal therapy (see glossary, p 221) versus no treatment over 5 weeks.[19] It found that imagery rehearsal therapy significantly improved PTSD symptoms at 3 or 6 months compared with no treatment (AR for symptoms improving by at least 1 level of clinical severity 65% with imagery rehearsal v 31% with no treatment; ARR 34%; NNT 3, CI not reported; P < 0.001). The fourth subsequent RCT (171 female victims of sexual assault) compared three treatments: cognitive processing therapy; prolonged exposure (see glossary, p 221); or minimal attention (telephone call every 2 weeks) for 6 weeks.[20] It found that, immediately after treatment, both cognitive processing therapy and prolonged exposure significantly reduced rates of PTSD compared with minimal attention (AR of not having PTSD assessed by several measures including Clinician Administered PTSD Scale: 33/62 [53%] with cognitive processing v 33/62 [53%] with prolonged exposure v 1/45 [2%] with minimal attention; P < 0.001 for either intervention v placebo). The fifth subsequent RCT (78 people with PTSD or severe sub-syndromal PTSD 6 months after a road traffic accident) compared three interventions: 8–12 sessions of cognitive behavioural therapy, 8–12 sessions of supportive psychotherapy (see glossary, p 221), and waiting list control.[21] It found that, immediately after treatment, cognitive behavioural therapy significantly increased the proportion of people who responded compared with supportive psychotherapy or waiting list control (20/27 [74%] with cognitive behavioural therapy v 14/27 [52%] with supportive psychotherapy v 4/24 [17%] with waiting list control; P < 0.05 for cognitive behavioural therapy v either comparison). These results were maintained at 3 months' follow up. **Versus eye movement desensitisation and reprocessing:** See benefits of eye movement desensitisation and reprocessing, p 213.

Harms: The systematic review[16] and subsequent RCTs[17–21] gave no information on adverse effects. Overall, cognitive behavioural therapy seems well tolerated. However, there have been case reports of worsening symptoms in some people receiving imaginal flooding (see glossary, p 221), leading to calls for caution when evaluating people for treatment.[22]

Comment: None.

OPTION	EYE MOVEMENT DESENSITISATION AND REPROCESSING

RCTs have found that eye movement desensitisation and reprocessing improves symptoms compared with no treatment, and have found no significant difference in symptoms between eye movement desensitisation and reprocessing and cognitive behavioural therapy.

Benefits: **Versus no treatment:** We found one systematic review (search date 2000), which identified nine RCTs (number of people not reported) in people with post-traumatic stress disorder.[23] It found that eye movement desensitisation and reprocessing (EMDR) (see glossary, p 221) was significantly more effective than no treatment in reducing symptoms of post-traumatic stress disorder (effect size 0.39, CI not reported; P < 0.05; see comment below). **Versus cognitive behavioural therapy:** We found one systematic review[23] and one subsequent RCT.[24] The review found no significant difference between EMDR and cognitive behavioural therapy (see glossary, p 221) (effect size for EMDR v cognitive behavioural therapy −0.44, CI not reported; reported as non-significant) or between EMDR with eye movements and EMDR without eye movements (effect size 0.22, CI not reported; reported as non-significant; see comment below).[23] The subsequent RCT (24 people with PTSD) found no significant difference between stress inoculation training plus prolonged exposure and eye movement desensitisation and reprocessing (see glossary, p 221) in the proportion of people with PTSD immediately after 8–12 weeks' treatment (assessed by structured interview: 9/12 [75%] with stress inoculation training plus prolonged exposure v 10/12 [83%] with eye movement desensitisation and reprocessing; RR 0.60, 95% CI 0.08 to 4.45) or at 3 months' follow up (10/12 [83%] in each group; RR 1.00, 95% CI 0.12 to 8.56).[24]

Harms: The systematic review and subsequent RCT gave no information on adverse effects. [23,24]

Comment: The review did not report duration of treatment or state when the outcome of improvement in symptoms was measured.[23]

OPTION   **OTHER PSYCHOLOGICAL TREATMENTS**

RCTs provided insufficient evidence to assess affect management, eclectic psychotherapy, group therapy, interapy, or psychodynamic psychotherapy. We found no RCTs of drama therapy or inpatient treatment programmes.

Benefits: **Affect management:** We found no systematic review, but found one RCT (48 women) comparing 15 weeks of affect management (see glossary, p 220) treatment (in addition to drug treatment) versus waiting list control.[25] It found that, compared with waiting list control, affect management improved post-traumatic stress disorder symptoms (assessed by the Davidson Trauma Scale: 45.8 with affect management v 73.1 with waiting list control; P = 0.02) and dissociative symptoms (see glossary, p 221) from baseline (assessed by the Dissociative Experiences Scale: 11.9 with affect management v 25.2 with waiting list control; P = 0.02). **Eclectic psychotherapy:** We found no systematic review but found one RCT (42 police officers) comparing brief eclectic psychotherapy (combining components of cognitive behavioural therapy and psychodynamic psychotherapy [see glossary, p 221]) versus waiting list control over 16 sessions of treatment.[26] It found that eclectic psychotherapy significantly reduced the proportion of people with post-traumatic stress disorder immediately after treatment (AR for post-traumatic stress disorder assessed by assessed by Structured Clinical Interview using DSM-IV criteria for PTSD: 9% with eclectic psychotherapy v 50% with waiting list control; P < 0.01) and at 3 months (AR 4% with eclectic psychotherapy v 65% with waiting list control; P < 0.01). **Group therapy:** We found no systematic review but found one RCT (55 female survivors of childhood sexual abuse with post-traumatic stress disorder) comparing three treatments: trauma focused group therapy; present focused group therapy (see glossary, p 221); or waiting list control.[27] Group therapy was undertaken in 90 minute sessions for 24 weeks. The RCT found that either type of group therapy significantly improved symptoms of dissociation and sexual abuse trauma (P < 0.05 for both outcomes) compared with waiting list control. It found no significant difference in overall symptoms (symptoms assessed using the Trauma Symptom Checklist 40: mean difference in score 8.1 with group therapy v 3.8 with wait list control; reported as nonsignificant; no further data reported). The RCT prospectively defined three groups, but combined results for both active treatment groups in its analysis. This makes the results difficult to interpret. It is likely to have been underpowered to detect a clinically important difference in outcomes. **Interapy:** We found no systematic review but found one RCT (25 people) that compared interapy (see glossary, p 221) versus waiting list control for 5 weeks.[28] It found that, at 5 weeks, interapy significantly improved intrusive symptom score from baseline compared with waiting list control (mean reduction 11.0 with interapy v 3.6 with waiting list control; P < 0.04) and reduced avoidance score (mean reduction 9.6 with interapy v 2.9 with waiting list control; P < 0.03). **Psychodynamic psychotherapy:** The systematic review of a range of psychological treatments[16] identified one RCT (112 people, search date not stated) that compared four interventions: psychodynamic psychotherapy, prolonged exposure, hypnotherapy (see glossary, p 221), and waiting list control.[29] It found that symptoms were improved from baseline significantly more within all active groups compared with waiting list control. However, the trial did not test the significance of comparative results. **Drama therapy; inpatient treatment programmes; supportive psychotherapy:** See glossary, p 221. We found no RCTs.

Harms: The systematic review[16] and RCTs[25-29] gave no information on adverse effects.

Comment: None.

| OPTION | SELECTIVE SEROTONIN REUPTAKE INHIBITORS AND RELATED ANTIDEPRESSANTS |

RCTs found that sertraline or paroxetine reduced symptoms at 3–7 months compared with placebo. RCTs found more limited evidence from the systematic review and one subsequent RCT that fluoxetine may reduce symptoms at 3 months compared with placebo. RCTs provided insufficient evidence to compare mirtazapine versus placebo or sertraline versus nefazodone.

Benefits: **Versus placebo:** We found one systematic review (search date 1999)[30] and seven subsequent RCTs (3 evaluating sertraline,[31-33] 2 evaluating paroxetine,[34,35] 1 evaluating fluoxetine,[36] and one evaluating mirtazapine.[37] The review identified 4 RCTs (375 people) comparing selective serotonin reuptake inhibitors versus placebo that used the Clinical Global Impression Scale change item or close equivalent as the primary outcome measure.[30] Response was defined as a Clinical Global Impression Scale score of 1 [very much improved] or 2 [much improved]. Two RCTs (183 people) found that sertraline significantly increased the proportion of people who responded after 3 months (OR 0.44, 95% CI 0.24 to 0.78). One RCT (280 people) found no significant difference between paroxetine and placebo in the proportion of people who responded after 3 months (OR 0.64, 95% CI 0.40 to 1.02) and another RCT (53 people) found no significant difference between fluoxetine and placebo in the proportion of people who reponded after 3 months (OR 0.30, 95% CI 0.09 to 1.02).[30] Five of the subsequent placebo-controlled RCTs found improved symptoms with selective serotonin reuptake inhibitors. The first subsequent RCT (208 people) found that sertraline 50–200 mg daily significantly improved symptoms at 12 weeks compared with placebo (mean reduction in post-traumatic stress disorder [PTSD] symptom score on the Clinician Administered PTSD Scale −33.0 with sertraline v −26.2 with placebo; P = 0.04).[31] The second subsequent RCT (96 people who had previously responded to sertraline for acute treatment of PTSD) found that sertraline significantly reduced PTSD relapse after 28 weeks compared with placebo (AR 5% with sertraline v 26% with placebo; ARR 21%; NNT 5; CI not reported; P < 0.02).[32] The third subsequent RCT (42 veteran male soldiers) found no significant difference between sertraline 50–200 mg daily and placebo in symptoms of PTSD after 10 weeks of treatment (mean reduction in Clinician Administered PTSD score −18.7 with sertraline v −13.5

with placebo; P = 0.53; see comment below).[33] The fourth subsequent RCT (307 people) found that paroxetine 20–50 mg daily significantly increased response rate at 12 weeks compared with placebo (response defined as "very much improved" or "much improved" on the Clinical Global Impression Scale; AR 59% with paroxetine v 38% with control; ARR 21%; NNT 5; CI not reported; P = 0.008).[34] The fifth subsequent RCT (551 people) found that paroxetine 20 or 40 mg daily significantly improved response rate (using the same definition) at 12 weeks compared with placebo (AR for response 62% with 20 mg paroxetine v 54% with 40 mg paroxetine v 37% with placebo; P < 0.001 for both paroxetine groups compared with placebo).[35] The sixth subsequent RCT (301 people, primarily male soldiers) found that fluoxetine 50–80 mg daily significantly improved symptoms compared with placebo after 12 weeks' treatment (mean reduction in Clinician Administered PTSD score −34.6 with fluoxetine v −29.6 with placebo; P = 0.021).[36] The clinical importance of this difference in symptoms is unclear. The seventh subsequent RCT (26 people with PTSD) compared mirtazapine 45 mg daily (17 people) versus placebo (9 people) for 8 weeks' treatment.[37] It found no significant difference in the proportion of people with global improvement in symptoms immediately after treatment (as assessed by the Short PTSD Rating Interview: 11/17 [65%] with mirtazapine v 2/9 [22%] with placebo; RR 6.42, 95% CI 0.99 to 41.21; results not intention to treat). The RCT is likely to have been underpowered to detect clinically important differences in outcomes. **Versus each other:** We found one systematic review[30] and one subsequent RCT.[38] Two RCTs identified by the review found no significant difference in response at 10–12 weeks between sertraline, paroxetine, or fluoxetine (sertraline, 42 people: OR 0.44, 95% CI 0.12 to 1.60; paroxetine, 280 people: OR 0.64, 95% CI 0.40 to 1.02; fluoxetine, 53 people: OR 0.30, 95% CI 0.09 to 1.02). These RCTs may have been underpowered to detect a clinically important difference in outcomes. The subsequent RCT compared sertraline 50–100 mg daily versus nefazodone 200–400 mg daily.[38] It found no significant difference in symptoms at 5 months (mean total eight item PTSD scale [TOP-8] score 5.23 with sertraline v 4.35 with nefazodone; P = 0.36). However, the results of that RCT should be interpreted with caution because, despite randomisation, people taking sertraline had significantly higher baseline TOP-8 scores than people taking nefazodone.

Harms: The systematic review gave no information on adverse effects, although it found no significant difference between antidepressants and placebo in the proportion of people who withdrew for any cause (7 RCTs; 712 people; RR 0.85, 95% CI 0.63 to 1.14).[30] The first subsequent RCT found that, compared with placebo, sertraline significantly increased insomnia (35% with sertraline v 22% with placebo; P = 0.04), diarrhoea (28% with sertraline v 11% with placebo; P = 0.003), and nausea (23% with sertraline v 11% with placebo; P = 0.03), and decreased appetite (12% with sertraline v 1% with placebo; P = 0.001).[31] The fourth subsequent RCT comparing paroxetine versus placebo found that adverse effects with an incidence of at least 10% and twice that of placebo were nausea (19.2% with paroxetine v 8.3% with placebo), somnolence (17.2%

with paroxetine v 3.8% with placebo), dry mouth (13.9% with paroxetine v 4.5% with placebo), asthenia (13.2% with paroxetine v 5.2% with placebo), and abnormal ejaculation (11.8% with paroxetine v 3.7% with placebo).[34] In the seventh subsequent RCT four people taking mirtazapine withdrew because of adverse effects, including sedation, panic attacks, increased anxiety, and irritability.[37] One person taking placebo withdrew because of pain. The RCT found that significantly more people taking placebo had palpitations (3/9 [33%] with placebo v 0/17 [0%] with mirtazapine; P = 0.03) and more people taking mirtazapine had increased appetite (6 with mirtazapine v 1 with placebo; P value not reported). A further RCT (65 people) assessing the harms of fluoxetine in people with PTSD found that fluoxetine was associated with significantly higher rates of nausea, diarrhoea, and thirst compared with placebo (P < 0.05 for all outcomes).[39] Known adverse effects of selective serotonin reuptake inhibitors include nausea and headache (see harms of prescription antidepressant drugs under depressive disorders, p 114).

Comment: The veteran soldiers in the third subsequent RCT evaluating sertraline had higher baseline Clinician Administered PTSD scores (mean baseline score 94.3) than people in the other RCTs of sertraline (mean baseline score about 74); this may explain the lack of significant improvement in symptoms between sertraline and placebo.[33]

OPTION   **TRICYCLIC ANTIDEPRESSANTS**

RCTs provided insufficient evidence to assess imipramine or amitriptyline in people with post-traumatic stress disorder.

Benefits: We found one systematic review (search date 1999) of antidepressant drugs for post-traumatic stress disorder.[30] The review identified two RCTs (81 people) comparing tricyclic antidepressants versus placebo that used the Clinical Global Impression Scale change item or close equivalent as the primary outcome measure.[30] One RCT (41 people) identified by the review found that the proportion of non-responders at 2 months was significantly lower with imipramine than with placebo (response defined as Clinical Global Impression score of 1 [very much improved] or 2 [much improved]; OR 0.21, 95% CI 0.05 to 0.78). The other RCT (40 people) identified by the review found no significant difference between amitriptyline and placebo in the proportion of people who responded after 2 months (OR 0.41, 95% CI 0.12 to 1.42).[30]

Harms: The systematic review gave no information on adverse effects, although it found no significant difference between antidepressants and placebo in the proportion of people who withdrew for any cause (7 RCTs; 712 people; RR 0.85, 95% CI 0.63 to 1.14).[30] Known adverse effects of tricyclic antidepressants include anticholinergic effects (see harms of prescription antidepressant drugs under depressive disorders, p 114).

Comment: None.

OPTION	MONOAMINE OXIDASE INHIBITORS

RCTs provided insufficient evidence to assess brofaromine or phenelzine in people with post-traumatic stress disorder.

Benefits: We found one systematic review (search date 1999) of antidepressant drugs for post-traumatic stress disorder.[30] The review identified three RCTs (247 people) comparing monoamine oxidase inhibitors versus placebo that used the Clinical Global Impression Scale change item or close equivalent as the primary outcome measure.[30] Two RCTs found no significant difference between brofaromine and placebo in the proportion of non-responders at 14 weeks (response defined as Clinical Global Impression Scale of 1 [very much improved] or 2 [much improved]: 114 people: OR 0.94, 95% CI 0.45 to 1.99; 64 people: OR 0.40, 95% CI 0.15 to 1.08). One RCT (37 people) found that phenelzine significantly increased the proportion of responders at 2 months compared with placebo (OR 0.21, 95% CI 0.06 to 0.73).[30]

Harms: The systematic review gave no information on adverse effects, although it found no significant difference between antidepressants and placebo in the proportion of people who withdrew for any cause (7 RCTs; 712 people; RR 0.85, 95% CI 0.63 to 1.14).[30] Known adverse effects of monoamine oxidase inhibitors include possible hypertensive crisis. Monoamine oxidase inhibitors may also require a need for dietary restriction (see harms of prescription antidepressant drugs under depressive disorders, p 114).

Comment: None.

OPTION	CARBAMAZEPINE

We found no RCTs of carbamazepine in people with post-traumatic stress disorder.

Benefits: We found no systematic review or RCTs.

Harms: We found no RCTs.

Comment: None.

OPTION	RISPERIDONE

We found no RCTs of risperidone in people with post-traumatic stress disorder.

Benefits: We found no systematic review or RCTs.

Harms: We found no RCTs.

Comment: None.

One RCT provided insufficient evidence to assess lamotrigine in people with post-traumatic stress disorder.

Benefits: We found one systematic review (search date 1999), which identified one small RCT (14 people) comparing lamotrigine versus placebo that used the Clinical Global Impression Scale change item or close equivalent as the primary outcome measure.[30] The RCT found no significant difference between lamotrigine and placebo in the proportion of non-responders at 2 months (response defined as Clinical Global Impression Scale score of 1 [very much improved] or 2 [much improved]; OR 0.39, 95% CI 0.04 to 3.71). However, it is likely to have been underpowered to detect a clinically important difference between groups.

Harms: The systematic review gave no information on adverse effects, although it found no significant difference between antidepressants and placebo in the proportion of people who withdrew for any cause (7 RCTs; 712 people; RR 0.85, 95% CI 0.63 to 1.14).[30]

Comment: None.

One systematic review identified no RCTs of sufficient quality in people with post-traumatic stress disorder.

Benefits: We found one systematic review (search date 1999), which identified no RCTs of sufficient quality.[30]

Harms: We found no RCTs.

Comment: None.

We found no RCTs of propranolol in people with post-traumatic stress disorder.

Benefits: We found no systematic review or RCTs.

Harms: We found no RCTs.

Comment: None.

GLOSSARY

Affect management A type of group treatment focusing on regulation of mood.

Anxiety management Involves teaching techniques to reduce anxiety levels. Examples include muscular relaxation in which individuals are taught to alternatively tense and relax specific muscle groups and breathing retraining to avoid overbreathing.

Cognitive behavioural therapy Covers a variety of techniques. *Imaginal exposure* entails exposure to a detailed account or image of what happened. *Real life exposure* involves confronting real life situations that have become associated with the trauma and cause fear and distress. *Cognitive therapy* entails challenging distorted thoughts about the trauma, the self, and the world. *Imaginal flooding* involves the intense reliving of the traumatic experience. *Memory structuring* involves listening to and clarifying the individual's narrative and structuring it for them to repeat to friends and family. *Prolonged exposure* entails repeated exposure to memories of the trauma, and to non-dangerous real life situations that are avoided because of trauma related fear. *Stress inoculation* entails instruction in coping skills and some cognitive techniques such as restructuring. *Supportive listening* involves actively listening to the individual's narrative and clarifying factual, sensory, and affective details.

Cognitive processing therapy Includes elements of cognitive therapy and writing and reading about the traumatic event.

Collaborative care Entails counselling, liaison, and coordination of care after discharge.

Dissociative symptoms Involve a disruption to memory or perception of the environment, e.g. an inability to recall details of a traumatic event that cannot be accounted for by ordinary forgetfulness or an organic cause such as head injury.

Drama therapy Entails using drama as a form of expression and communication.

Eye movement desensitisation and reprocessing (EMDR) Entails asking the person to focus on the traumatic event, a negative cognition associated with it, and the associated emotions.[40] The person is then asked to follow the therapist's finger as it moves from side to side.

Hypnotherapy Entails hypnosis to allow people to work through the traumatic event.

Imagery rehearsal therapy Involves encouraging participants to practice pleasant imagery exercises and employ cognitive behavioural tools to deal with unpleasant images.

Interapy A protocol driven treatment delivered through the internet, which includes psychoeducation and cognitive reappraisal. For further information, see http://www.interapy.nl.

Present focused group therapy A group intervention that involves identifying and modifying patterns of behaviour that have arisen from their past traumatic experience.

Psychodynamic psychotherapy Entails analysis of defence mechanisms, interpretations, and pre-trauma experiences.

Psychological debriefing A technique that entails detailed consideration of the traumatic event and the normalisation of psychological reactions.

Relaxation treatment A technique involving imagination of relaxing situations to induce muscular and mental relaxation.

Supportive counselling A non-directive intervention dealing with current issues rather than the trauma itself.

Supportive psychotherapy A non-directive intervention that involves helping an individual to explore their thoughts, feelings, and behaviour with the aim of achieving clearer understanding of self and the ability to cope with situations more effectively.

Trauma focused group therapy A group intervention that involves reconstructing a past traumatic event, identifying and modifying negative self images associated with it, and integrating memories of the event into the individual's conscious awareness of self and others.

REFERENCES

1. American Psychiatric Association. *Diagnostic and statistical manual of mental disorders*. 4th ed. Washington: APA, 1994.

2. Kessler RC, Sonnega A, Bromet E, et al. Posttraumatic stress disorder in the national comorbidity survey. *Arch Gen Psychiatry* 1995;52:1048–1060.

3. O'Brien S. *Traumatic events and mental health*. Cambridge: Cambridge University Press, 1998.

4. Rose S, Bisson J, Wessely S. Psychological debriefing for preventing post traumatic stress disorder (PTSD). In: The Cochrane Library, Issue 2, 2003. Oxford: Update Software. Search date 2001; primary sources Medline, Embase, Psychlit, Pilots, Biosis, Pascal, Occupational Safety and Health, Sociofile, Cinahl, Psycinfo, Psyndex, Sigle, Lilacs, Cochrane Controlled Clinical Trials, National Research Register, hand searches of *Journal of Traumatic Stress*, and contact with leading researchers.

5. Campfield KM, Hills AM. Effect of timing of critical incident stress debriefing (CISD) on posttraumatic symptoms. *J Traum Stress* 2001;14:327–340.

6. Brom D, Kleber RJ, Hofman MC. Victims of traffic accidents: incidence and prevention of post-traumatic stress disorder. *J Clin Psychol* 1993;49:131–140.

7. Andre C, Lelord F, Legeron P, et al. Controlled study of outcomes after 6 months to early intervention of bus driver victims of aggression [in French]. *Encephale* 1997;23:65–71.

8. Bryant RA, Harvey AG, Basten C, et al. Treatment of acute stress disorder: a comparison of cognitive behavioural therapy and supportive counselling. *J Consult Clin Psychol* 1998;66:862–866.

9. Bryant RA, Sackville T, Dang ST, et al. Treating acute stress disorder: an evaluation of cognitive behavior therapy and supportive counselling techniques. *Am J Psychiatry* 1999;156:1780–1786.

10. Gidron Y, Gal R, Freedman S, et al. Translating research findings to PTSD prevention: results of a randomised controlled pilot study. *J Trauma Stress* 2001;14:773–780.

11. Bordow S, Porritt D. An experimental evaluation of crisis intervention. *Soc Sci Med* 1979;13A:251–256.

12. Zatzick DF, Roy-Byrne P, Russo JE, et al. Collaborative interventions for physically injured trauma survivors: a pilot randomized effectiveness trial. *Gen Hosp Psychiatry* 2001;23:114–123.

13. Schelling G, Briegel J, Roozendaal B, et al. The effect of stress doses of hydrocortisone during septic shock on posttraumatic stress disorder in survivors. *Biol Psychiatry* 2001;50:978–985.

14. Pitman RK, Sanders KM, Zusman RM, et al. Pilot study of secondary prevention of posttraumatic stress disorder with propranolol. *Biol Psychiatry* 2002;51:189–192.

15. Mellman TA, Bustamante V, David D, et al. Hypnotic medication in the aftermath of trauma. *J Clin Psychiatry* 2002;63:1183–1184.

16. Sherman JJ. Effects of psychotherapeutic treatments for PTSD: a meta-analysis of controlled clinical trials. *J Trauma Stress* 1998;11:413–436. Search date not reported; primary sources Psychlit, Eric, Medline, Cinahl, Dissertation Abstracts, and Pilots Traumatic Stress Database.

17. Marks I, Lovell K, Noshirvani H, et al. Treatment of posttraumatic stress disorder by exposure and/or cognitive restructuring: a controlled study. *Arch Gen Psychiatry* 1998;55:317–325.

18. Tarrier N, Sommerfield C, Pilgrim H, et al. Cognitive therapy or imaginal exposure in the treatment of post-traumatic stress disorder. *Br J Psychiatry* 1999;175:571–575.

19. Krakow B, Hollifield M, Johnston L, et al. Imagery rehearsal therapy for chronic nightmares in sexual assault survivors with posttraumatic stress disorder: a randomized controlled trial. *JAMA* 2001;286:537–545.

20. Resick A, Nishith P, Weaver TL, et al. A comparison of cognitive-processing therapy with prolonged exposure and a waiting condition for the treatment of chronic posttraumatic stress disorder in female rape victims. *J Consult Clin Psychol* 2002;70:867–879.

21. Blanchard EB, Hickling EJ, Devineni T, et al. A controlled evaluation of cognitive behavioral therapy for posttraumatic stress in motor vehicle accident survivors. *Behav Res Ther* 2003;41:79–96.

22. Pitman RK, Altman B, Greenwald E, et al. Psychiatric complications during flooding therapy for posttraumatic stress disorder. *J Clin Psychiatry* 1991;52:17–20.

23. Eye movement desensitisation and reprocessing (EMDR): a meta-analysis. *J Consult Clin Psychol* 2001;69:305–316. Medline and Psychinfo searched from 1988 to April 2000, and Current Contents searched from 1997 to March 2000, plus reference lists from articles found in these searches.

24. Lee C, Gavriel H, Drummond P, et al. Treatment of PTSD: stress inoculation training with prolonged exposure compared to EMDR. *J Clin Psychol* 2002;58:1071–1089.

25. Zlotnick C, Shea T, Rosen K, et al. An affect-management group for women with posttraumatic stress disorder and histories of childhood sexual abuse. *J Trauma Stress* 1997;10:425–436.

26. Gersons BPR, Carlier IVE, Lamberts RD, et al. Randomised clinical trial of brief eclectic psychotherapy for police officers with posttraumatic stress disorder. *J Trauma Stress* 2000;13:333–348.

27. Classen C, Koopman C, Nevill-Manning K, et al. A preliminary report comparing trauma-focused and present-focused group therapy against a wait-listed condition among childhood sexual abuse survivors with PTSD. *J Aggress Maltreat Trauma* 2001;14:265–288.

28. Lange A, Van de Ven JP, Schrieken B, et al. Interapy: treatment of posttraumatic stress through the Internet: a controlled trial. *J Behav Ther Exp Psychiatry* 2001;32:73–90.

29. Brom D, Kleber RJ, Defares PB. Brief psychotherapy of posttraumatic stress disorders. *J Consult Clin Psychol* 1989;57:607–612.

30. Stein DJ, Zungu-Dirwayi N, Van der Linden GJ, et al. Pharmacotherapy for posttraumatic stress disorder. In: The Cochrane Library, Issue 2, 2003. Oxford: Update Software. Search date 1999; primary sources Medline, Psychlit, Pilots Traumatic Stress Database, Dissertation Abstracts, trials register of the Cochrane Depression, Anxiety and Neurosis Controlled Group, hand searches of reference lists, and personal contact with post-traumatic stress disorder researchers and pharmaceutical companies.

31. Davidson JR, Rothbaum BO, van der Kolk BA, et al. Multicenter, double blind comparison of sertraline and placebo in the treatment of posttraumatic stress disorder. *Arch Gen Psychiatry* 2001;58:485–492.

32. Davidson J, Pearlstein T, Londborg P, et al. Efficacy of sertraline in preventing relapse of posttraumatic stress disorder: results of a 28-week double-blind, placebo-controlled study. *Am J Psychiatry* 2001;158:1974–1981.

33. Zohar J, Amital D, Miodownik C. Double-blind placebo-controlled pilot study of sertraline in military veterans with posttraumatic stress disorder. *J Clin Psychopharmacol* 2002;22:190–195.

34. Tucker P, Zaninelli R, Yehuda R, et al. Paroxetine in the treatment of chronic posttraumatic stress disorder: results of a placebo-controlled, flexible-dosage trial. *J Clin Psychiatry* 2001;62:860–868.

35. Marshall RD, Beebe KL, Oldham M, et al. Efficacy and safety of paroxetine treatment for chronic PTSD: a fixed-dose, placebo-controlled study. *Am J Psychiatry* 2001;158:1982–1988.

36. Martenyi F, Brown EB, Zhang H, et al. Fluoxetine versus placebo in posttraumatic stress disorder. *J Clin Psychiatry* 2002;63:199–206.

37. Davidson JRT, Weisler RH, Butterfield MI, et al. Mirtazapine vs. placebo in posttraumatic stress disorder: a pilot trial. *Biol Psychiatry* 2003;53:188–191.

38. Saygin MZ, Sungur MZ, Sabol EU, et al. Nefazodone versus sertraline in treatment of posttraumatic stress disorder. *Bull Clin Psychopharmacol* 2002;12:1–5.

39. Barnett SD, Tharwani HM, Hertzberg MA, et al. Tolerability of fluoxetine in posttraumatic stress disorder. *Prog Neuropsychopharmacol Biol Psychiatry* 2002;26:363–367.

40. Shapiro F. Eye movement desensitisation: a new treatment for post-traumatic stress disorder. *J Behav Ther Exp Psychiatry* 1989;20:211–217.

Jonathan Bisson
Consultant Liaison Psychiatrist
Cardiff and Vale NHS Trust
Cardiff
UK

Competing interests: None declared.

Search date December 2002

Zia Nadeem, Andrew McIntosh, and Stephen Lawrie

Key Messages

- Most evidence is from systematic reviews of RCTs that report disparate outcomes. There is a need for larger RCTs, over longer periods, with well designed end points, including standardised, validated symptom scales. No intervention has been found to consistently reduce negative symptoms.

- **Continuation of antipsychotic drugs for 6–9 months after an acute episode to reduce relapse rates** Systematic reviews have found that continuing antipsychotic drugs for at least 6 months after an acute episode reduces relapse rates compared with no treatment or placebo, and that some benefit of continuing antipsychotics is apparent for up to 2 years.

- **Multiple session family interventions to reduce relapse rates** One systematic review found that multiple session family interventions reduced relapse rates at 12 months compared with usual care, single session family interventions, or psychoeducational interventions.

- **Psychoeducational interventions to reduce relapse rates** One systematic review has found that psychoeducation reduces relapse rates at 9–18 months compared with a control intervention.

- **Behavioural therapy to improve adherence** One RCT found that behavioural interventions improved adherence to antipsychotic medication over 3 months compared with usual treatment. Two RCTs found limited evidence that behavioural interventions may improve adherence more than psychoeducational therapy.

- **Compliance therapy to improve adherence** Two RCTs found limited evidence that compliance therapy may increase adherence to antipsychotic drugs at 6 and 18 months compared with non-specific counselling.

- **Psychoeducational interventions to improve adherence** One systematic review found limited evidence that psychoeducation improved adherence to antipsychotic medication compared with usual care. Two RCTs found limited evidence that psychoeducational may improve adherence less than behavioural therapy.

- **Chlorpromazine** One systematic review has found that, compared with placebo, chlorpromazine reduces the proportion of people who have no improvement, or have marked or worse severity of illness at 6 months on a psychiatrist rated scale. The review found that chlorpromazine caused more adverse effects, such as sedation, acute dystonia, and parkinsonism, than placebo.

- **Clozapine** Two systematic reviews found that clozapine improved symptoms over 4–10 weeks compared with standard antipsychotic drugs. However, RCTs found that clozapine may be associated with blood dyscrasias. Three systematic reviews of small RCTs provided insufficient evidence to compare clozapine versus other new antipsychotic drugs. One systematic review in people resistant to standard treatment found that clozapine improved symptoms after 12 weeks and after 2 years compared with standard antipsychotic drugs. RCTs provided insufficient evidence to compare clozapine versus other newer antipsychotics in people resistant to standard antipsychotic drugs.

- **Depot bromperidol decanoate** RCTs found no significant difference in the proportion of people who needed additional medication, left the trial early, or had movement disorders over 6–12 months between depot bromperidol decanoate and haloperidol or fluphenazine decanoate.

- **Depot haloperidol decanoate** One systematic review of one small RCT found no significant difference in global clinical state at 4 months between depot haloperidol decanoate and oral haloperidol, but it may have been too small to exclude a clinically important difference. Haloperidol is associated with acute dystonia, akathisia, and parkinsonism.

- **Haloperidol** One systematic review has found that haloperidol increases physician rated global improvement at 6 and 24 weeks compared with placebo but is associated with acute dystonia, akathisia, and parkinsonism.

- **Thioridazine** One systematic review has found that thioridazine improves global mental state over 3–12 months compared with placebo.

- **Cognitive behavioural therapy to reduce relapse rates** Limited evidence from a systematic review of two RCTs found no significant difference in relapse rates between cognitive behavioural therapy plus standard care and standard care alone.

- **Multiple session family interventions to improve adherence** One systematic review found that "compliance with medication" over 9–24 months was higher in people who received multiple family interventions compared with usual care, single family interventions, or psychoeducational interventions, but the difference did not quite reach significance.
- **Perazine** RCTs provided insufficient evidence to assess perazine.
- **Social skills training to reduce relapse rates** One systematic review of small RCTs provided insufficient evidence to assess social skills training.
- **Amisulpride; loxapine; molindone; olanzapine; pimozide; quetiapine; risperidone; sulpiride; ziprasidone; zotepine** Systematic reviews have found that these newer antipsychotic drugs are as effective in improving symptoms as standard antipsychotic drugs, and have different profiles of adverse effects.

DEFINITION Schizophrenia is characterised by the positive symptoms (see glossary, p 249) of auditory hallucinations, delusions, and thought disorder, and by the negative symptoms (see glossary, p 249) of demotivation, self neglect, and reduced emotion.[1] People are defined as being resistant to standard antipsychotic drugs if, over the preceding 5 years, they have not had a clinically important improvement in symptoms after 2–3 regimens of treatment with standard antipsychotic drugs for at least 6 weeks (from at least 2 classes at doses equivalent to or greater than 1000 mg/day chlorpromazine) and they have had no period of good functioning.[2,3] Approximately 30% (10–45%) of people with schizophrenia meet these criteria.[3]

INCIDENCE/ PREVALENCE Onset of symptoms typically occurs in early adult life (average age 25 years) and is earlier in men than in women.[4,5] Prevalence worldwide is 2–4/1000. One in 100 people will develop schizophrenia in their lifetime.

AETIOLOGY/ RISK FACTORS Risk factors include a family history (although no major genes have been identified), obstetric complications, developmental difficulties, central nervous system infections in childhood, cannabis use, and acute life events.[4] The precise contributions of these factors and ways in which they may interact are unclear.

PROGNOSIS About three quarters of people suffer recurrent relapse and continued disability, although the proportion of people who improved significantly increased after the mid-1950s (mean 48.5% from 1956–1985 v 35.4% from 1895–1956).[6] Outcome may be worse in people with insidious onset and delayed initial treatment, social isolation, or a strong family history; in people living in industrialised countries; in men; and in people who misuse drugs.[5] Drug treatment is generally successful in treating positive symptoms, but up to a third of people derive little benefit and negative symptoms are notoriously difficult to treat. About half of people with schizophrenia do not adhere to treatment in the short term. The figure is even higher in the longer term.[7]

AIMS OF INTERVENTION To relieve symptoms and to improve quality of life, with minimal adverse effects of treatment.

OUTCOMES	Severity of positive and negative symptoms; global clinical improvement; global clinical impression (a composite measure of symptoms and everyday functioning); rate of relapse; adherence to treatment; adverse effects of treatment.
METHODS	*Clinical Evidence* search and appraisal December 2002. Most RCTs were small, short term, with high withdrawal rates, and employed many different outcome measures.[8] There were a large number of good systematic reviews. Therefore, if possible, we focused primarily on systematic reviews and included only the outcomes that we thought were the most clinically relevant. Because each treatment is associated with different benefits and harms, we used estimates of global effectiveness if they were available. We searched for placebo controlled RCTs of standard antipsychotic medication and comparative RCTs of newer antipsychotic drugs.

QUESTION What are the effects of drug treatments?

OPTION CHLORPROMAZINE

One systematic review has found that, compared with placebo, chlorpromazine reduces the proportion of people who have no improvement, or marked or worse severity of illness at 6 months on a psychiatrist rated scale. The review found that chlorpromazine caused more adverse effects, such as sedation, acute dystonia, and parkinsonism, than placebo.

Benefits:
Versus placebo: We found one systematic review (search date 1999, 45 RCTs, 3116 people, mean dose 511 mg/day, range 25–2000 mg/day).[9] It found that, compared with placebo, chlorpromazine significantly reduced the proportion of people who had no improvement on a psychiatrist rated global impression scale at 6 months (13 RCTs; 583/921 [63%] with chlorpromazine v 609/790 [77%] with placebo; RR of failing to improve 0.72, 95% CI 0.62 to 0.83; NNT 7, 95% CI 5 to 10) and significantly reduced the proportion of people who had marked or worse severity of illness on a psychiatrist rated scale at 1 week to 6 months (5 RCTs; 323/493 [66%] with chlorpromazine v 231/285 [81%] with placebo; RR of increased severity of illness 0.77, 95% CI 0.71 to 0.84; NNT 5, 95% CI 4 to 8).

Harms:
Versus placebo: The systematic review found that, compared with placebo, chlorpromazine caused significantly higher rates of sedation (218/698 [31%] with chlorpromazine v 65/490 [13%] with placebo; RR 2.4, 95% CI 1.7 to 3.3; NNH 6, 95% CI 4 to 8), acute dystonia (28/439 [6%] with chlorpromazine v 5/234 [2%] with placebo; RR 3.1, 95% CI 1.3 to 7.6; NNH 24, 95% CI 14 to 77), parkinsonism (123/723 [17%] with chlorpromazine v 40/542 [7%] with placebo; RR 2.6, 95% CI 1.2 to 5.4; NNH 10, 95% CI 8 to 16), weight gain (31/75 [41%] with chlorpromazine v 7/90 [8%] with placebo; RR 4.4, 95% CI 2.1 to 9.0; NNH 3, 95% CI 2 to 5), skin photosensitivity (81/496 [16%] with chlorpromazine v 9/303 [3%] with placebo; RR 5.2, 95% CI 3 to 10; NNH 7, 95% CI 6 to 10), dizziness caused by hypotension (112/688 [16%] with chlorpromazine v 38/504 [7%] with placebo; RR 1.9, 95% CI 1.3 to 2.6;

NNH 12, 95% CI 8 to 20), and dry mouth (32/473 [7%] with chlorpromazine v 4/283 [1%] with placebo; RR 4.0, 95% CI 1.6 to 10.0; NNH 19, 95% CI 12 to 37).[9] Chlorpromazine was also associated with higher rates of seizures (19/450 [4%] with chlorpromazine v 4/245 [2%] with placebo; RR 2.4, 95% CI 0.4 to 16) and blood dyscrasias (10/207 [5%] with chlorpromazine v 2/187 [1%] with placebo; RR 2.0, 95% CI 0.7 to 6.0), although the differences did not reach significance. We found no long term data on the risk of tardive dyskinesia or the rare but potentially fatal neuroleptic malignant syndrome. Despite the frequent adverse effects, the review found that people taking chlorpromazine were more likely to stay in RCTs in both the short and the medium term than people taking placebo.

Comment: The review did not categorise symptoms as positive or negative because this information was rarely available from included RCTs.[9] It found significant heterogeneity among RCTs, but found that the analysis of global improvement over 9 weeks to 6 months remained significant after removal of the heterogeneous RCTs (RR 0.65, 95% CI 0.5 to 0.9).

OPTION   HALOPERIDOL

One systematic review has found that haloperidol increases the proportion of people with psychiatrist rated global improvement at 6 and 24 weeks compared with placebo, but is associated with acute dystonia, akathisia, and parkinsonism.

Benefits: **Versus placebo:** We found one systematic review (search date 1998, 20 RCTs, 1001 people).[10] It found that haloperidol (over a wide range of doses) significantly increased psychiatrist rated global improvement at 6 weeks (3 RCTs, 159 people; 61/88 [69%] with haloperidol v 23/71 [32%] with placebo; RR 2.3, 95% CI 1.7 to 3.3; NNT 3, 95% CI 2 to 5) and at 24 weeks (8 RCTs; 72/163 [44%] v 21/150 [14%]; RR 3.5, 95% CI 2.3 to 5.6; NNT 3, 95% CI 3 to 5) compared with placebo.

Harms: **Versus placebo:** The systematic review found that, compared with placebo, haloperidol significantly increased the risk of acute dystonia (2 RCTs; RR 4.7, 95% CI 1.7 to 44; NNH 5, 95% CI 3 to 9), akathisia (3 RCTs: RR 6.5, 95% CI 1.5 to 28; NNH 6, 95% CI 4 to 14), and parkinsonism (4 RCTs; RR 8.9, 95% CI 2.6 to 31; NNH 3, 95% CI 2 to 5).[10] People taking haloperidol were significantly more likely to be treated with anticholinergic drugs than people taking placebo (4 RCTs; RR 4.9, 95% CI 1.01 to 24; NNH 2, 95% CI 1 to 3).

Comment: The median size of RCTs in the review was 38 people, but the quality of the RCTs was higher than average for schizophrenia trials.[10] Although the dose range was very wide, most RCTs used 4–20 mg daily and adjusted dose according to need. The review found evidence of publication bias for the 6–24 months global outcome ratings.[10]

OPTION   THIORIDAZINE

One systematic review has found that thioridazine improves global mental state over 3–12 months compared with placebo.

Benefits: **Versus placebo:** We found one systematic review (search date 1999, 11 RCTs, 560 people).[11] It found that thioridazine significantly reduced the proportion of people who were "no better or worse" in global clinical impression at 3–12 months compared with placebo (5 RCTs; 27/84 [32%] with thioridazine v 57/81 [70%] with placebo; RR 0.5, 95% CI 0.37 to 0.68; NNT 3, 95% CI 3 to 5).

Harms: **Versus placebo:** The review found no significant difference in adverse effects between thioridazine and placebo, but may have lacked power to detect a clinically important difference.[11]

Comment: None.

OPTION   DEPOT BROMPERIDOL DECANOATE

RCTs found no significant difference in the proportion of people who needed additional medication, left the trial early, or had movement disorders over 6–12 months between depot bromperidol decanoate and haloperidol or fluphenazine decanoate.

Benefits: **Versus standard antipsychotic drugs:** One systematic review (search date 1999, 3 RCTs, 97 people) found no significant difference between depot bromperidol and haloperidol or fluphenazine decanoate in the proportion of people who needed additional antipsychotics or benzodiazepines over 6–12 months (19/48 [39%] with bromperidol v 18/49 [37%] with haloperidol or fluphenazine; RR 1.08, 95% CI 0.68 to 1.70) or who left the trial early (10/48 [21%] with bromperidol v 5/49 [10%] with haloperidol or fluphenazine; RR 1.92, 95% CI 0.80 to 4.60).[12]

Harms: **Versus standard antipsychotic drugs:** The review found no significant difference in movement disorders over 6–12 months between bromperidol and haloperidol or fluphenazine (2 RCTs: 16/38 [42%] with bromperidol v 22/39 [56%] with haloperidol or fluphenazine; RR 0.74, 95% CI 0.47 to 1.17).[12]

Comment: None.

OPTION   DEPOT HALOPERIDOL DECANOATE

One systematic review of one small RCT found no significant difference in global clinical state at 4 months between depot haloperidol decanoate and oral haloperidol, but it may have been too small to exclude a clinically important difference. Haloperidol is associated with acute dystonia, akathisia, and parkinsonism.

Benefits: **Versus standard antipsychotic drugs:** We found one systematic review (search date 1998) that identified one small RCT (22 people) comparing depot haloperidol versus oral haloperidol.[13] It found no significant difference in the proportion of people with "no improvement" in global clinical impression at 4 months (8/11 [73%] with depot haloperidol v 9/11 [82%] with oral haloperidol; RR of no improvement 0.89, 95% CI 0.56 to 1.40). The RCT may have been too small to detect a clinically important difference.

Mental health

Harms: **Versus standard antipsychotic drugs:** The RCT found no significant difference between depot and oral haloperidol in the proportion of people who needed anticholinergic drugs for movement disorders (3/11 [27%] with depot haloperidol v 1/11 [9%] with oral haloperidol; RR 3.00, 95% CI 0.37 to 24.58).[13] Also see harms of haloperidol, p 228.

Comment: Depot injection is believed to ensure adherence, but we found no evidence from RCTs to support this.

OPTION **CLOZAPINE**

One systematic review found that clozapine improved symptoms over 4–10 weeks compared with standard antipsychotic drugs. However, RCTs found that clozapine may be associated with blood dyscrasias. One systematic review of small RCTs provided insufficient evidence to compare clozapine versus other newer antipsychotic drugs.

Benefits: **Versus standard antipsychotic drugs:** We found one systematic review (search date 1999, 31 RCTs, 2589 people), which compared clozapine versus standard antipsychotic drugs, such as chlorpromazine and haloperidol.[14] It found that clozapine significantly reduced the proportion of people with no clinical improvement over 4–10 weeks compared with standard antipsychotic drugs (14 RCTs; 267/561 [48%] with clozapine v 377/570 [66%] with standard antipsychotics; RR of no important improvement 0.75, 95% CI 0.66 to 0.84). This means that, on average, six people will need to be treated for one to improve (NNT 6, 95% CI 5 to 7). The review found that, despite the requirement for regular blood tests, significantly fewer people withdrew from treatment with clozapine over 7–24 months compared with standard antipsychotic drugs (111/750 [15%] with clozapine v 140/763 [18%] with standard antipsychotics; RR 0.76, 95% CI 0.66 to 0.92). **Versus other new antipsychotic drugs:** We found one systematic review (search date 1999, 8 RCTs, 795 people).[15] Five of the RCTs identified by the review were in people with treatment resistant schizophrenia (see benefits of clozapine in people who are resistant to standard antipsychotic drugs, p 245).

Harms: **Versus standard antipsychotic drugs:** The review found that, compared with standard antipsychotic drugs, clozapine was significantly more likely to cause hypersalivation (351/699 [50%] with clozapine v 161/720 [22%] with standard antipsychotics; RR 2.23, 95% CI 1.95 to 2.57; NNH 3, 95% CI 3 to 4), increased temperature (129/560 [23%] with clozapine v 86/587 [15%] with standard antipsychotics; RR 1.57, 95% CI 1.27 to 1.98; NNH 11, 95% CI 7 to 25), and sedation (392/751 [52%] with clozapine v 332/776 [43%] with standard antipsychotics; RR 1.23, 95% CI 1.13 to 1.34; NNH 10, 95% CI 6 to 22), but that it was less likely to cause dry mouth (40/397 [10%] with clozapine v 111/402 [28%] with standard antipsychotics; RR 0.36, 95% CI 0.26 to 0.51; NNT 6, 95% CI 4 to 8) and extrapyramidal adverse effects (202/614 [33%] with clozapine v 304/621 [49%] with standard antipsychotics; RR 0.67, 95% CI 0.58 to 0.77; NNT 6, 95% CI 5 to 9).[14] A large case series found leucopenia in 3% of 99 502 people taking clozapine over 5 years.[16] However, it found that monitoring white cell (neutrophil) counts was associated with a lower rate of cases of agranulocytosis in people taking clozapine (382 v 995; AR 0.38% v 1%) and deaths (12 v 149).[16] The review found that clozapine significantly increased blood problems, including leucopenia and neutropenia compared with standard antipsychotic drugs (24/637 [4%] with clozapine v 12/656 [2%] with standard antipsychotics; RR 1.85, 95% CI 0.99 to 3.47).[14] We found one systematic review (search date 1996, 12 RCTs, all included in the first review) that performed a meta-regression analysis combining results with various new antipsychotic drugs and comparing them with results with haloperidol.[17] It found that the difference in withdrawal rates did not persist after controlling for dose of haloperidol.

Comment: Some of the benefits of clozapine were more apparent in the long term, depending on which drug was used for comparison in the RCTs.

OPTION   AMISULPRIDE

Three systematic reviews found limited evidence that amisulpride may improve symptoms more than standard antipsychotic drugs, although one of the reviews suggested that effects may be attributable to differences in dose. The reviews found that extrapyramidal adverse effects were less likely with amisulpride than with standard antipsychotic drugs. RCTs found no significant difference in symptoms between amisulpride and olanzapine or risperidone.

Benefits: **Versus standard antipsychotic drugs**: We found three systematic reviews.[17-19] The first systematic review (search date 2000) identified four RCTs (651 people), which compared amisulpride versus a standard antipsychotic (haloperidol [3 RCTs] or flupentixol [1 RCT]), and used the Clinical Global Impression scale to assess outcomes.[18] It found that amisulpride significantly reduced the proportion of people who were less than "much improved" in global clinical impression compared with standard antipsychotic drugs (107/324 [33%] with amisulpride v 163/327 [50%] with standard antipsychotics; RR of failing to improve 0.66, 95% CI 0.55 to 0.80; NNT 6, 95% CI 5 to 11). It also found that amisulpride significantly reduced the proportion of people who left the study early (14 RCTs; 282/881 [32%] with amisulpride v 242/631 [38%] with standard antipsychotics; RR 0.72, 95% CI 0.62 to 0.83; NNT 9, 95% CI 7 to 16). The second systematic review (search date 1998, 4 RCTs, including 2 RCTs identified by the first review, duration 4–6 weeks, 683 people) compared amisulpride versus standard antipsychotic drugs, usually haloperidol.[17] It is unclear whether allocation concealment was adequately performed in all included RCTs. It found that symptom reduction was greater with amisulpride than with standard antipsychotic drugs (standardised effect size –0.35, 95% CI –0.52 to –0.18), indicating that about 64% (95% CI 57% to 70%) of people do worse with standard antipsychotic drugs than with amisulpride. It also found that, compared with standard antipsychotic drugs, amisulpride significantly reduced the proportion of people who withdrew from the trial (NNH 9, 95% CI 5 to 22). All four short term RCTs identified by the review included people randomised to relatively high doses of amisulpride (estimated equivalent to 20 mg haloperidol), which may have exaggerated results in favour of amisulpride.[17] The review performed a meta-regression analysis and found that, after adjustment for dose differences in standard antipsychotics (usually haloperidol or chlorpromazine), newer antipsychotic drugs (amisulpride, olanzapine, quetiapine, risperidone) lose their therapeutic advantage over standard antipsychotic drugs. Meta-regression was not available for amisulpride alone. The third systematic review (11 RCTs, 6 of which were included in the first or second review) found that amisulpride improved Brief Psychiatric Rating Scale (BPRS) scores compared with haloperidol or flupentixol (mean effect size 0.11; CI not stated; no further data provided).[19] It also found that people taking amisulpride were less likely to withdraw from the study early. **Versus olanzapine:** We found no systematic review but found one RCT (377 people) comparing amisulpride versus olanzapine for 2 months' treatment.[20] It found no significant difference in symptoms at 2 months assessed by BPRS score (mean reduction 17.6 with amisulpride v 16.3 with olanzapine; reported as non-significant; CI not stated). **Versus risperidone:** The first review identified one RCT (228 people), which found no significant difference between amisulpride and risperidone in BPRS symptom scores.[18]

Harms: **Versus standard antipsychotic drugs:** The first review found that, compared with standard antipsychotic drugs, amisulpride significantly reduced the proportion of people who had at least one adverse effect (6 RCTs; 261/373 [70%] with amisulpride v 308/378 [81%] with standard antipsychotics; RR 0.85, 95% CI 0.79 to 0.92; NNT 9, 95% 5% CI 6 to 17).[18] It also found that people taking amisulpride were significantly less likely to experience at least one extrapyramidal symptom (7 RCTs; 161/383 [42%] with amisulpride v 234/388 [60%] with standard antipsychotics; RR 0.68, 95% CI 0.60 to 0.79; NNT 5, 95% CI 4 to 8). The second review found that movement disorders, measured by the Simpson Angus scale, were significantly less frequent with amisulpride compared with standard antipsychotic drugs (SMD −0.44, 95% CI −0.26 to −0.61).[17] The reduction in extrapyramidal adverse effects remained significant despite adjustment for dose differences in standard antipsychotics.[17] The third systematic review found that people taking amisulpride experienced fewer movement disorders than people taking standard antipsychotic drugs.[19] It found that amisulpride significantly reduced the use of antiparkinsonian medication compared with standard antipsychotic drugs (effect size 0.25, 95% CI 0.17 to 0.32). **Versus olanzapine:** The RCT found that significantly fewer people had clinically important weight gain (more than 7% total body weight) with amisulpride than with olanzapine (27/189 [14%] with amisulpride v 48/188 [25%] with olanzapine; P = 0.007).[20] **Versus risperidone:** The RCT identified by the first review found no significant difference in adverse effects, extrapyramidal symptoms, or withdrawal rate between amisulpride and risperidone.[18]

Comment: None.

OPTION	LOXAPINE

One systematic review comparing loxapine versus standard antipsychotic drugs found no significant difference in global improvement or adverse effects.

Benefits: **Versus standard antipsychotic drugs:** We found one systematic review (search date 1999, 22 RCTs, 1073 people), which compared loxapine (dose range 25–250 mg/day) versus standard antipsychotic drugs, primarily chlorpromazine.[21] It found no significant difference in clinical global improvement between loxapine and standard antipsychotic drugs (9 RCTs; 59/206 [29%] with loxapine v 65/205 [32%] with standard antipsychotics; RR of no improvement 0.82, 95% CI 0.52 to 1.31).

Harms: The review found no significant difference in adverse effects between loxapine and standard antipsychotic drugs (11 RCTs; 164/255 [64%] with loxapine v 166/251 [66%] with standard antipsychotics; RR 0.90, 95% CI 0.57 to 1.41).[21]

Comment: All of the RCTs identified by the review were conducted in the USA or India and none lasted longer than 12 weeks.[21]

OPTION	MOLINDONE

One systematic review found no significant difference in global clinical improvement or in the proportion of people who had adverse effects over 4–12 weeks between molindone and standard antipsychotic drugs.

Benefits: **Versus standard antipsychotic drugs:** We found one systematic review (search date 1999, 9 RCTs, 4 CCTs, 150 people) comparing molindone versus standard antipsychotic drugs, primarily haloperidol or chlorpromazine.[22] It found no significant difference between molindone and standard antipsychotic drugs in global clinical improvement over 4–12 weeks as assessed by a physician (4 RCTs; 25/84 [29.8%] with molindone v 20/66 [30.3%] with standard antipsychotics; RR of no improvement 1.10, 95% CI 0.68 to 1.78).

Harms: **Versus standard antipsychotic drugs:** The review found no significant difference between molindone and standard antipsychotic drugs in movement disorders (rigidity, tremor, akasthesia, use of antiparkinsonian medication) or in the proportion of people who had adverse effects (2 RCTs, 1 CCT; 24/42 [57%] with molindone v 25/42 [59%] with standard antipsychotics; RR 0.96, 95% CI 0.73 to 1.27).[22] One RCT identified by the review found that significantly more people taking molindone compared with standard antipsychotic drugs experienced confusion (9/14 [64%] with molindone v 6/30 [20%] with standard antipsychotics; RR 3.21, 95% CI 1.42 to 7.26). The review also found that significantly more people had weight loss with molindone than with standard antipsychotic drugs (2 RCTs; 12/30 [40%] with molindone v 4/30 [13%] with standard antipsychotics; RR 2.78, 95% CI 1.10 to 6.99) and

Mental health

that fewer people had weight gain with molindone than with standard antipsychotic drugs (2 RCTs; 4/30 [13%] with molindone *v* 11/30 [37%] with standard antipsychotics; RR 0.39, 95% CI 0.95 to 1.00).

Comment: None.

OPTION   OLANZAPINE

Systematic reviews found limited evidence that olanzapine may improve symptoms more than standard antipsychotic drugs and good evidence that olanzapine has fewer adverse effects, although one of the reviews suggested that effects may be attributable to differences in dose. Systematic reviews found no clear difference in symptoms or adverse effects among olanzapine, amisulpride, risperidone, and clozapine.

Benefits: **Versus standard antipsychotic drugs:** We found three systematic reviews.[17,23,24] The first review (search date 1999, 15 RCTs, 3282 people) compared olanzapine versus standard antipsychotic drugs, usually haloperidol.[23] It found no significant difference in psychotic symptoms over 6–8 weeks between olanzapine (2.5–25 mg/day) and standard antipsychotic drugs (4 RCTs; 1056/1926 [55%] with olanzapine *v* 596/852 [70%] with standard antipsychotics; RR for no important response [defined as a 40% reduction on any scale] 0.90, 95% CI 0.76 to 1.06). The second review (search date 1998, 4 RCTs, all included in the first review, 2846 people) performed a meta-regression analysis comparing newer versus standard antipsychotics, which adjusted for dose of standard antipsychotic (see benefits of amisulpride, p 231).[17] Meta-regression analysis was not available for olanzapine alone. The third review (search date 1998, 3 RCTs, all included in the previous review, 2606 people) also found no significant difference in the mean change on a combined rating of positive and negative symptoms (Positive and Negative Syndrome Scale [PANSS]) between olanzapine and haloperidol.[24] However, it conducted a subsequent meta-regression analysis to control for confounding variables (e.g. age and duration of illness, among others) and found limited evidence that olanzapine significantly improved mean PANSS rating scale score compared with standard antipsychotics (WMD −5.9, 95% CI −11.1 to −0.6). The meta-regression analysis did not appear to take account of the dose of haloperidol.[24] **Versus clozapine:** See benefits of clozapine, p 230. **Versus amisulpride:** See benefits of amisulpride, p 231. **Versus risperidone:** We found two systematic reviews[25,26] and one subsequent RCT.[27] The first review (search date 1999, 3 RCTs) found that olanzapine improved mean PANSS scores at 28–30 weeks compared with risperidone (2 RCTs, 392 people; WMD 7.5 points, 95% CI 2.9 to 12.0 on a scale of 210 points), although it found no significant difference at 54 weeks (1 RCT, 435 people; WMD 6.1, 95% CI 1.9 to 10.3).[25] Olanzapine was also associated with significantly fewer withdrawals for any cause at 28–30 weeks than risperidone (2 RCTs; 85/204 [42%] with olanzapine *v* 109/200 [54%] with risperidone; RR 0.76, 95% CI 0.62 to 0.94).[25] The second review (search review 2000, 2 RCTs, including 1 RCT identified by the first review) found similar results but did not quantify its conclusions.[26] The subsequent RCT

(377 people) found no significant difference between olanzapine and risperidone in the proportion of people who responded at 8 weeks (response defined as a < 20% reduction in PANSS score: 48% with olanzapine v 51% with risperidone; reported as non-significant; no further data provided).[27]

Harms:
Versus standard antipsychotic drugs: The first review found no significant difference between olanzapine and standard antipsychotic drugs in the proportion of people who withdrew from the trial for any cause at 4–8 weeks (9 RCTs; 744/2068 [36%] with olanzapine v 464/952 [49%] with standard antipsychotics; RR 0.85, 95% CI 0.65 to 1.10) or at 1 year (4 RCTs; 1577/1905 [83%] v 748/833 [90%]; RR 0.90, 95% CI 0.75 to 1.08).[23] It found that, compared with standard antipsychotic drugs, olanzapine significantly reduced the proportion of people who required anticholinergic drugs for extrapyramidal adverse effects (293/1884 [15%] with olanzapine v 401/810 [49%] with standard antipsychotics; RR 0.26, 95% CI 0.17 to 0.40) and caused significantly less nausea (174/1576 [11%] with olanzapine v 117/771 [15%] with standard antipsychotics; RR 0.74, 95% CI 0.59 to 0.92; NNT 25, 95% CI 14 to 85), vomiting (97/1336 [7%] with olanzapine v 81/660 [12%] with standard antipsychotics; RR 0.59, 95% CI 0.45 to 0.78; NNT 20, 95% CI 12 to 46), or drowsiness (443/1576 [28%] with olanzapine v 268/771 [34%] with standard antipsychotics; RR 0.82, 95% CI 0.72 to 0.92; NNT 15, 95% CI 9 to 38). Olanzapine was associated with a significantly greater increase in appetite (1 RCT; 343/1336 [26%] with olanzapine v 103/660 [16%] with standard antipsychotics; RR 1.65, 95% CI 1.35 to 2.01; NNH 10, 95% CI 7 to 15) and weight gain than standard antipsychotic drugs.[23] The second review found that fewer people withdrew from the trial with olanzapine than with haloperidol, but the difference did not persist after adjustment for dose.[17] It found that dystonia and akathisia were significantly less frequent with olanzapine than with haloperidol, even after adjustment for dose (ARR for dystonia with olanzapine v haloperidol 14%, 95% CI 11% to 17%; ARR for akathisia with olanzapine v haloperidol 4.8%, 95% CI 3.1% to 6.5%). Olanzapine was associated with a 12% (95% CI 8% to 15%) increase in excessive appetite compared with haloperidol.[17]
Versus clozapine: See harms of clozapine, p 230. **Versus amisulpride:** See harms of amisulpride, p 232. **Versus risperidone:** The first review found that olanzapine was associated with significantly fewer extrapyramidal adverse effects compared with risperidone (1 RCT; 32/172 [19%] with olanzapine v 52/167 [31%] with risperidone; RR 0.60, 95% CI 0.41 to 0.88; NNT 8, 95% CI 5 to 28), less parkinsonism (1 RCT; 22/172 [13%] with olanzapine v 37/167 [22%] with risperidone; RR 0.58, 95% CI 0.37 to 0.94; NNT 11, 95% CI 6 to 77), and less need for antiparkinsonian medication (1 RCT; 34/172 [20%] with olanzapine v 55/167 [33%] with risperidone; RR 0.60, 95% CI 0.41 to 0.87; NNT 8, 95% CI 4 to 25).[25] People taking olanzapine had greater weight gain, but the difference was not significant either at 28–30 weeks (2 RCTs: WMD +2.86, 95% CI −0.68 to +6.34) or at 54 weeks (WMD +3.56, 95% CI −0.20 to +6.90). The second review found similar results but did not perform a meta-analysis.[26] The subsequent RCT found

no significant difference between olanzapine and risperidone in severity of extrapyramidal adverse effects, need for anticholinergics, or withdrawals from the trial.[27] Fewer people on risperidone experienced clinically important weight gain (AR for ≥ 7% weight gain 27.3% with olanzapine v 11.6% with risperidone).

Comment: **Versus standard antipsychotic drugs:** The results of the reviews are dominated by one large multicentre RCT reported by drug company employees.[17,23,24] Benefits seem to be highest at a dose of 15 mg daily, and higher doses may be associated with more harms. Results depended on the statistical test used, and their reliability may be compromised by heterogeneity.

OPTION	PERAZINE

Two weak RCTs found no significant difference in global clinical impression over 28 days between perazine and haloperidol. Two RCTs provided insufficient evidence to assess perazine compared with zotepine, and one RCT found no significant difference in mental state at 28 days between perazine and amisulpride. Three RCTs found no significant difference in extrapyramidal effects over 28 days between perazine and zotepine or amisulpride.

Benefits: **Versus standard antipsychotic drugs:** We found one systematic review (search date 2001), which identified two RCTs (71 people) comparing perazine versus haloperidol.[28] It could not perform a meta-analysis because of poor reporting in one of the RCTs. One of the RCTs (32 people) found no significant difference between perazine and haloperidol in the proportion of people who were "no better or worse" in global clinical impression at 28 days (8/17 [47%] with perazine v 6/15 [60%] with haloperidol; RR 1.18, 95% CI 0.53 to 2.62). **Versus other new antipsychotic drugs:** The review identified two RCTs comparing perazine versus zotepine.[28] It could not perform a meta-analysis because of methodological differences between the RCTs. The first RCT (34 people) found that perazine was significantly less effective than zotepine in improving symptoms as assessed by mean Brief Psychiatric Rating Scale score at 28 days (WMD 7.9, 95% CI 1.1 to 14.7). The second RCT (40 people), which used a different method to calculate mean Brief Psychiatric Rating Scale score, found that perazine was significantly more effective than zotepine in improving symptoms at the end of the trial (trial duration not specified: WMD −0.4, 95% −0.7 to −0.1). One RCT identified by the review found no significant difference between perazine and amisulpride in the proportion of people whose mental state was "no better or worse" at 28 days (4/15 [27%] with perazine v 3/15 [20%] with amisulpride; RR 1.33, 95% CI 0.36 to 4.97).[28]

Harms: **Versus standard antipsychotic drugs:** The review gave no information about the adverse effects of perazine compared with haloperidol.[28] **Versus other new antipsychotic drugs:** The review (3 RCTs) found no significant difference between perazine and zotepine or amisulpride in the risk of akathisia (3/56 [5%] with

perazine v 10/55 [18%] with zotepine or amisulpride; RR 0.30, 95%
CI 0.09 to 1.00), dyskinesia (1/56 [2%] v 3/55 [5%]; RR 0.42, 95%
CI 0.06 to 2.74), or parkinsonism over 28 days (10/41 [24%] with
perazine v 8/40 [20%] with zotepine or amisulpride; RR 1.22, 95%
CI 0.54 to 2.78).[28]

Comment: None.

OPTION   PIMOZIDE

**One systematic review comparing pimozide versus standard antipsychotic
drugs found no significant difference in global clinical impression, and
found that pimozide decreased sedation but increased tremor. It found no
overall difference in cardiovascular adverse effects such as rise or fall in
blood pressure or dizziness between pimozide and standard antipsychotic
drugs.**

Benefits: **Versus standard antipsychotic drugs:** We found one systematic
review (search date 1999) comparing pimozide (mean dose
7.5 mg/day, range 1–75 mg/day) versus standard antipsychotic
drugs, including chlorpromazine, haloperidol, fluphenazine, and
carpipramine.[29] It found no significant difference in global clinical
impression between pimozide and standard antipsychotics at 1–3
months (3 RCTs; 18/50 [36%] with pimozide v 22/50 [44%] with
standard antipsychotics; RR 0.82, 95% CI 0.52 to 1.29) or at 4–6
months (6 RCTs; 57/104 [55%] with pimozide v 55/102 [54%] with
standard antipsychotics; RR 1.01, 95% CI 0.80 to 1.28).

Harms: **Versus standard antipsychotic drugs:** The review found that,
over 1–3 months, pimozide caused significantly less sedation than
standard antipsychotic drugs (53/117 [45%] with pimozide v
68/115 [59%] with standard antipsychotics; RR 0.77, 95% CI 0.61
to 0.98; NNT 7, 95% CI 4 to 61), but that it was more likely to cause
tremor (43/97 [44%] with pimozide v 27/95 [28%] with standard
antipsychotics; RR 1.57, 95 CI 1.07 to 2.29; NNH 6, 95% CI 3 to
44).[29] It found similar cardiovascular symptoms such as rise or fall
in blood pressure and dizziness between pimozide and standard
antipsychotic drugs. There was little usable ECG data. One RCT in
the review found no significant difference in ECG changes between
pimozide and standard antipsychotic drugs, but it may have been
too small to detect a clinically important difference (2/28 [7%] with
pimozide v 3/28 [11%] with standard antipsychotics; RR 0.67, 95%
CI 0.1 to 3.7).

Comment: Sudden death has been reported in a number of people taking
pimozide at doses over 20 mg daily, but we found no evidence from
RCTs that pimozide is more likely to cause sudden death than other
antipsychotic drugs.[29] The manufacturer recommends periodic ECG
monitoring in all people taking more than 16 mg daily pimozide and
avoidance of other drugs known to prolong the QT interval on an
ECG or cause electrolyte disturbances (other antipsychotic drugs,
antihistamines, antidepressants, and diuretics).

Schizophrenia

OPTION	QUETIAPINE

Three systematic reviews comparing quetiapine versus standard antipsychotic drugs found no significant difference in symptoms, but two of the reviews found that quetiapine reduced akathisia, parkinsonism, and the proportion of people who left the trial early.

Benefits: **Versus standard antipsychotic drugs:** We found two systematic reviews.[17,30] The first review (search date 2000, 7 RCTs) compared quetiapine (50–800 mg/day) versus standard antipsychotic drugs (usually haloperidol).[30] It found no significant difference in mental state over 6 weeks between quetiapine and standard antipsychotic drugs (Brief Psychiatric Rating Scale or Positive and Negative Syndrome Scale score not improved, 4 RCTs; 367/723 [51%] with quetiapine v 283/524 [54%] with standard antipsychotics; RR 0.91, 95% CI 0.73 to 1.13). The second review (search date 1998, 2 RCTs, both included in the first review, 511 people) performed a meta-regression analysis comparing newer versus standard antipsychotics, which adjusted for dose of standard antipsychotic (see benefits of amisulpride, p 231).[17] Meta-regression was not available for quetiapine alone.

Harms: **Versus standard antipsychotic drugs:** The first review found that, compared with standard antipsychotic drugs, quetiapine was associated with significantly fewer people leaving trials early for any cause over 6 weeks (6 RCTs; 334/913 [36.5%] with quetiapine v 254/711 [35.7%] with standard antipsychotics; RR 0.86, 95% CI 0.75 to 0.98), less dystonia (3 RCTs; 4/580 [0.69%] with quetiapine v 19/379 [5%] with standard antipsychotics; RR 0.24, 95% CI 0.04 to 0.49), less akathisia (3 RCTs; 19/580 [3%] with quetiapine v 68/379 [18%] with standard antipsychotics; RR 0.24, 95% CI 0.15 to 0.38), and less parkinsonism (2 RCTs; 31/479 [6%] with quetiapine v 92/279 [33%] with standard antipsychotics; RR 0.22, 95% CI 0.15 to 0.33), but more dry mouth (2 RCTs: 31/322 [10%] with quetiapine v 11/327 [3%] with standard antipsychotics; RR 2.85, 95% CI 1.46 to 5.57).[30]

Comment: The RCTs in the review had substantial withdrawal rates and did not conduct intention to treat analyses.[30]

OPTION	RISPERIDONE

Systematic reviews found limited evidence that risperidone may improve symptoms more than standard antipsychotic drugs (mainly haloperidol) and found good evidence that, at lower doses, risperidone has fewer adverse effects, although one of the reviews suggested that effects may be attributable to differences in dose. Systematic reviews found no significant difference in symptoms between risperidone and other new antipsychotic drugs.

Benefits: **Versus standard antipsychotic drugs:** We found three systematic reviews[17,24,31] and one additional RCT.[32] The first review (search date 1997, 14 RCTs, 3401 people) found that, at 12 weeks, risperidone (mean dose range 6.1–12 mg/day) significantly increased the proportion of people who had "clinical improvement" compared with standard antipsychotic drugs, usually haloperidol.[31]

"Clinical improvement" was variably defined but usually as a 20% reduction in symptoms (11 RCTs; 894/2088 [43%] with risperidone v 482/893 [54%] with standard antipsychotics; RR of no clinical improvement 0.81, 95% CI 0.75 to 0.88; NNT 10, 95% CI 7 to 16). The review did not find significant heterogeneity among RCTs. The second review (search date 1998, 8 RCTs, all included in the first review) found "substantial heterogeneity" among six RCTs of 4–12 weeks' treatment.[17] It found that risperidone improved symptom scores over 12 months compared with standard antipsychotic drugs (2 RCTs; WMD –0.40, 95% CI –0.27 to –0.54, indicating that about 66% of people taking standard antipsychotics had worse composite symptom scores than with risperidone). Meta-regression analysis suggested that this difference did not persist after controlling for dose of standard antipsychotic (see benefits of amisulpride, p 231). The third review (search date 1998, 11 RCTs, including 8 identified by the first review, 1208 people) found that risperidone significantly improved negative and positive symptoms, as measured using the Positive and Negative Syndrome Scale, compared with haloperidol (WMD –8.3, 95% CI –13.8 to –2.7).[24] The additional RCT (99 people) comparing a range of doses of risperidone versus haloperidol found no significant difference in the proportion of people who responded over 8 weeks (response defined as ≥ 20% reduction in Positive and Negative Syndrome Scale; reported as non-significant; results presented graphically).[32] **Versus olanzapine:** See benefits of olanzapine, p 234. **Versus amisulpride:** See benefits of amisulpride, p 231. **Versus clozapine:** See benefits of clozapine, p 230.

Harms: **Versus standard antipsychotic drugs:** The first review found no significant difference between risperidone and standard antipsychotic drugs in the proportion of people who withdrew from treatment because of adverse effects (139/1585 [9%] with risperidone v 70/591 [12%] with standard antipsychotics; RR 0.78, 95% CI 0.58 to 1.05).[31] It found that, compared with people taking standard antipsyschotic drugs, people taking risperidone developed significantly fewer extrapyramidal effects (347/1728 [20%] with risperidone v 234/551 [42%] with standard antipsychotics; RR 0.63, 95% CI 0.55 to 0.72; NNT 5, 95% CI 5 to 10), required less antiparkinsonian medication (444/1810 [24%] with risperidone v 274/626 [44%] with standard antipsychotics; RR 0.64, 95% CI 0.57 to 0.73; NNT 7, 95% CI 5 to 10), and were less likely to develop daytime somnolence (481/1509 [32%] with risperidone v 197/589 [33%] with standard antipsychotics; RR 0.87, 95% CI 0.76 to 0.99; NNT 22, 95% CI 11 to 500). However, it found that risperidone was associated with significantly more weight gain than standard antipsychotics (398/1290 [31%] with risperidone v 71/362 [20%] with standard antipsychotics; RR 1.37, 95% CI 1.10 to 1.71; NNH 13, 95% CI 8 to 36). The second review found no significant difference between risperidone and haloperidol in the proportion of people who withdrew from treatment, but found that risperidone reduced symptoms of dystonia (WMD –0.26, 95% CI –0.39 to –0.12), parkinsonism (WMD –0.39, 95% CI –0.51 to –0.27), and dyskinesia (WMD –0.16, 95% CI –0.28 to –0.04).[17] Differences persisted after controlling for dose. The third review found that, compared with haloperidol, risperidone significantly reduced the proportion of people who required medication for extrapyramidal side effects (OR 0.42, 95% CI 0.19 to 0.96; absolute numbers presented graphically).[24] The additional RCT found no significant difference in the rate of overall adverse effects between risperidone and haloperidol.[32] **Versus olanzapine:** See harms of olanzapine, p 235 **Versus amisulpride:** See harms of amisulpride, p 232. **Versus clozapine:** See harms of clozapine, p 230.

Comment: The first review found evidence of publication bias.[31] Sensitivity analyses found that benefits in clinical improvement and continuing treatment of risperidone compared with standard antipsychotic drugs were no longer significant if RCTs using more than 10 mg haloperidol daily were excluded. This could be because of loss of power. Exclusion of the higher dosage RCTs did not remove the difference in rate of extrapyramidal adverse effects.[31]

OPTION   SULPIRIDE

One systematic review found no significant difference in global clinical impression over 4–10 weeks between sulpiride and standard antipsychotic drugs. The review found that the use of antiparkinson drugs over 4–10 weeks was less frequent with sulpiride compared with standard antipsychotic drugs.

Benefits: **Versus standard antipsychotic drugs:** One systematic review (search date 1998, 7 RCTs, 366 people) found no significant difference in the proportion of people who had no improvement in global clinical impression over 4–10 weeks between sulpiride and standard antipsychotic drugs, usually haloperidol chlorpromazine, or perphenazine (74/248 [30%] with sulpiride v 96/266 [36%] with standard antipsychotics; RR of no important improvement 0.82, 95% CI 0.64 to 1.05).[33]

Harms: **Versus standard antipsychotic drugs:** The review found that the use of antiparkinson drugs over 4–10 weeks was significantly less frequent with sulpiride compared with standard antipsychotic drugs (84/253 [33%] v 115/258 [44%]; RR 0.73, 95% CI 0.59 to 0.90).[33]

Comment: The review stated that the other two RCTs it identified reported improvement in mental state with sulpiride compared with placebo, but that no raw data could be obtained because of poor reporting in the RCTs.[33] Observational evidence and clinical experience suggest that sulpiride may be associated with galactorrhoea, but RCT data did not quantify the risk.[34]

OPTION   ZIPRASIDONE

One systematic review found no significant difference in mental state improvement between ziprasidone and haloperidol, and found that ziprasidone reduced akathisia and acute dystonia but increased nausea and vomiting.

Benefits: **Versus standard antipsychotic drugs:** We found one systematic review comparing ziprasidone versus standard antipsychotic drugs.[35] The review (search date 1999, 4 RCTs, 690 people) identified one RCT (301 people) that provided sufficient data to assess clinically important improvement in mental state (≥20% reduction in Positive and Negative Syndrome Scale score). It found no significant difference in mental state between ziprasidone and haloperidol (95/148 [64%] with ziprasidone v 114/153 [74%] with haloperidol; RR of no important improvement in mental state 0.86, 95% CI 0.74 to 1.00).

Harms: **Versus standard antipsychotic drugs:** The review found no clear difference in overall adverse effects between ziprasidone and haloperidol.[35] It found that, compared with haloperidol, ziprasidone was significantly less likely to cause akathisia over 1 week (2 RCTs; 19/296 [6%] with ziprasidone v 27/142 [19%] with haloperidol; RR 0.34, 95% CI 0.20 to 0.59; NNH 8, 95% CI 5 to 18) and over 28 weeks (1 RCT; 7/148 [5%] with ziprasidone v 25/153 [16%] with haloperidol; RR 0.3, 95% CI 0.1 to 0.7; NNH 9, 95% CI 5 to 21), and that it was less likely to cause acute dystonia over 1 week (2 RCTs; 13/296 [4%] with ziprasidone v 15/142 [10%] with haloperidol; RR 0.42, 95% CI 0.20 to 0.85; NNH 16, 95% CI 9 to 166). Ziprasidone was associated with significantly more nausea and vomiting both over 1 week (59/206 [29%] with ziprasidone v 8/100 [8%] with haloperidol; RR 3.58, 95% CI 1.78 to 7.20; NNH 5, 95% CI 4 to 8) and over 28 weeks (1 RCT; 31/148 [21%] with ziprasidone v 15/153 [10%] with haloperidol; RR 2.14, 95% CI 1.20 to 3.79; NNH 9, 95% CI 5 to 33) compared with haloperidol.

Comment: The duration of RCTs in the review was less than 6 weeks.[35] Most RCTs reported a withdrawal rate of over 20% and no RCT clearly described adequate precautions for the blinding of treatment allocation.

OPTION ZOTEPINE

One systematic review found weak evidence that zotepine increased the proportion of people with a clinically important improvement in symptoms compared with standard antipsychotic drugs, and reduced akasthesia, dystonia, and rigidity. This finding was not robust because removal of a single RCT from the analysis meant that the difference between zotepine and standard antipsychotics was no longer significant.

Benefits: **Versus standard antipsychotic drugs:** We found one systematic review (search date 1999, 8 RCTs, 356 people) comparing zotepine (75–450 mg/day) versus standard antipsychotic drugs, usually haloperidol.[36] It found that zotepine was significantly more likely than standard antipsychotic drugs to bring about "clinically important improvement" at 4–12 weeks, as defined by a pre-stated cut off point on the Brief Psychiatric Rating Scale (4 RCTs; 89/179 [50%] with zotepine v 62/177 [35%] with standard antipsychotics; RR 1.25, 95% CI 1.1 to 1.4; NNT 7, 95% CI 4 to 22; see comment below).

Harms: The review found that, compared with standard antipsychotic drugs, zotepine caused significantly less akathisia (67/199 [34%] with zotepine v 91/197 [46%] with standard antipsychotics; RR 0.73, 95% CI 0.58 to 0.93; NNT 8, 95% CI 5 to 34), dystonia (7/35 [20%] with zotepine v 15/35 [43%] with standard antipsychotics;

RR 0.47, 95% CI 0.24 to 0.93; NNT 4, 95% CI 2 to 56), and rigidity (19/83 [23%] with zotepine v 30/81 [37%] with standard antipsychotics; RR 0.63, 95% CI 0.40 to 0.98; NNT 7, 95% CI 4 to 360).[36] Two RCTs found abnormal ECG results in people taking zotepine, but few additional details were given.

Comment: All but one RCT identified by the review were of 12 weeks' or less duration and all were conducted in Europe.[36] Only one RCT favoured zotepine over standard antipsychotic drugs, and removal of this RCT from the analysis renders the results non-significant.

QUESTION Which interventions reduce relapse rates?

OPTION CONTINUED TREATMENT WITH ANTIPSYCHOTIC DRUGS

Systematic reviews have found that continuing antipsychotic drugs for at least 6 months after an acute episode reduces relapse rates compared with no treatment or placebo, and that some benefit of continuing antipsychotics is apparent for up to 2 years. Eight systematic reviews found no significant difference in relapse rates among antipsychotic drugs. One systematic review found that clozapine reduces relapse rates over 12 weeks compared with standard antipsychotic drugs. Another review found that fewer people taking depot zuclopenthixol decanoate relapsed over 12 weeks to 1 year compared with people taking other depot preparations. A third review found that bromperidol increased the proportion of people who relapsed compared with haloperidol or fluphenazine. One additional RCT found that risperidone reduced relapse over 2.2 years compared with haloperidol.

Benefits: **Versus no treatment or placebo:** We found three systematic reviews.[9,10,37] The first review (search date not stated, 66 studies, 4365 people taking antipsychotic drugs, mean dose 630 mg chlorpromazine equivalents daily, mean follow up of 6.3 months) included 29 controlled trials with a mean follow up of 9.7 months (see comment below).[37] It found that continuing compared with withdrawing antipsychotic drugs significantly reduced the proportion of people who relapsed (28 controlled studies, 2448 people; 16% with continued treatment v 51% with withdrawing treatment; ARR 35%, 95% CI 33% to 38%; NNT 3, 95% CI 3 to 4). Over time, the relapse rate in people maintained on antipsychotic treatment approached that in those withdrawn from treatment, but was still lower in those on treatment at 2 years. The second review (search date 1997, 5 RCTs, 2 included in the first review) found that continuing chlorpromazine significantly reduced relapse rates over 6–24 months compared with placebo (3 RCTs; 106/264 [40%] with chlorpromazine v 176/248 [71%] with placebo; RR 0.57, 95% CI 0.48 to 0.67; NNT 3, 95% CI 3 to 4).[9] The third review (search date 1998, 2 RCTs, neither included in the previous reviews, 70 people currently in remission) compared haloperidol versus placebo over 1 year.[10] It found that haloperidol significantly reduced relapse over 1 year compared with placebo (32/47 [68%] with haloperidol v 23/23 [100%] with placebo; RR 0.67, 95% CI 0.54 to 0.83, NNT 4, 95% CI 2 to 7). **Choice of drug:** We found 11 systematic reviews[12–14,23,29,38–43] and one additional RCT[44] evaluating the effects of newer versus older antipsychotics, newer antipsychotics versus each other, and oral versus intramuscular administration of antibiotics on relapse rates (see table 1, p 253). Eight reviews found no significant difference between antipsychotics in relapse rates,[13,23,29,38–42] but in two of the reviews[23,29] the number of people studied was too small to rule out a clinically important difference. A ninth review (search date 1998) found that clozapine significantly reduced relapse rates over 12 weeks compared with standard antipsychotics (19 RCTs; RR 0.6, 95% CI 0.5 to 0.8).[14] A tenth review (search date 1998) found that significantly fewer people taking depot zuclopenthixol decanoate relapsed over 12 weeks to 1 year compared with people taking other depot preparations (3 RCTs; 296 people: RR 0.7, 95% CI 0.6 to 1.0; NNT 9, 95% CI 5 to 53).[43] An eleventh review (search date 1999) found that bromperidol significantly increased the proportion of people who relapsed compared with haloperidol or fluphenazine (2 RCTs; RR 3.92, 95% CI 1.05 to 14.6; NNH 5, 95% CI 3 to 28).[12] The additional RCT (365 people) found that risperidone versus haloperidol significantly reduced relapse over 2.2 years (NNT 5, 95% CI 4 to 10).[44]

Harms: **Versus no treatment or placebo:** The first review found that mild transient nausea, malaise, sweating, vomiting, insomnia, and dyskinesia were reported in an unspecified number of people after sudden drug cessation, but were usually acceptable with gradual dose reduction.[37] The other reviews gave no information on adverse effects of continuing treatment with antipsychotic drugs.[9,10] **Choice of drug:** The review comparing different depot antipsychotic drugs found that the annual incidence of tardive dyskinesia was 5%.[43]

Comment: In the systematic review of continued treatment versus withdrawal of treatment, meta-analysis of the 29 controlled trials gave similar results to those obtained when all 66 studies were included.[37] A commentary of the review suggested that it was weakened because all RCT results were used rather than weighted comparisons, no length of time was given since the last acute episode, and no distinction was made between people experiencing a first episode and those with chronic illness.[45] Some clinicians use depot antipsychotic drugs in selected people to ensure adherence to medication. We found no evidence from RCTs to support this practice.

| OPTION | COGNITIVE BEHAVIOURAL THERAPY |

Limited evidence from a systematic review of two RCTs found no significant difference in relapse rates between cognitive behavioural therapy plus standard care and standard care alone.

Benefits: We found one systematic review (search date 2001), which identified two RCTs (123 people) comparing the effects of cognitive behavioural therapy plus standard care versus standard care alone on relapse rates.[46] Both RCTs identified by the review incorporated challenging key beliefs, problem solving, and enhancement of coping. The review found no significant difference between cognitive behavioural therapy plus standard care and standard care alone in relapse or readmission to hospital over 10 weeks (1 RCT; 0/33 [0%] with cognitive behavioural therapy plus standard care *v* 4/28 [14%] with standard care alone; RR 0.09, 95% CI 0.01 to 1.69) or over 9–24 months (2 RCTs; 36/63 [57%] with cognitive behavioural therapy plus standard care *v* 31/60 [52%] with standard care alone; RR 1.13, 95% CI 0.82 to 1.56).[46]

Harms: The systematic review gave no information on harms.[46]

Comment: None.

OPTION   FAMILY INTERVENTIONS

One systematic review found that multiple session family interventions reduced relapse rates at 12 months compared with usual care, single session family interventions, or psychoeducational interventions.

Benefits: We found one systematic review (search date 1999) that compared multiple family interventions versus usual care, single family interventions, or psychoeducational interventions.[47] Family interventions consisted mainly of education about the illness and training in problem solving over at least six weekly sessions. The review found that multiple family interventions significantly reduced relapse rates at 12 months compared with other interventions (11 RCTs, 729 people; OR 0.52, 95% CI 0.31 to 0.89; absolute numbers not provided). On average, eight families would have to be treated to avoid one additional relapse (and likely hospitalisation) at 12 months in the family member with schizophrenia (NNT 8, 95% CI 6 to 18).[47]

Harms: The review gave no information on harms.[47]

Comment: These results may overestimate the effect of family interventions because of the difficulty of blinding people and investigators.[47] Although no harms were reported, illness education could possibly have adverse consequences on morale and outlook. The mechanism for the effects of family intervention remains unclear. It is thought to work by reducing "expressed emotion" (hostility and criticism) in relatives of people with schizophrenia. The time consuming nature of this intervention, which must normally take place at evenings or weekends, can limit its availability. It cannot be applied to people who have little contact with home based carers.

OPTION   PSYCHOEDUCATIONAL INTERVENTIONS

One systematic review has found that psychoeducation reduces relapse rates at 9–18 months compared with usual care.

Benefits: **Versus usual treatment:** We found one systematic review (search date 2002), which identified one RCT of a brief individual intervention (10 sessions or less), six RCTs of brief group psychoeducational interventions, and four RCTs of standard length group psychoeducational interventions (11 sessions or more).[48] It found that standard length group psychoeducational interventions were significantly more effective than usual care in preventing relapse without readmission over 9–18 months (2 RCTs; 14/57 [24%] with psychoeducation *v* 24/57 [42%] with usual care; RR 0.58, 95% CI 0.34 to

0.99). It also found that brief group psychoeducational interventions were significantly more effective than usual care in preventing relapse or readmission over 1 year (5 RCTs; 153/326 [47%] with psychoeducation v 162/296 [55%] with usual care; RR 0.85, 95% CI 0.74 to 0.98; NNT 12, CI 6 to 83). The review found that any form of psychoeducation significantly reduced relapse with or without readmission to hospital over 9–18 months compared with usual care (6 RCTs; 176/383[46%] with psychoeducation v 192/337 [57%] with usual care; RR 0.78, 95% CI 0.62 to 0.98; NNT 9, 95% CI 6 to 22; see comment below).

Harms: The systematic review gave no information on harms.[48]

Comment: The systematic review found few good RCTs.[48] There was significant heterogeneity of both interventions and outcomes.

OPTION   **SOCIAL SKILLS TRAINING**

One systematic review of small RCTs provided insufficient evidence to assess social skills training.

Benefits: We found one systematic review (search date not stated 1999), which identified nine RCTs (471 people) comparing the effect of social skills training versus standard care or psychoeducational interventions on relapse rates.[49] It found no significant difference in relapse rates over 1 year of treatment between social skills training and other interventions (4 RCTs, 125 people; OR 0.74, 95% CI 0.43 to 1.29; absolute numbers not provided), but found that social skills training reduced relapse over 2 years of treatment (2 RCTs, 264 people; OR 3.03, 95% CI 1.11 to 8.33; absolute numbers not provided).

Harms: The review gave no information on harms.[49]

Comment: None.

QUESTION   **Which interventions are effective in people who are resistant to standard antipsychotic drugs?**

OPTION   **INTERVENTIONS IN PEOPLE WHO ARE RESISTANT TO STANDARD ANTIPSYCHOTIC DRUGS**

Systematic reviews in people resistant to standard antipsychotic drugs found that clozapine or olanzapine improved symptoms after 12 weeks and after 2 years compared with standard antipsychotic drugs. RCTs provided insufficient evidence to compare newer antipsychotics in people resistant to standard antipsychotic drugs.

Benefits: **Clozapine versus standard antipsychotic drugs:** We found one systematic review (search date 1999, 6 RCTs) comparing clozapine versus standard antipsychotic drugs in people who were resistant to standard treatment.[14] It found that, compared with standard antipsychotic drugs, clozapine significantly increased the proportion of people who improved at 6–12 weeks (4 RCTs, 370 people; RR for no improvement compared with standard antipsychotic drugs 0.7, 95% CI 0.6 to 0.8) and at 12–24 months (2 RCTs, 648 people;

RR 0.8, 95% CI 0.6 to 1.0). It found no difference in relapse rates at 12 weeks. **Clozapine versus other new antipsychotic drugs:** We found one systematic review (search date 1988, 8 RCTs, 5 in people with treatment resistant schizophrenia, 595 people), which compared clozapine versus olanzapine, risperidone, and zotepine.[15] It found no significant difference between clozapine and other new antipsychotics in global clinical impression (Clinical Global Impression [CGI] score: WMD −0.09, 95% CI −0.34 to +0.15) or mental state (Brief Psychiatric Rating Scale or Positive and Negative Syndrome Scale < 20% improved: 83/173 [48%] with clozapine v 81/178 [45%] with olanzapine or risperidone; RR 1.05, 95% CI 0.84 to 1.32). However, the number of people studied was too small to rule out a clinically important difference. **Olanzapine versus standard antipsychotic drugs:** One systematic review (search date 1999, 1 RCT, 84 people) found no significant difference in psychotic symptoms over 8 weeks between olanzapine (25 mg/day) and chlorpromazine (39/42 [93%] with olanzapine v 42/42 [100%]; RR for no important response defined as a 40% reduction on the CGI scale 0.93, 95% CI 0.85 to 1.01).[23] The RCT is likely to have been too small to exclude a clinically important difference. **Olanzapine versus other new antipsychotic drugs:** We found one systematic review (search date 1999, 1 RCT, 180 people) comparing olanzapine versus clozapine, which found no significant difference in psychotic symptoms over 8 weeks (45/90 [50%] with olanzapine v 55/90 [61%] with clozapine; RR for no important response [defined as a 40% reduction on the CGI scale] 0.82, 95% CI 0.63 to 1.07).[23] The RCT is likely to have been too small to exclude a clinically important difference. **Other interventions:** We found no RCTs examining the effects of other interventions in people resistant to standard treatment.

Harms: **Clozapine versus standard antipsychotic drugs:** See harms of clozapine, p 230. **Clozapine versus other new antipsychotic drugs:** The review found that, compared with other new antipsychotic drugs (mainly olanzapine and risperidone), clozapine was significantly less likely to cause extrapyramidal adverse effects (305 people; RR 0.3, 95% CI 0.1 to 0.6; NNT 6, 95% CI 4 to 9).[15] It also found that clozapine may be less likely to cause dry mouth and more likely to cause fatigue, nausea, dizziness, hypersalivation, and hypersomnia than other new antipsychotic drugs, but these findings were from one or at most two RCTs. It found that people taking clozapine tended to be more satisfied with their treatment than those taking other new antipsychotic drugs, but also tended to withdraw from RCTs more often. It found no significant difference in rates of blood dyscrasias between clozapine and other new antipsychotic drugs, but the number of people studied was too small (558) to rule out a clinically important difference.[15]

Comment: Some RCTs in the reviews included people who were partial responders to neuroleptic drugs and people unable to take some neuroleptic medication because of adverse effects.[14,15,23] The reviews did not specify the duration of treatment resistant illness of the participants in the RCTs. RCTs are underway to clarify the mode of action of cognitive behavioural therapy and establish its effects in people who are resistant to standard treatments.

| QUESTION | Which interventions improve adherence to antipsychotic medication? |

| OPTION | BEHAVIOURAL THERAPY |

One RCT found that behavioural interventions improved adherence to antipsychotic medication compared with usual treatment. Two RCTs found limited evidence that behavioural interventions may improve adherence more than psychoeducational therapy.

Benefits:
We found no systematic review. **Versus usual treatment:** We found one RCT (36 men).[50] The behavioural training method comprised being told the importance of adhering to antipsychotic medication and instructions on how to take medication. Each participant was given a self monitoring spiral calendar, which featured a dated slip of paper for each dose of antipsychotic. Adherence was estimated by pill counts (see comment below). After 3 months fewer people had high pill adherence after usual treatment compared with behaviour therapy (figures not provided). **Versus psychoeducational therapy:** See benefits of psychoeducational interventions, p 248.

Harms:
None reported.

Comment:
Assessing adherence by pill count has potential confounders in that people may throw pills away.[50]

| OPTION | COMPLIANCE THERAPY |

Two RCTs found limited evidence that compliance therapy may increase adherence to antipsychotic drugs at 6 and 18 months compared with non-specific counselling.

Benefits:
We found no systematic review, but found two RCTs.[51,52] The first RCT (47 people with acute psychoses, most of whom fulfilled criteria for schizophrenia or had been admitted with the first episode of a psychotic illness) compared compliance therapy (see glossary, p 249) versus supportive counselling.[51] It found that, compared with non-specific counselling, compliance therapy significantly increased the proportion of people with improved adherence at 4–6 weeks (improved adherence defined as a score ≥ 5 on a scale from 1–7, where 1 is complete refusal and 7 active participation, ready acceptance, and taking some responsibility for adhering to antipsychotic medication; OR 6.3, 95% CI 1.6 to 24.6) and at 6 month follow up (OR 5.2, 95% CI 1.5 to 18.3; absolute numbers not provided; see comment below).[51] The second RCT (74 people with acute psychoses, most of whom fulfilled criteria for schizophrenia and had been admitted to hospital with relapse of symptoms) found that compliance therapy significantly improved compliance over 18 months measured on a 7 point scale of medication adherence compared with non-specific counselling (mean difference 1.4, 95% CI 0.9 to 1.6).[52]

Harms:
The RCTs gave no information on harms.[51,52]

Comment: Other trials have examined the potential benefits of compliance therapy but either did not employ a standardised measure of adherence or did not assess adherence in a blind fashion. In the first RCT, about a third of each group did not complete the RCT, and missing data are estimated from the mean scores in each group.[51]

OPTION   FAMILY INTERVENTIONS

One systematic review found that "compliance with medication" over 9–24 months was higher in people who received multiple family interventions compared with usual care, single family interventions, or psychoeducational interventions, but the difference did not quite reach significance.

Benefits: We found one systematic review (search date 1999) that compared multiple family interventions versus usual care, single family interventions, or psychoeducational interventions.[47] Family interventions consisted mainly of education about the illness and training in problem solving over at least six weekly sessions. The review found that "compliance with medication" over 9–24 months was higher in people who received multiple family interventions compared with other interventions, but the difference did not quite reach significance (5 RCTs, 393 people; OR 0.63, 95% CI 0.40 to 1.01; no further data provided).[47]

Harms: The review gave no information on harms.[47]

Comment: Although no harms were reported, illness education could possibly have adverse consequences on morale and outlook. The mechanism for the effects of family intervention remains unclear. It is thought to work by reducing "expressed emotion" (hostility and criticism) in relatives of people with schizophrenia. The time consuming nature of this intervention, which must normally take place at evenings or weekends, can limit its availability. It cannot be applied to people who have little contact with home based carers.

OPTION   PSYCHOEDUCATIONAL INTERVENTIONS

One systematic review found limited evidence that psychoeducation improved adherence to antipsychotic medication compared with usual care. Two RCTs found limited evidence that psychoeducation may improve adherence less than behavioural therapy.

Benefits: **Versus usual treatment:** We found one systematic review (search date 2002), which identified four RCTs that assessed adherence with medication.[48] The RCTs compared individual or group psychoeducation of either standard length (11 sessions or more) or brief length (10 sessions or less) versus usual care. The first RCT (67 people) found no significant difference in adherence between brief individual psychoeducation and usual care measure on a continuous scale of medication compliance. The second RCT (82 people) found no significant difference in adherence over 18 months between standard length group interventions and usual care. However, two further RCTs identified by the review comparing brief group psychoeducational interventions versus control suggested that psychoeducation was more effective in improving adherence. The third

RCT (236 people) found that a brief group psychoeducational intervention significantly improved adherence compared with control (measured on a continuous scale of "medication concordance"; WMD −0.4, 95% CI −0.6 to −0.2). The fourth RCT (46 people) comparing a brief psychoeducational intervention versus usual care found limited evidence that psychoeducational interventions may improve adherence over 1 year (mean number of non-compliant episodes 0.38 with psychoeducation v 1.14 with usual care).[48]

Versus behavioural therapy: We found two RCTs.[50,53] The first RCT (36 men) compared three interventions: psychoeducation, behavioural therapy, or usual treatment.[50] The behavioural training method comprised being told the importance of complying with antipsychotic medication and instructions on how to take medication. Each participant was given a self monitoring spiral calendar, which featured a dated slip of paper for each dose of antipsychotic. Adherence was estimated by pill counts (see comment below). The RCT found that, after 3 months, fewer people had high pill adherence after psychoeducation compared with behavioural therapy, but the difference was not significant (3/11 [27%] with psychoeducation v 8/11 [72%] with behavioural therapy had pill adherence scores of 80% measured by pill counts; RR of high pill adherence score 0.37, 95% CI 0.13 to 1.05). The RCT is likely to have been too small to detect a clinically important difference.[50] The second RCT (39 people) compared a psychoeducational intervention, a behavioural intervention given individually, and a behavioural intervention involving the person with schizophrenia and their family.[53] The individual behavioural intervention consisted of specific written guidelines, and oral instructions given to people to use a pill box consisting of 28 compartments for every medication occasion during a week. The behavioural intervention, when given to the individual and their family, contained additional instructions for the family members to compliment the person with schizophrenia for taking their prescribed medication. The primary outcome measure was pill count at 2 months (see comment below). The RCT found that medication adherence was significantly more likely with behavioural interventions than with psychoeducation (> 90% adherence at 2 months, 25/26 [96%] with behavioural interventions v 6/13 [46%] with psychoeducation; RR 2.08, 95% CI 1.15 to 3.77, NNT 2, 95% CI 2 to 5).

Harms: None reported.

Comment: Assessing adherence by pill count has potential confounders in that people may throw pills away.[50,53] Each psychoeducational intervention varied in the protocol used and few employed the same outcome measurements.

GLOSSARY

Compliance therapy A treatment based on cognitive behavioural therapy and motivational interviewing techniques with a view to improving adherence to medication.

Negative symptoms This generally refers to qualities that are abnormal by their absence (e.g. loss of drive, motivation, and self care).

Positive symptoms This refers to symptoms that characterise the onset or relapse of schizophrenia, usually hallucinations and delusions, but sometimes including thought disorder.

REFERENCES

1. Andreasen NC. Symptoms, signs and diagnosis of schizophrenia. *Lancet* 1995;346:477–481.

2. Kane JM, Honigfeld G, Singer J, et al. Clozapine for the treatment-resistant schizophrenic. *Arch Gen Psychiatry* 1988;45:789–796.

3. Meltzer HY. Treatment-resistant schizophrenia: the role of clozapine. *Curr Med Res Opin* 1997;14:1–20.

4. Cannon M, Jones P. Neuroepidemiology: schizophrenia. *J Neurol Neurosurg Psychiatry* 1996;61:604–613.

5. Jablensky A, Sartorius N, Ernberg G, et al. Schizophrenia: manifestations, incidence and course in different cultures. A World Health Organisation ten-country study. *Psychol Med* 1992;monograph supplement 20:1–97.

6. Hegarty JD, Baldessarini RJ, Tohen M, et al. One hundred years of schizophrenia: a meta-analysis of the outcome literature. *Am J Psychiatry* 1994;151:1409–1416.

7. Johnstone EC. Schizophrenia: problems in clinical practice. *Lancet* 1993; 341:536–538.

8. Thornley B, Adams C. Content and quality of 2000 controlled trials in schizophrenia over 50 years. *BMJ* 1998;317:1181–1184. Search date 1997; primary sources hand searching of conference proceedings, Biological Abstracts, Cinahl, The Cochrane Library, Embase, Lilacs, Psychlit, Pstndex, Medline, and Sociofile.

9. Thornley B, Adams CE, Awad G. Chlorpromazine versus placebo for those with schizophrenia. In: The Cochrane Library, Issue 2, 2002. Oxford: Update Software. Search date 1999; primary sources Biological Abstracts, Embase, Medline, Psychlit, SciSearch, Cochrane Library, Cochrane Schizophrenia Group's Register, hand searches of reference lists, and personal contact with pharmaceutical companies and authors of trials.

10. Joy CB, Adams CE, Lawrie SM. Haloperidol versus placebo for schizophrenia. In: The Cochrane Library, Issue 2, 2002. Oxford: Update Software. Search date 1998; primary sources Biological Abstracts, The Cochrane Schizophrenia Group's Register, Embase, Medline, Psychlit, SciSearch, hand searches of references, and contact with authors of trials and pharmaceutical companies.

11. Sultana A, Reilly J, Fenton M. Thioridazine for schizophrenia. In: The Cochrane Library, Issue 2, 2002. Oxford: Update Software. Search date 1999; primary sources Biological Abstracts, Cinahl, The Cochrane Library, The Cochrane Schizophrenia Group's Register, Embase, Medline, Psychlit, Sociofile, reference lists, pharmaceutical companies, and authors of trials.

12. Quraishi S, David A, Adams, CE. Depot bromperidol decanoate for schizophrenia. In: The Cochrane Library, Issue 2, 2002. Search date 1999; primary sources Biological Abstracts, Cochrane Library, Cochrane Schizophrenia Group's Register, Embase, Medline, PsycLIT, hand searches of reference lists and personal contact with Janssen Cilag.

13. Quraishi S, David A. Depot haloperidol decanoate for schizophrenia. In: The Cochrane Library, Issue 2, 2002. Oxford: Update Software. Search date 1998; primary sources Biological Abstracts, Embase, Medline, Psychlit, SciSearch, The Cochrane Library, reference lists, authors of studies, and pharmaceutical companies.

14. Wahlbeck K, Cheine M, Essali MA. Clozapine versus typical neuroleptic medication for schizophrenia. In: The Cochrane Library, Issue 2, 2002. Oxford: Update Software. Search date 1999; primary sources Biological Abstracts, Cochrane Schizophrenia Group's Register, Cochrane Library, Embase, Lilacs, Medline, Psychlit, SciSearch Science Citation Index, hand searches of reference lists, and personal communication with pharmaceutical companies.

15. Tuunainen A, Gilbody SM. Newer atypical antipsychotic medication versus clozapine for schizophrenia. In: The Cochrane Library, Issue 2, 2002. Oxford: Update Software. Search date 1998; primary sources Biological Abstracts, Cochrane Schizophrenia Group's Register, Cochrane Library, Embase, Lilacs, Medline, Psychlit, hand searches of reference lists and personal contact with authors of trials and pharmaceutical companies.

16. Honigfeld G, Arellano F, Sethi, et al. Reducing clozapine-related morbidity and mortality: five years experience of the clozaril national registry. *J Clin Psychiatry* 1998;59(suppl 3):3–7.

17. Geddes J, Freemantle N, Harrison P, et al, for the National Schizophrenia Development Group. Atypical antipsychotics in the treatment of schizophrenia: systematic review and meta-regression analysis. *BMJ* 2000;321:1371–1377. Search date 1998; primary sources Medline, Embase, Psychlit, and Cochrane Controlled Trials Register.

18. Mota Neto JIS, Lima MS, Soares BGO. Amisulpride for schizophrenia. In: The Cochrane Library, Issue 2, 2002. Oxford: Update Software. Search date 2000, Biological Abstracts Cinahl, Cochrane Library, Cochrane Schizophrenia Group's Register, Embase, Lilacs, Psyclit, Science Citation Index, hand searches of reference lists and personal contact with the manufacturer of amisulpride.

19. Leucht S, Pitschel-Walz G, Engel RR, et al. Amisulpride, an unusual "atypical" antipsychotic: a meta-analysis of randomized controlled trials. *Am J Psychiatry* 2002;159:177–179. Search date 2000; primary sources Medline, Current Contents, hand searches of reference lists and personal contact with the manufacturer of amisupride.

20. Martin S, Ljo H, Peuskens J, et al. A double blind, randomised comparative trial of amisulpiride versus olanzapine in the treatment of schizophrenia: short term results at two months. *Curr Med Res Opin* 2002;18:355–362.

21. Fenton M, Murphy B, Wood J, et al. Loxapine for schizophrenia. In: The Cochrane Library, Issue 2, 2002. Oxford: Update Software. Search date 1999; primary sources Biological Abstracts, The Cochrane Library, The Cochrane Schizophrenia Group's Register, Embase, Lilacs, Psyndex, Psychlit, and hand searches of reference lists.

22. Bagnall AM, Fenton M, Lewis R, et al. Molindone for schizophrenia and severe mental illness. In: The Cochrane Library, Issue 2, 2002. Oxford: Update Software. Search date 1999; primary sources Biological Abstracts, The Cochrane Library, The Cochrane Schizophrenia Group's Register, Cinahl, Embase, Psychlit, pharmaceutical databases, hand searches of reference lists, and personal contact with authors of trials.

23. Duggan L, Fenton M, Dardennes RM, et al. Olanzapine for schizophrenia. In: The Cochrane Library, Issue 2, 2002. Oxford: Update Software. Search date 1999; primary sources Biological Abstracts, Embase, Medline, Psychlit, Cochrane Library, hand searches of reference lists and conference abstracts, and personal communication with authors of trials and pharmaceutical companies.

24. Peuskens J, de Hert M, Jones, M. The clinical value of risperidone and olanzapine: a

meta-analysis of efficacy and safety. *Int J Psych Clin Prac* 2001;5:170–187. Search date 1998, primary sources Medline, Embase, Psychlit 1991–1998.

25. Gilbody SM, Bagnall AM, Duggan L, et al. Risperidone versus other atypical antipsychotic medication for schizophrenia. In: The Cochrane Library, Issue 2, 2002. Oxford: Update Software. Search date 1999; primary sources Biological Abstracts, Cochrane Library, Cochrane Schizophrenia Group's Register, Embase, Medline, Lilacs, Psyindex, Psychlit, pharmaceutical databases on the Dialog Corporation Datastar and Dialog services, hand search of reference lists, and contact with pharmaceutical companies and authors of trials.

26. De Rossi M, Donda P, Bellantuono C. Efficacy and tolerability of olanzapine: a critical review of the international literature. *Rivista di Psichiatria* 2001;36:183–203.

27. Conley RR, Mahmoud R. A randomized double-blind study of risperidone and olanzapine in the treatment of schizophrenia or schizoaffective disorder. *Am J Psychiatry* 2001;158:765–774.

28. Leucht S, Hartung B. Perazine for schizophrenia. In: The Cochrane Library, Issue 2, 2002. Search date 2001; primary sources Cochrane Schizophrenia Group's register (January 2001) , Biological Abstracts, CINAHL, The Cochrane Library, Embase, Medline, Psyclit, Lilacs, Psyndex, Sociological Abstracts, Sociofile, hand searches of reference lists and personal contact with pharmaceutical companies and authors.

29. Sultana A, McMonagle T. Pimozide for schizophrenia or related psychoses. In: The Cochrane Library, Issue 2, 2002. Oxford: Update Software. Search date 1999; primary sources Biological Abstracts, The Cochrane Schizophrenia Group's Register, Embase, Janssen-Cilag UK's register of studies, Medline, hand searches of reference lists, and personal contact with pharmaceutical companies.

30. Srisurapanont M, Disayavanish C, Taimkaew K. Quetiapine for schizophrenia. In: The Cochrane Library, Issue 2, 2002. Oxford: Update Software. Search date 2000; primary sources Biological Abstracts, Embase, Medline, Psychlit, The Cochrane Library, Cinahl, Sigle, Sociofile, hand searches of journals, and personal communication with authors of studies and pharmaceutical companies.

31. Kennedy E, Song F, Hunter R, et al. Risperidone versus typical antipsychotic medication for schizophrenia. In: The Cochrane Library, Issue 2, 2002. Oxford: Update Software. Search date 1997; primary sources Biological Abstracts, The Cochrane Trials Register, Embase, Medline, Psychlit, hand searches of reference lists, and personal communication with pharmaceutical companies.

32. Lopez Ibor JJ, Ayuso JL, Gutierrez M, et al. Risperidone in the treatment of chronic schizophrenia: multicenter study comparative to haloperidol. *Actas Luso Esp Neurol Psiquiatr Cienc Afines* 1996;24:165–172.

33. Soares BGO, Fenton M, Chue P. Sulpiride for schizophrenia. In: The Cochrane Library, Issue 2, 2002. Oxford: Update Software. Search date 1998; primary sources Biological Abstracts, Cinahl, Cochrane Schizophrenia Group's Register, The Cochrane Library, Embase, Medline, Psychlit, Sigle, and Sociofile.

34. Harnryd C, Bjerkenstedt L, Bjork K, et al. Clinical evaluation of sulpiride in schizophrenic

35. Bagnall AM, Lewis RA, Leitner ML, et al. Ziprasidone for schizophrenia and severe mental illness. In: The Cochrane Library, Issue 2, 2002. Oxford: Update Software. Search date 1999; primary sources Biological Abstracts, The Cochrane Library, The Cochrane Schizophrenia Group's Register, Embase, Lilacs, Psyndex, Psychlit, pharmaceutical databases, hand searches of reference lists, and personal contact with authors of trials.

36. Fenton M, Morris F, De Silva P, et al. Zotepine for schizophrenia. In: The Cochrane Library, Issue 2, 2002. Oxford: Update Software. Search date 1999; primary sources Biological Abstracts, The Cochrane Library, The Cochrane Schizophrenia Group's Register, Embase, Dialog Corporation Datastar service, Medline, Psychlit, hand searches of reference lists, and personal contact with authors of trials and pharmaceutical companies.

37. Gilbert PL, Harris MJ, McAdams LA, et al. Neuroleptic withdrawal in schizophrenic people: a review of the literature. *Arch Gen Psychiatry* 1995;52:173–188. Search date not stated; primary source Medline.

38. Quraishi S, David A. Depot pipothiazine palmitate and undeclynate for schizophrenia. In: The Cochrane Library, Issue 2, 2002. Oxford: Update Software. Search date 1998; primary sources Biological Abstracts, Cochrane Library, Cochrane Schizophrenia Group's Register, Embase, Medline, Psychlit, hand searches of reference lists, and personal communication with pharmaceutical companies.

39. Adams CE, Eisenbruch M. Depot fluphenazine versus oral fluphenazine for those with schizophrenia. In: The Cochrane Library, Issue 2, 2002. Oxford: Update Software. Search date 1995; primary sources Biological Abstracts, The Cochrane Library, Cochrane Schizophrenia Group's Register, Embase, Medline, Psychlit, Science Citation Index, hand searches of reference lists, and personal communication with pharmaceutical companies.

40. Quraishi S, David A. Depot flupenthixol decanoate for schizophrenia or similar psychotic disorders. In: The Cochrane Library, Issue 2, 2002. Oxford: Update Software. Search date 1998; primary sources Biological Abstracts, The Cochrane Library, Cochrane Schizophrenia Group's Register, Embase, Medline, Psychlit, SciSearch, references, and personal communication with authors of trials and pharmaceutical companies.

41. Quraishi S, David A. Depot fluspirilene for schizophrenia. In: The Cochrane Library, Issue 2, 2002. Oxford: Update Software. Search date 1998; primary sources Biological Abstracts, The Cochrane Library, The Cochrane Schizophrenia Group's Register, Embase, Medline, Psychlit, and hand searches of reference lists.

42. Quraishi S, David A. Depot perphenazine decanoate and enanthate for schizophrenia. In: The Cochrane Library, Issue 2, 2002. Oxford: Update Software. Search date 1998; primary sources Biological Abstracts, The Cochrane Library, The Cochrane Schizophrenia Group's Register, Embase, Medline, Psychlit, hand searches of reference lists, and personal communication with pharmaceutical companies.

43. Coutinho E, Fenton M, Quraishi S. Zuclopenthixol decanoate for schizophrenia and other serious mental illnesses. In: The Cochrane Library, Issue 2, 2002. Oxford: Update Software. Search date 1998; primary sources Biological Abstracts, Cinhal, The Cochrane Library, The Cochrane

Schizophrenia Group's Register, Embase, Medline, and Psychlit. References of all eligible studies were searched for further trials. The manufacturer of zuclopenthixol was contacted.

44. Csernansky JG, Mahmoud R, Brenner R; The Risperidone-USA-79 Study Group. A comparison of risperidone and haloperidol for the prevention of relapse in patients with schizophrenia. *New Engl J Med* 2002;346:1:16–22.

45. Jeste D, Gilbert P, McAdams L, et al. Considering neuroleptic maintenance and taper on a continuum: need for an individual rather than dogmatic approach. *Arch Gen Psychiatry* 1995;52:209–212.

46. Cormac I, Jones C, Campbell C. Cognitive behavioural therapy for schizophrenia. In: The Cochrane Library, Issue 2, 2002. Oxford: Update Software. Search date 2001, primary sources Biological Abstracts, Cochrane Schizophrenia Group's Register, Cinahl, The Cochrane Library, Medline, Embase, Psychlit, Sigle, Sociofile, reference lists of articles, and personal communication with authors of trials.

47. Pilling S, Bebbington P, Kuipers E, et al. Psychological treatments in schizophrenia: I. Meta-analysis of family interventions and cognitive behaviour therapy. *Psychol Med* 2002;32:763–782.

48. Pekkala E, Merinder L. Psychoeducation for schizophrenia. In: The Cochrane Library, Issue 2, 2002. Oxford: Update Software. Search date 2002; primary sources Cinahl, The Cochrane Library, Cochrane Schizophrenia Group's Register, Embase, Medline, Psychlit, Sociofile, hand searched reference lists, and personal contact with authors.

49. Pilling S, Bebbington P, Kuipers E, et al. Psychological treatments in schizophrenia: II. Meta-analysis of randomised controlled trials of social skills training and cognitive remediation. *Psychol Med* 2002;32:783–791.

50. Boczkowski JA, Zeichner A, DeSanto N. Neuroleptic compliance among chronic schizophrenic outpeople: an intervention outcome report. *J Consult Clin Psychol* 1985;53:666–671.

51. Kemp R, Kirov G, Everitt B, et al. Randomised controlled trial of compliance therapy. 18-month follow-up. *Br J Psychiatry* 1998;172:413–419.

52. Kemp R, Hayward P, Applewhaite G, et al. Compliance therapy in psychotic people: randomised controlled trial. *BMJ* 1996;312:345–349.

53. Azrin NH, Teichner G. Evaluation of an instructional program for improving medication compliance for chronically mentally ill outpatients. *Behaviour Res Ther* 1998;36:849–861.

Zia Nadeem
Research Fellow
Department of Psychiatry

Andrew McIntosh
Lecturer in Psychiatry
Department of Psychiatry

Stephen Lawrie
Senior Clinical Research Fellow and
Honorary Consultant Psychiatrist
University of Edinburgh
UK

Competing interests: SL has been paid for speaking about critical appraisal by employees of the manufacturers of olanzapine, quetiapine, risperidone, and ziprasidone, and has been paid to speak about the management of schizophrenia by employees of the manufacturers of amisulpiride, olanzapine, risperidone, and clozapine. AM and ZN none declared.

TABLE 1   Continued treatment with antipsychotic drugs: choice of drugs (see text, p 242).

Review	Search date	Number of RCTs	Comparisons	Main Conclusion
39	1995	6	Oral v depot fluphenazine	No significant difference
13	1998	7	Haloperidol decanoate v other depots	No significant difference
40	1999	8	Flupenthixol decanoate v other depots	No significant difference
38	1999	7	Pipotiazine (pipothiazine) palmitate v other depots	No significant difference
38	1999	2	Pipotiazine (pipothiazine) palmitate v oral antipsychotics	No significant difference
41	1999	1	Fluspirilene decanoate v oral chlorpromazine	No significant difference
41	1999	3	Fluspirilene decanoate v other depots	No significant difference
42	1999	1	Perphenazine enanthate v clopenthixol decanoate	No significant difference
29	2000	11	Pimozide v standard antipsychotics	No significant difference
23	1999	1	Olanzapine v standard antipsychotics	No significant difference
43	1998	3	Zuclopenthixol decanoate v other depots	People taking zuclopenthixol had lower relapse rates over 12 weeks to 1 year
14	1999	19	Clozapine v standard antipsychotics	Relapse rates up to 12 weeks were lower with clozapine
12	1999	2	Bromperidol v haloperidol or fluphenazine	Relapse rates over 6–12 months were lower with haloperidol or fluphenazine

Note

When looking up a class of drug, the reader is advised to also look up specific examples of that class of drug where additional entries may be found. The reverse situation also applies.

INDEX

The number needed to treat: adjusting for baseline risk

Adapted with permission from Chatellier et al, 1996[1]

BACKGROUND

The number needed to treat (NNT) to avoid a single additional adverse outcome is a meaningful way of expressing the benefit of an active treatment over a control. It can be used both to summarise the results of a therapeutic trial or series of trials and to help medical decision making about an individual patient.

If the absolute risk of adverse outcomes in a therapeutic trial is ARC in the control group and ART in the treatment group, then the absolute risk reduction (ARR) is defined as (ARC − ART). The NNT is defined as the inverse of the ARR:

$$NNT = 1/(ARC − ART)$$

Since the Relative Risk Reduction (RRR) is defined as (ARC − ART)/ARC, it follows that NNT, RRR, and ARC are related by their definitions in the following way:

$$NNT \times RRR \times ARC = 1$$

This relationship can be used to estimate the likely benefits of a treatment in populations with different levels of baseline risk (that is different levels of ARC). This allows extrapolation of the results of a trial or meta-analysis to people with different baseline risks. Ideally, there should be experimental evidence of the RRR in each population. However, in many trials, subgroup analyses show that the RRR is approximately constant in groups of patients with different characteristics. Cook and Sackett therefore proposed that decisions about individual patients could be made by using the NNT calculated from the RRR measured in trials and the baseline risk in the absence of treatment estimated for the individual patient.[2]

The method may not apply to periods of time different to that studied in the original trials.

USING THE NOMOGRAM

The nomogram shown on the next page allows the NNT to be found directly without any calculation: a straight line should be drawn from the point corresponding to the estimated absolute risk for the patient on the left hand scale to the point corresponding to the relative risk reduction stated in a trial or meta-analysis on the central scale. The intercept of this line with the right hand scale gives the NNT. By taking the upper and lower limits of the confidence interval of the RRR, the upper and lower limits of the NNT can be estimated.

REFERENCES

1. Chatellier G, Zapletal E, Lemaitre D, *et al*. The number needed to treat: a clinically useful nomogram in its proper context. *BMJ* 1996;312:426–429.
2. Cook RJ, Sackett DL. The number needed to treat: a clinically useful measure of treatment effect. *BMJ* 1995;310:452–454.

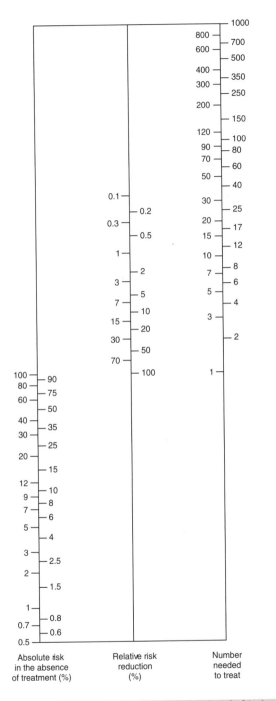

FIGURE Nomogram for calculating the number needed to treat. Published with permission.[1]

Abbreviations

AR	Absolute risk	**NS**	Not significant
ARR	Absolute risk reduction	**OR**	Odds ratio
ARI	Absolute risk increase	**P**	P value
CI	Confidence interval	**RCT**	Randomised controlled trial
CCT	Controlled clinical trial	**RR**	Relative risk
HR	Hazard ratio	**RRI**	Relative risk increase
NNH	Number needed to harm	**RRR**	Relative risk reduction
NNT	Number needed to treat	**WMD**	Weighted mean difference

How to calculate risk

AR = # events (good or bad) in treated or control groups/ # people in that group

ARC = AR of events in the control group

ART = AR of events in the treatment group

ARR = ARC − ART

RR = ART/ARC = 1 − RRR

RRR = (ARC − ART)/ARC = 1 − RR

NNT = 1/ARR

To express decimals as percentages, multiply by 100.

If:

the RR (or OR) = 1, or the CI includes 1, there is no significant difference between treatment and control groups

the RR > 1 and the CI does not include 1, events are significantly more likely in the treatment than the control group

the RR < 1 and the CI does not include 1, events are significantly less likely in the treatment than the control group

RR of 0.8 means a RRR of 20% (meaning a 20% reduction in the relative risk of the specified outcome in the treatment group compared with the control group).

RRR is usually constant across a range of absolute risks. But the ARR is higher and the NNT lower in people with higher absolute risks.

Example: If a person's AR of stroke, estimated from his age and other risk factors (see appendix 1), is 0.25 without treatment but falls to 0.20 with treatment, the ARR is 25%−20% = 5%; the RRR is (25%−20%)/25% = 20%;
and the NNT is 1/0.05 = 20. In a person with an AR of stroke of only 0.025 without treatment, the same treatment will still produce a 20% RRR, but treatment will reduce her AR of stroke to 0.020, giving a much smaller ARR of 2.5%−2% = 0.5%, and a NNT of 200.

We are pleased to provide you with this copy of
Clinical Evidence Mental Health.

We at United Health Foundation support you in your efforts
to provide the best quality of health care for your patients.

For more information on United Health Foundation,
please visit our website at:

www.unitedhealthfoundation.org.

Clinical Evidence Mental Health Questionnaire

As a recipient of *Clinical Evidence Mental Health* your feedback is
important to help us serve your needs. We hope you will take a
moment to answer and return this brief survey.

1 How relevant is the content of this book to your practice?
   ☐ Very useful   ☐ Somewhat useful
   ☐ Useful   ☐ Not at all useful

2 Do you find *Clinical Evidence Mental Health* easy to use?
   ☐ Yes   ☐ No

3 Has receiving *Clinical Evidence* helped you alter, modify or
   confirm any aspect of your clinical practice?
   ☐ Yes   ☐ No

4 Are you aware you have free access to the online version at
   www.clinicalevidence.com as part of this distribution by
   United Health Foundation?
   ☐ Yes   ☐ No   ☐ Don't Know/Didn't Use

5 Have you found the *Clinical Evidence* website user friendly?
   ☐ Yes   ☐ No   ☐ Don't Know/Didn't Use

6 Would you be interested in a PDA version of *Clinical
   Evidence Mental Health*?
   ☐ Yes   ☐ No

7 Have you shared information from *Clinical Evidence Mental Health*
   with your patients as part of your patient/clinical relationship?
   ☐ Yes   ☐ No

Name ....

Address ....

....

City...........................State ....Zip.......................

United Health Foundation

P.O. Box 1459
Minneapolis, Minnesota 55440
www.unitedhealthfoundation.org
e-mail: ce@unitedhealthfoundation.org

United Health Foundation
MN008-W375
P.O. Box 1459
Minneapolis, MN 55440

United Health Foundation
Clinical Evidence
MN008-W375
P.O. Box 1459
Minneapolis, MN 55440-1459